# English-French Medical Dictionary and Phrasebook

# French-English

first edition 2010

ISBN is 1450589685
EAN-13 is 9781450589680

by A.H. Zemback

# Contents

| English | French |
|---|---|
| **abdomen** *The portion of the body bordered by the diaphragm and the pelvis.* | abdomen |
| **abdominal reflex** *Elicited by stroking the abdomen lightly from mid-axillary line to umbilicus. A normal response is contraction of the umbilicus toward the stimulated side.* | réflexe cutané abdominal |
| **abducens nerve** *A motor nerve (6th cranial nerve) that controls the lateral rectus muscle of the eye.)* | 1. nerf abducens 2. moteur oculaire externe nerf |
| **abducent** *Abducting or to separate.* | abducteur |
| **aberrant** *Different than normal.* | aberrant |
| **abnormal** | anormal |
| **ABO system** *The system using human blood antigens to determine blood type.* | système ABO |
| **abortion** *Premature expulsion of the fetus from the uterus.* | avortement |
| **above normal** | au-dessus de la normale |
| **abrade, to** *To scrape away with friction.* | ronger |
| **abruptio placentae** *The premature detachment of a normally implanted placenta resulting in maternal decompensation.* | hématome rétroplacentaire |
| **abscess** *A localized collection of pus.* | abcès |
| **absence** | absence |
| **absolute** | absolu |
| **abuse** | abus |
| **acalculia** *The inability to perform mathematical calculations.* | acalculie |
| **acanthoma** *An adult cornyfying squamous carcinoma.* | acanthome |
| **acanthosis** *Hypertrophy of the prickle cell layer of the skin.* | acanthose |
| **acapnia** *A condition of lower than normal carbon dioxide level in the blood.* | acapnie |
| **acariasis** *Mite infestation.* | acariase |
| **acaricide** *A treatment for mite infestation.* | acaricide |
| **acarus** *A mite.* | acarien |
| **acatalasia** *A condition characterized by the congenital absence of the enzyme catalase.* | acatalasie |
| **acathisia** *The inability to sit quietly or to have motor restlessness.* | acathisie |
| **access** | 1. abord 2. base de données |
| **accessory** *Complimentary or concomitant.* | accessoire |
| **accessory nerve (XI)** *Supplies motor innervation to the sternocleidomastoid and trapezius.* | nerf onzième paire crânienne |
| **accident** | accident |
| **acclimatization** *The process of becoming adapted to a new environment.* | acclimatation |

| English | French |
|---|---|
| **accommodation** *A term used to describe the ability of the eye to adjust to various distances.* | accommodation |
| **according to** | selon |
| **accretion** *The expected growth of tissue from the intake of nutrients.* | accrétion |
| **acephalous** *A absence of a head.* | acéphale |
| **acetabular** *Referring to the acetabulum.* | acétabulaire |
| **acetabulum** *The cup-shaped cavity with which the head of the femur articulates.* | cavité cotyloïdien |
| **acetaminophen** *Mild analgesic drug used for pain relief.* | paracétamol |
| **acetonemia** *The presence of acetone in the blood.* | acétonémie |
| **acetonuria** *The presence of acetone in the urine.* | acétonurie |
| **acetylcholine** *A reversible acetic acid ester of choline.* | acétylcholine |
| **acetylsalicylic acid** *The chemical name for common aspirin.* | acétylsalicylique (acide) |
| **achalasia** *Inability to relax the smooth muscle fibers of the gastrointestinal tract. In the case of esophageal achalasia one has dilatation and hypertrophy of the esophagus.* | achalasie |
| **achieved** | accompli |
| **Achilles tendon reflex** *The normal response to tapping the achilles tendon with a reflex hammer is the plantar flexion of the foot.* | réflexe achilléen |
| **achlorhydria** *The absence of hydrochloric acid in gastric secretions.* | achlorhydrie |
| **acholia** *The lack of bile.* | acholie |
| **achondroplasia** *A congenital inadequacy of enchondral bone formation resulting in a type of dwarfism.* | achondroplasie |
| **achromatic spindle** *The threads between the poles of the spindle in karyokinesis.* | fuseau achromatique |
| **achromatopsia** *Inability to differentiate yellow, blue, red or their intermediates.* | achromatopsie |
| **achylia** *The absence of chyle.* | achylie |
| **acid phosphatase** *A phosphate derived chemical that is optimally active in an acidic environment.* | phosphatase acide |
| **acid** *Substance with a pH less than 7.* | acide |
| **acid-base balance** *The equilibrium of the electrolytes in the body.* | équilibre acido-basique |
| **acidemia** *A lower than normal pH in the blood.* | acidémie |
| **acidity** *Referring to an acid state.* | acidité |
| **acinitis** *The inflammation of the acini.* | acinite |
| **acne** *Inflamed or infected sebaceous glands.* | acné |
| **acne rosacea** *A chronic disease characterized by the presence of flushing of the skin of the nose, forehead and cheeks.* | 1. acné rosacée 2. couperose |
| **acorea** *The absence of the pupil of the eye.* | acorée |
| **acoustic crest** *A prominence on ampulla of the semicircular ducts.* | crête ampullaire |
| **acoustic neuroma** *A nonmalignant tumor that can cause deafness, tinnitus and vertigo.* | neurinome de l'acoustique |
| **acoustic** *Referring to the auditory system.* | acoustique |

| English | French |
|---|---|
| **Acquired Immunodeficiency Syndrome (AIDS)** *Presence of an AIDS defining illness or having a CD4 of less than 200/mm3.* | syndrome d'immunodéficience acquise (SIDA) |
| **acrocephaly** *A condition characterized by a pointed head.* | acrocéphalie |
| **acrocyanosis** *A benign condition in which the feet and hands are cyanotic, cold and sweating.* | acrocyanose |
| **acrodermatitis** *Inflammation of the skin of the hands and/or feet.* | acrodermatite |
| **acrodynia** *An infantile condition exhibited by swollen bluish-red extremities and later polyarthritis..* | acrodynie |
| **acromegaly** *Hyperplasia of the nose, jaw, fingers and toes.* | acromégalie |
| **acromioclavicular** *Referring to the junction of the acromion and clavicle.* | acromio-claviculaire |
| **acrotic** *Referring to the surface.* | acrotique |
| **actin** *A protein in the muscle that, along with myosin, facilitates muscle contraction and relaxation.* | actine |
| **actinic dermatosis** *A skin disease caused by exposure to radiation from the sun, ultraviolet waves or gamma radiation.* | acinodermatose |
| **actinon** *A radioactive element, radon-219.* | radon 219 |
| **action potential** *The alteration in electrical potential associated with the movement along a nerve cell.* | potentiel d'action |
| **activity** | activité |
| **actomyosin** *Myosin and actin complex present in muscles.* | actomyosine |
| **acuity** *1. Relating to accuracy of hearing, as in hearing acuity. 2. Severity of illness as in, "What is the patient's acuity?"* | acuité |
| **acupuncture** *Traditionally an aspect of Chinese medicine involving insertion of needles into the skin.* | acupuncture |
| **acute** *Abrupt onset.* | aigu |
| **acyesis** *Feminine sterility.* | stérilité féminine |
| **adactylia** *A congenital condition exhibited by the absence of toes and fingers.* | adactylie |
| **Adam's apple** *A prominence on the anterior neck caused by the thyroid cartilage of the larynx.* | pomme d'Adam |
| **add, to** | ajouter |
| **addiction** | 1. addiction 2. toxicomanie |
| **Addison's disease** *A disease of the adrenal gland exhibited by anemia, hypotension and a bronze tone to the skin.* | Addison, maladie d' |
| **adduction** *To bring toward the midline.* | adduction |
| **adductor** *A muscle that brings a part to the midline.* | adducteur |
| **adenectomy** *The removal of a gland.* | adénectomie |
| **adenitis** *The inflammation of a gland.* | adénite |
| **adenocarcinoma** *Cancer from glandular tissue.* | adénocarcinome |
| **adenofibroma** *Connective tissue with glands that form a tumor.* | adénofibrome |
| **adenohypophysis** *The anterior portion of the pituitary gland.* | antéhypophyse |

| English | French |
|---|---|
| **adenoid** *Referring to a gland.* | adénoïde |
| **adenoidectomy** *Removal of the adenoids.* | adénoïdectomie |
| **adenoiditis** *Inflammation of the adenoids.* | adénoïdite |
| **adenoids** *Pharyngeal tonsils.* | végétations adénoïdes |
| **adenolymphoma** *A salivary gland tumor, also called Warthin's tumor.* | adénolymphome |
| **adenomyoma** *A tumor characterized by the overgrowth of endometrial and uterine muscle tissue.* | adénomyome |
| **adenomyosis** *A condition characterized by the overgrowth of endometrial and uterine muscle tissue.* | adénomyose |
| **adenopathy** *Generally referring to a condition of the lymphatic glands.* | adénopathie |
| **adenosine triphosphate (ATP)** *A chemical that represents the energy reserve of the muscle.* | adénosine triphosphate (ATP) |
| **adenosine diphosphate** *A product of hydrolysis of ATP.* | adénosine diphosphate (ADP) |
| **adenosine monophosphate** *A nucleotide, it is produced when ATP is converted to ADP.* | adénosine monophosphate (AMP) |
| **adenovirus** *A type of a virus that can cause upper respiratory tract infections.* | 1. adénovirus 2. virus APC |
| **adephagia** *Insatiable hunger.* | boulimie |
| **adequate** | 1. adéquat 2. convenable |
| **adherence** | adhérence |
| **adhesion** *The abnormal adherence of tissue exposed to inflammation or after surgery.* | adhésion |
| **adhesive tape** *Tape used to secure dressings or intravenous lines to the body.* | sparadrap |
| **adiadochokinesia** *The inability to perform rapid alternating movements.* | adiadococinésie |
| **adipose** *Referring to fat.* | adipeux |
| **aditus** *The entrance to an organ or part.* | aditus |
| **adjustment** | ajustement |
| **adjuvant** *Term used to describe the medical treatment after initial therapy, as in adjuvant radiation therapy after initial chemotherapy.* | adjuvant |
| **admission** | entrée |
| **adnexa** *The appendages, for example, of the uterus are the ovaries, fallopian tubes and the ligaments of the uterus.* | annexes |
| **adolescence** | adolescence |
| **adrenal** *Referring to being near the kidney.* | surrénalien |
| **adrenal cortex** *The outer layer of the adrenal gland.* | corticosurrénale |
| **adrenal gland** *A gland located on the superior aspect of both kidneys.* | surrénale glande |
| **adrenal medulla** *The innermost part of the adrenal gland.* | médullosurrénale |
| **adrenalectomy** *Excision of the adrenal gland.* | 1. adrénalectomie 2. surrénalectomie |

| English | French |
|---|---|
| **adrenaline (epinephrine)** *A hormone secreted by the adrenal glands and a synthetic medication used for treatment of allergic reactions and cardiac arrest.* | adrénaline |
| **adrenergic** *That which is activated or transmitted by epinephrine.* | adrénergique |
| **adrenocorticotrophic hormone (ACTH)** *A hormone that influences the cortex of the adrenal glands.* | adrénocorticotrope hormone |
| **advanced** | 1.avancé 2. évolué |
| **adventitia** *Outermost.* | adventice |
| **adverse effect** *In reference to medication use, it is an undesirable consequence of the drug.* | effet indésriable |
| **advise, to** | conseiller |
| **aerobe** *An organism that grows in the presence of oxygen.* | aérobie |
| **aerodontalgia** *The dental pain that occurs with low atmospheric pressure, like during airflight.* | aérodontalgie |
| **aerophagy** *A condition associated with hysteria in which one swallow repeatedly swallows air and then belches.* | aérophagie |
| **afebrile** *Absence of fever.* | 1. afébrile 2. aprétique |
| **affect** | affect |
| **affected** | atteint |
| **affective disorder** *Manic-depressive psychosis.* | trouble thymique |
| **afferent loop syndrome** *The obstruction of the duodenum or jejunum after gastrojejunostomy, resulting in duodenal distention.* | anse afférente, syndrome de l' |
| **afferent** *Moving toward the center.* | afférent |
| **affinity** *To have a natural liking for.* | affinité |
| **aflatoxin** *A toxin produced by Aspergillus flavus.* | aflatoxine |
| **after-birth** *The tissue expelled after the birth of a child that includes the placenta and allied membranes.* | 1. arrière-faix 2. délivre |
| **after-load** *Referring to the amount of pressure the heart needs to pump against. If one has left heart failure it is beneficial to reduce after-load.* | post-charge |
| **after-pains** *The pain experienced after childbirth caused by uterine contractions.* | tranchées utérines |
| **after-taste** | arrière-goût |
| **agar** *Media used for bacterial cultures.* | 1. gélose 2. agar |
| **age** | âge |
| **agenesis** *The absence of an organ.* | agénésie |
| **agglutination** *The process of adherence of a mass.* | agglutination |
| **aggression** | agression |
| **aging** | vieillissement |
| **agitation** | agitation |
| **aglutition** *The inability to swallow.* | impossibilité d'avaler |
| **agnathia** *Congenital abnormality characterized by the absence of the mandible.* | agnathie |
| **agnosia** *A condition exhibited by the loss of sensory stimuli.* | agnosie |

| English | French |
|---|---|
| **agonist** *A synthetic compound that activates cells normally activated by natural chemicals.* | agoniste |
| **agony** *Anguish or torment.* | agonie |
| **agoraphobia** *The fear of being in a large open space.* | agoraphobie |
| **agranulocytosis** *A condition characterized by leukopenia and neutropenia.* | agranulocytose |
| **agraphia** *The inability to express one's thoughts in writing.* | agraphie |
| **agreement** | accord |
| **ague** *A term used to describe recurrent fever typically associated with malaria.* | fièvre intermittente |
| **AIDS** | SIDA |
| **air embolism** *The blockage of an artery or vein by an air bubble.* | aéroembolisme |
| **air flow** | écoulement gazeux |
| **akathisia** *A condition exhibited by motor restlessness and inability to sit quietly.* | akathisie |
| **akinesia** *An absence of movement or sparsity of movement.* | akinésie |
| **albinism** *Congenital absence of pigment in the eyes, skin and hair.* | albinisme |
| **albino** *A person who lacks pigment in the eyes, skin and hair.* | albinos |
| **albumin** *A protein that is soluble in water and coagulates if heated.* | albumine |
| **albuminuria** *The presence of albumin in the urine.* | albuminurie |
| **alcohol** | alcool |
| **alcoholic** *Referring to alcohol.* | 1. alcoolique 2. éthylique |
| **alcoholism** *An addiction to alcohol.* | alcoolisme |
| **aldehyde** *A substance derived by oxidizing and containing a CHO group from alcohol.* | aldéhyde |
| **aldosterone** *A steroid secreted by the adrenal cortex that regulates electrolytes.* | aldostérone |
| **aldosteronism** *A condition characterized by the excessive secretion of aldosterone.* | 1. aldostéronisme 2. hyperaldostéronisme |
| **alert** | attentif |
| **alexia** *Inability to read due to a central brain lesion.* | alexie |
| **alga** *Singular form of algae.* | algue |
| **algid** *cold* | algide |
| **algogenic** *Pain causing.* | algogène |
| **alimentary** | alimentaire |
| **alkali** *A class of compounds that form soluble carbonates.* | alcali |
| **alkaline** *Referring to something with properties of an alkali.* | alcalin |
| **alkalinuria** *The urine in an alkaline state.* | alcalinurie |
| **alkaloid** *Plant derived nitrogenous organic compound.* | alcaloïde |
| **alkalosis** *A condition in which the pH is increased.* | alcalose |
| **alkaptonuria** *A condition exhibited by the urine turning dark upon standing because of the presence of alkapton bodies in it.* | alcaptonurie |

| English | French |
|---|---|
| **allantois** *A posterior portion of the hind-gut of an embryo.* | allantoïde |
| **allele** *A type of a gene; in humans there are two alleles per chromosome pair.* | allèle |
| **allergen** *A compound that causes an allergic reaction.* | allergène |
| **allergy** *An immune response by the body to a compound it is hypersensitive to.* | allergie |
| **alleviate** | atténuer |
| **allograft** *A tissue transplant of from someone of the same species but different genotype.* | allogreffe |
| **allopathy** *Treatment of disease with minute amounts of natural substances.* | allopathie |
| **alopecia** *The absence of hair in areas where it normally exists.* | 1. alopécie 2. calvitie |
| **alpha wave** *Electroencephalographic waves with a frequency of 8-13 per second.* | onde alpha |
| **alpha-fetoprotein** *A glycoprotein that has a high serum level in hepatocellular and nonseminomatous germ cell tumors.* | alpha-fœtoprotéine (AFP) |
| **alteration** | changement |
| **altitude sickness** *A general term used for an illness that occurs at high altitude.* | mal des montagnes |
| **alveolar** *Referring to the alveolus.* | alvéolaire |
| **alveolus** *A small sac like structure commonly used for the pulmonary alveolus.* | alvéole pulmonaire |
| **Alzheimer's disease** *A dementia of unknown cause or pathogenesis.* | Alzheimer, maladie d' |
| **amalgam** *An alloy that includes mercury as one ingredient.* | amalgame |
| **amastia** *A development condition exhibited by the absence of breasts.* | amastie |
| **amaurosis** *Blindness that occurs without an ocular lesion but may include the optic nerve.* | amaurose |
| **ambidextrous** *Ability to use both hands equal ability.* | ambidextre |
| **amblyopia** *Decreased vision without an ocular lesion.* | amblyopie |
| **ambulation** *A walk.* | ambulation |
| **ambulatory electrocardiographic monitoring** *A continuous recording of the electrocardiogram used to detect occult dysrhythmias.* | Holter ECG |
| **ambulatory** *Referring to one's ability to walk.* | ambulatoire |
| **ameba** *A one-celled protozoan.* | amibe |
| **amebiasis** *A condition in which one is infected with amebae, mostly commonly Entamoeba histolytica.* | amibiase |
| **amebicide** *A compound used to treat amebiasis.* | amoebicide |
| **ameboma** *A mass caused by inflammation as seen in amebiasis.* | amoebome |
| **amelia** *A congenital anomaly exhibited by the absence of limbs.* | amélie |
| **amelioration** *Resolution of a problem.* | amélioration |
| **amenorrhea** *The absence of menses.* | aménorrhée |
| **amentia** *The absence of mental ability.* | arriération profonde |
| **ametria** *Congenital absence of the uterus.* | 1. absence d'utérus 2. amétrie |

| English | French |
|---|---|
| **ametropia** *Abnormal refractive ability of the eyes resulting in hypermetropia, myopia or astigmatism.* | amétropie |
| **amino acid** *A compound containing a carboxyl and an amino group.* | aminé acide |
| **ammonia** *A colorless alkaline gas.* | ammoniac |
| **amnesia** *The inability to remember past events.* | amnésie |
| **amnesia, antegrade** *The inability to remember events which occurred after the insult that caused the condition.* | amnésie antérograde |
| **amnesiac stroke** *Cerebral infarct exhibited by loss of memory.* | ictus amnésique |
| **amniocentesis** *Transabdominal aspiration of amniotic fluid.* | amniocentèse |
| **amniography** *X-ray of the gravid uterus after insertion of opaque dye.* | amniographie |
| **amnion** *The membrane lining the placenta which produces the amniotic fluid.* | amnios |
| **amniotic fluid** *The fluid surrounding the fetus.* | liquide amniotique |
| **amorphous** *A fetus with no heart and no definitive shape.* | amorphe |
| **amount** | montant |
| **ampulla** *The dilated end of a duct.* | ampoule |
| **ampulla chyli** *Also called cisterna chyli; it is a dilated area of the thoracic duct that collects lymph from several areas.* | citerne de Pecquet |
| **amylase** *An enzyme involved in the hydrolysis of starch.* | amylase |
| **amyloidosis** *The accumulation of amyloid in body tissues.* | amyloïdose |
| **amyotonia** *A condition associated with the lack of muscle tone.* | amyotonie |
| **amyotrophic lateral sclerosis** *A progressive neurodegenerative disorder.* | sclérose latérale amyotrophique |
| **amyotrophy** *Atrophy of muscle tissue.* | amyotrophie |
| **anabolism** *The formation of molecules in organisms from simpler molecules.* | anabolisme |
| **anacrotic** *Referring to a prominent bulge on the ascending portion of a pulse recording.* | anacrote |
| **anaerobe** *An organism that lives in the absence of oxygen.* | anaérobie |
| **analeptic** *A medication used as a stimulant to the central nervous system.* | analeptique |
| **analgesia** *The absence of pain.* | analgésie |
| **analgesic** *A medication used to remove pain.* | analgésique |
| **analogous** *To resemble or be similar to.* | analogue |
| **anaphase** *A stage in mitosis following metaphase.* | anaphase |
| **anaphoresis** *Reduced activity of the sweat glands.* | anaphorèse |
| **anaphylaxis** *An exaggerated response to a foreign substance.* | anaphylaxie |
| **anaplasia** *The loss of normal differentiation of tumor cells.* | anaplasie |
| **anastomosis** *Surgical formation of a connection between two previously separate parts.* | anastomose |
| **anatomical chart** *A pictorial diagram of part of the anatomy.* | planche anatomique |
| **anatomical** *Referring to the anatomy.* | anatomique |

| English | French |
|---|---|
| **anatomical snuff-box** *The area on the back of the hand near the base of the thumb that is between the extensor pollicus longus and extensor pollicus brevis.* | tabatière anatomique |
| **anatomy** *The study of body structure.* | anatomie |
| **ancylostomiasis** *A type of nematode parasite, also called hookworm.* | ankylostomiase |
| **androgen** *A compound that produces masculinizing characteristics.* | androgène |
| **android pelvis** *A pelvis shaped like a man's.* | bassin androïde |
| **androsterone** *A hormone excreted in the urine of men and women.* | androstérone |
| **anemia** *Lower than normal red blood cell count.* | anémie |
| **anencephaly** *The congenital absence of the cranial vault and cerebral hemispheres.* | anencéphalie |
| **aneroid** *The absence of liquid.* | anéroïde |
| **anesthesia** *Loss of sensation.* | anesthésie |
| **anesthetic** *A chemical that produces anesthesia.* | anesthésique |
| **anesthetist** *A person who administers anesthesia.* | anesthésiste |
| **aneurysm** *A condition exhibited by the dilatation of the walls of an artery or vein to form a blood-filled sac.* | anévrisme |
| **angiectasia** *Dilation of a blood or lymph vessel.* | angiectasie |
| **angiitis** *The inflammation of a lymph or blood vessel.* | angéite |
| **angina pectoris** *Exercise induced myocardial ischemia.* | angine de poitrine |
| **angiogram** *Radiologic imaging of blood vessels.* | angiogramme |
| **angiography** *Roentgenographic imaging of blood vessels.* | angiographie |
| **angioma** *A tumor comprised of blood or lymph vessels.* | angiome |
| **angioneurotic** *Caused by a neurosis affecting the blood vessels, like vasospasm.* | angioneurotique |
| **angioneurotic edema** *A condition exhibited by sudden edema of skin and mucous membranes.* | œdème de Quincke |
| **angioplasty** *Surgical alteration of blood vessels.* | angioplastie |
| **angiosarcoma** *A sarcoma comprised of blood vessels.* | angiosarcome |
| **angiospasm** *A spasm of a blood vessel.* | angiospasme |
| **angiotensin** *A blood protein that increases aldosterone secretion.* | angiotensine |
| **angiotensin converting enzyme inhibitors (ACEI)** *A class of medicines that prevent conversion of angiotension I to angiotensin II, a potent vasoconstrictor.* | inhibiteurs de l'enzyme de conversion |
| **anguish** | angoisse |
| **anhidrosis** *A condition exhibited by reduced quantity of sweat.* | anhidrose |
| **anhidrotic** *Something the reduces the quantity of sweat.* | anhidrotique |
| **anhydrous** *Lacking water.* | anhydre |
| **aniseikonia** *A condition in which the ocular image of an object is viewed differently by each eye..* | aniséiconie |
| **anisocoria** *Pupillary diameter inequality.* | anisocorie |
| **anisocytosis** *Variation in size of erythrocytes.* | anisocytose |
| **anisomelia** *Unequal size of arms or legs.* | anisomélie |

| English | French |
|---|---|
| **anisometropia** *Refractive power inequality between the two eyes.* | anisométropie |
| **ankle** | cheville |
| **ankle clonus** *An abnormal response exhibited by alternating plantar- and dorsiflexion noted after the examiner rapidly dorsiflexes the foot.* | clonus du pied |
| **ankle edema** | œdème malléolaire |
| **ankle joint** | articulation tibio-astragalienne |
| **ankle support (device)** | chevillère |
| **ankle swelling** | œdème des chevilles |
| **ankyloglossia** *Limitation of tongue motion because of a short frenulum.* | ankyloglossie |
| **ankylosing spondylitis** *A type of arthritis found in the spine that is exhibited by bony fusion.* | spondylarthrite anklyosante |
| **ankylosis** *Abnormal immobility of a joint.* | ankylose |
| **annular** *Referring to a ring.* | annulaire |
| **anomia** *Inability to name or recognize familiar objects.* | anomie |
| **anonychia** *Congenital absence of fingernails or toenails.* | anonychie |
| **anoperineal** *Referring to the anus and perineum.* | anopérinéal |
| **anorchous** *The absence of testicles.* | anorchide |
| **anorectal** *Referring to the anus and rectum.* | anorectal |
| **anorexia nervosa** *A mental disorder characterized by the desire to avoid eating and to lose weight.* | anorexie mentale |
| **anorexia** *The loss of appetite.* | anorexie |
| **anosmia** *Lack of the sense of smell.* | anosmie |
| **anovulation** *Lack of ovulation.* | anovulation |
| **anovulatory cycle** *A menstrual cycle in which no ovum is released.* | cycle anovulatoire |
| **anoxemia** *Reduction in blood oxygen concentration.* | anoxémie |
| **anoxia** *Reduced oxygen levels in body tissues.* | anoxie |
| **antacid** *A medication, usually with a calcium or magnesium base that binds with acid in the stomach.* | antiacide |
| **antagonist** *A muscle or agent that acts in counteract to effects of another muscle or agent.* | antagoniste |
| **antemortem** *Refers to: before death.* | avant la mort |
| **antenatal** *Refers to events before birth.* | anténatal |
| **anterior root** *A motor nerve root that is in the anterior part of the spinal cord between the anterior and lateral funiculi.* | racine antérieure |
| **anterior** *Toward the front.* | antérieur |
| **anterograde** *Moving forward.* | antérograde |
| **anteroinferior** *Toward the front and lower part.* | antéro-inférieur |
| **anterolateral** *Toward the front and away from the midline.* | antérolatéral |
| **anteromedian** *Toward the front and toward the midline.* | antéromédian |
| **anteroposterior** *From front to the back. (An AP x-ray has the beam directed from the front to the back.)* | antéropostérieur |
| **anterosuperior** *Toward the front and the upper part.* | antérosupérieur |

| English | French |
|---|---|
| **anteversion** *The forward leaning of an organ.* | antéversion |
| **anthelmintic** *An agent used to destroy worms.* | 1. anthelminthique 2. vermifuge |
| **anthracosis** *Pneumoconiosis caused by coal dust.* | anthracose |
| **anthrax** *An infectious disease caused by Bacillus anthracis; there are cutaneous, inhalation and gastrointestinal syndromes.* | anthrax |
| **anti-inflammatory** *Medication used to reduce inflammation.* | anti-inflammatoire |
| **antibiotic** *A medication that inhibits or kills microorganisms.* | antibiotique |
| **antibody** *A protein that combines with and counteracts foreign substances.* | anticorps |
| **anticholinergic** *Parasympathetic blocker.* | anticholinergique |
| **anticholinesterase** *Cholinesterase blocker.* | anticholinestérase |
| **anticoagulant** *Medication used to inhibit coagulation.* | anticoagulant |
| **anticodon** *A series of three nucleotides that form a unit of genetic code for transfer RNA.* | anticodon |
| **anticonvulsant** *Medication used to treat seizures.* | anticonvulsivant |
| **antidepressant** *Medication used to treat depression.* | 1. antidépresseur 2. thymoanaleptique |
| **antidiuretic hormone** *Vasopressin.* | antidiurétique hormone |
| **antidote** *A medication that neutralizes a toxin.* | antidote |
| **antigen** *A foreign substance, like bacteria, that induces an immune response.* | antigène |
| **antiglobulin test (Coombs' test)** *Test used to detect erythroblastosis fetalis.* | test à l'antiglobuline |
| **antihemophilic factor** *Also called factor VIII. A deficiency of the factor causes hemophilia.* | facteur antihémophilique |
| **antihistamine** *Medication used to treat conditions exhibited by a histamine response* | antihistaminique |
| **antilymphocyte** *A serum globulin that has antibodies to lymphocytes.* | antilymphocytaire |
| **antilymphocyte globulin** *The gamma globulin portion of antilymphocyte serum.* | globuline antilymphocytaire |
| **antimalarial** *Medication used to treat malaria.* | antipaludique |
| **antimetabolite** *A substance that impedes metabolism.* | antimétabolite |
| **antimigraine** *Medication used to treat headaches.* | antimigraineux |
| **antimitotic** *Impeding mitosis.* | antimitotique |
| **antimycotic** *Inhibition of fungal growth.* | 1. antifongique 2. antimycosique |
| **antinuclear factor** *Also called antinucleic antibody (ANA); it is found in conditions such as lupus and rheumatoid arthritis.* | facteur antinucléaire |
| **antiperistaltic** *An agent that impedes normal peristalsis.* | antipéristaltique |
| **antipruritic** *Medication used to treat pruritus.* | antiprurigineux |
| **antipyretic** *Medication used to treat fever.* | antipyrétique |
| **antiseptic** *A substance that inhibits microorganism growth.* | antiseptique |
| **antiserum** *A substance that contains antibodies to specific antigens.* | antisérum |

| English | French |
|---|---|
| **antispasmodic** *Medication used to treat muscle spasm.* | antispasmodique |
| **antithrombin** *A substance that inhibits thrombin, thus decreasing the body's ability to coagulate.* | antithrombine |
| **antithyroid** *A substance inhibiting the effect of the thyroid.* | antithyroïdien |
| **antitoxin** *A substance that inhibits the effect of a toxin.* | antitoxine |
| **antitussive** *Medication used to diminish a cough.* | antitussif |
| **antivenin** *An antitoxin formulated for various types of snake bites.* | antivenin |
| **antrotomy** *To cut open the antrum.* | antrotomie |
| **antrum** *Referring to a cavity or chamber.* | antre |
| **anuria** *The lack of urine excretion.* | anurie |
| **anus** *The body opening distal to the rectum.* | anus |
| **anxiety** *Nervousness or unease.* | anxiété |
| **anxiety neurosis** *Abnormal presence of anxiety.* | névrosé d'angoisse |
| **anxious** *Experiencing nervousness or unease.* | anxieux |
| **aorta** *The large artery originating at the left ventricle and going to the pelvis where it bifurcates.* | aorte |
| **aortic insufficiency** *A dysfunction of the aortic valve allowing backflow of blood into the heart.* | insuffisance aortique |
| **aortic** *Referring to the aorta.* | aortique |
| **aortic stenosis** *Narrowing of the aortic orifice.* | rétrécissement aortique |
| **aortic valve** *The valve situated between the left ventricle and the aorta.* | valve aortique |
| **apart** | séparé |
| **apathy** | apathie |
| **aperistalsis** *Lack of intestinal peristalsis.* | apéristaltisme |
| **aperture** *An opening or hole, as in the hole the light passes through in a camera.* | ouverture |
| **apex** *The highest point of something.* | sommet |
| **apex of heart** *Normally found 8cm to the left of the midsternal line in the 5th intercostal space.* | pointe du cœur |
| **Apgar score** *A scoring system for newborns that utilizes heart rate, respiratory effort, muscle tone, responsiveness and skin color.* | Apgar, indice d' |
| **aphagia** *The lack of eating.* | aphagie |
| **aphakia** *The congenital absence of the lens of the eye.* | aphakie |
| **aphasia** *Diminished ability to communicate via speech or writing.* | aphasie |
| **aphid** *A minute insect that feeds on plants.* | puceron |
| **aphonia** *The loss of voice.* | aphonie |
| **aphthous stomatitis** *Grouped small lesions that occur on the tongue or in the mouth.* | 1. aphte buccal 2. muguet 3. stomatite aphteuse |
| **apicetomy** *Removal of the apex of the petrous portion of the temporal bone.* | apicectomie |
| **aplastic anemia** *Bone marrow failure causing a decrease in all types of blood cells.* | anémie aplasique |
| **apnea** *Absence of respiration.* | apnée |

| English | French |
|---|---|
| **apocrine gland** *A gland that releases some of its cytoplasm in secretions; an example is axillary sweat glands.* | gland apocrine |
| **aponeurosis** *A tendinous expansion that connects with muscle to move a part.* | aponévrose |
| **apophysis** *Generally a bony outgrowth that forms a process or tubercle.* | apophyse |
| **apoplexy** *Extravasation of blood within an organ.* | apoplexie |
| **appearance** | aspect |
| **appendectomy** *Surgical excision of the appendix.* | appendicectomie |
| **appendicitis** *Inflammation of the appendix.* | appendicite |
| **appendix** *An appendage of the cecum.* | appendice |
| **apperception** *The ability to interpret sensory impressions.* | aperception |
| **application** | application |
| **applicator** | applicateur |
| **appointment** | rendez-vous |
| **apprehension** *A fear that something unpleasant will happen.* | appréhension |
| **approval** | agrément |
| **approximate** | approximatif |
| **approximately** | approximativement |
| **apraxia** *The inability to carry out intentional movements when paralysis is not present.* | apraxie |
| **apron** | tablier |
| **apt** *Suitable in the circumstances.* | apte |
| **aptitude** *A natural talent for something.* | aptitude |
| **aptyalism** *Diminished or absence of saliva.* | aptylisme |
| **aqueous humor** *The fluid between the cornea and lens, anterior to the globe.* | humeur aqueuse |
| **aqueous** *Use of water as a solvent or medium.* | aqueux |
| **arachnodactyly** *A condition exhibited by abnormally long and slender fingers.* | arachnodactylie |
| **arachnoid** *Refers to that which resembles a spider web.* | arachnoïde |
| **arbovirus** *Virus that is transmitted by arthropods; responsible for diseases such as Yellow fever and dengue fever.* | arbovirus |
| **arcuate nucleus** *Small masses of gray matter found on the medulla oblongata.* | noyau arqué |
| **arcus** *Narrow opaque band.* | arc |
| **areola** *The pigmented skin surrounding a nipple.* | aréole |
| **areolar tissue** *The hyperpigmented tissue around the nipple.* | tissu conjonctif lâche |
| **argininosuccinicaciduria** *Presence of arginosuccinic acid in the urine; associated with mental retardation.* | argininosuccinurie |
| **argue, to** | 1. argumenter 2. discuter |
| **argyria** *The greyish discoloration of the skin and conjunctiva.* | argyrie |
| **arm** | bras |

| English | French |
|---|---|
| around | autour |
| arousal *Awaken an emotion.* | éveil |
| arousal response | réaction d'arrêt |
| arrhenoblastoma *An ovarian tumor that results in masculine secondary sex characteristics.* | arrhénoblastome |
| arrhythmia *An abnormal heart rhythm.* | arythmie |
| arterial blood gas *Measurement of the arterial concentration of carbon dioxide and oxygen.* | gazométrie artérielle |
| arterial *Referring to an artery.* | artériel |
| arteriectomy *Surgical excision of an artery.* | artériectomie |
| arteriography *Roentgenography of an artery after infusion of contrast media.* | artériographie |
| arterioplasty *Surgical repair of an artery.* | artérioplastie |
| arteriosclerosis *Hardening and thickening of arterial walls.* | artériosclérose |
| arteriotomy *Creation of an opening in an artery.* | artériotomie |
| arteriovenous aneurysm *A sac like structure created by the abnormal communication of an adjacent artery and vein.* | anévrisme atrério-veineux |
| arteritis *Inflammation of an artery.* | artérite |
| artery *Vessel that carries oxygenated blood from the heart to the periphery.* | artère |
| arthralgia *Joint pain.* | arthralgie |
| arthritis *Joint inflammation.* | arthrite |
| arthrochalasis *Abnormal laxity of a joint.* | hyperlaxité articulaire |
| arthrodesis *Surgical fusion of a joint.* | arthrodèse |
| arthrodynia *Joint pain.* | arthrodynie |
| arthrography *Joint roentgenography.* | arthrographie |
| arthroplasty *Plastic surgery involving a joint.* | arthroplastie |
| arthroscopy *Viewing of the inside of a joint with a specially designed scope.* | arthroscopie |
| arthrotomy *Surgical opening of a joint.* | arthrotomie |
| articular *Referring to a joint.* | articulaire |
| artifact *An aberration from the normal.* | artefact |
| artificial *Not natural produced.* | artificiel |
| arytenoid *Referring to the cartilage in the posterior larynx.* | aryténoïde |
| asbestos *A heat resistant silicate material.* | 1. asbeste 2. amiante |
| asbestosis *Lung disease caused by the inhalation of asbestos.* | asbestose |
| ascaricide *Agent that destroys ascaris.* | ascaricide |
| ascaris *A nematode from genus intestinal lumbricoid parasite, also called round worm.* | ascaris |
| ascending colon *The portion of the colon between the cecum and the right colic flexure.* | côlon ascendant |
| ascertain, to *Synonym of "to determine".* | déterminer |
| ascites *Serous fluid in the abdominal cavity.* | ascite |

| English | French |
|---|---|
| **ascorbic acid** *Commonly known as vitamin C; a deficiency of this vitamin causes scurvy.* | 1. ascorbique acide 2. vitamine C |
| **asepsis** *Lack of infection.* | asepsie |
| **aseptic** *Being free of septic matter.* | aseptique |
| **asexual** *Without sex or sex organs.* | asexué |
| **asleep** | endormi |
| **aspermia** *Absence of sperm.* | aspermie |
| **asphyxia** *A condition exhibited by a lack of oxygen and subsequent loss of consciousness or death.* | asphyxie |
| **aspiration** *Taking air or matter into the lungs. Removal of fluid from a cavity.* | aspiration |
| **aspirator** *A device used to remove fluid from a cavity.* | aspirateur |
| **aspirin** *Common name for acetylsalicylic acid.* | aspirine |
| **assay** *A procedure for measuring the activity of a biological sample.* | détermination |
| **assessment** *An evaluation.* | bilan |
| **assistance** | aide |
| **assisted ventilation** *The act of helping one breathe through artificial means.* | ventilation assistée |
| **asteatosis** *A condition exhibited by diminished sebaceous secretion.* | astéatose |
| **astereognosis** *Lack of ability to recognize objects by touching them.* | astéréognosie |
| **asthenia** *Diminished strength and energy.* | asthénie |
| **asthenopia** *Visual fatigue accompanied by ocular pain.* | asthénopie |
| **astragalus** *Synonym of talus.* | astragale |
| **astringent** *An agent causing contraction of the skin.* | astringent |
| **astrocytoma** *A tumor comprised of astrocytes.* | astrocytome |
| **astroglia** *The neurologic tissue which is composed of astrocytes..* | astroglie |
| **asymmetry** *Lack of symmetry.* | asymétrie |
| **asymptomatic** | asymptomatique |
| **asynclitism** *Oblique presentation of the head during delivery.* | asynclitisme |
| **at random** | hasard au |
| **atavism** *The inheritance of characteristics from remote rather than immediate ancestors.* | atavisme |
| **ataxia** *Lack of muscular coordination.* | ataxie |
| **atelectasis** *Incomplete expansion or collapse of a lung.* | atélectasie |
| **atherogenic** *Something that causes atheromatous lesions in arterial walls.* | athérogène |
| **atheroma** *Degenerative arteriosclerosis.* | athérome |
| **athetosis** *An involuntary symptom exhibited by continuous slow, writhing movements, mostly in the hands.* | athétose |
| **athlete's foot** *Common term for tinea pedis.* | athlète, pied d' |
| **atlas** *The first cervical vertebra.* | atlas |
| **atomizer** *A device for propelling a fine mist.* | atomiseur |
| **atony** *Absence of normal muscle tone.* | atonie |

| English | French |
|---|---|
| **atresia** *Closure of a body orifice as in atresia ani in which there is a congenital imperforate anus.* | atrésie |
| **atrial natriuretic factor** *A chemical secreted by the right atrium that promotes sodium excretion in the urine.* | facteur natriurétique auriculaire |
| **atrial** *Referring to the atrium.* | atrial |
| **atrial septal defect** *An abnormal communication between the atria of the heart.* | communication interauriculaire |
| **atrio-ventricular block** *An interruption of the electrical conduction at the atrio-ventricular node.* | bloc auriculo-ventriculaire |
| **atrioventricular bundle** *Also called bundle of His.* | faisceau atrio-ventriculaire |
| **atrioventricular** *Referring to the atrium and ventricle.* | atrioventriculaire |
| **atrium** *Referring to a chamber used as an entrance, as in the entrance to the heart.* | 1. atrium 2. oreillette |
| **atrophic** *Referring to atrophy.* | atrophique |
| **atrophy** *A diminution in the size of a part.* | atrophie |
| **atropine** *A parasympathetic agent derived from Atropa belladonna.* | atropine |
| **attack** *A fit or paroxysm.* | accès |
| **attack, seizure** *An episode of epilepsy.* | attaque |
| **atypical** *Not usual.* | atypique |
| **audiogram** *The recording of a one's hearing in decibels.* | audiogramme |
| **audiologist** *A specialist in the field of hearing.* | audiologiste |
| **audiometer** *A device used to measure hearing.* | audiomètre |
| **auditory** *Referring to hearing.* | auditif |
| **aural** *Referring to the ear.* | aural |
| **auricle** *The external portion of the ear.* | 1. auricule 2. pavillon de l'oreille |
| **auricular** *Referring to the auricle.* | auriculaire |
| **auriculotemporal** *The area of the ear and temple.* | auriculotemporal |
| **auscultation** *The act of listening to sounds emanating from the body.* | auscultation |
| **autism** *A mental condition exhibited by difficulty in forming relationships, communicating and uses abstract thought.* | autisme |
| **autistic** *Referring to autism.* | autiste |
| **autoantibody** *An antibody that acts against the organism's own tissue.* | auto-anticorps |
| **autoantigen** *A normal tissue constituent that prompts a cell-mediated response.* | auto-antigen |
| **autoclave** *A device used for sterilization with the use of steam under pressure.* | autoclave |
| **autogenous** *Self-generated.* | autogène |
| **autograft** *Grafting tissue from one part of person to another part of the same person.* | autogreffe |
| **autohypnosis** *Self-hypnosis.* | autohypnose |
| **autoimmunization** *The body's ability to promote an immune response without external resources.* | auto-immunisation |

19

| English | French |
|---|---|
| **autolysis** *A state of self destruction of cells within a body.* | autolyse |
| **autonomic nervous system** *Responsible for regulation of cardiac muscle, smooth muscle and glandular activity.* | système nerveux autonome |
| **autopsy** *Examination of a body post-mortem in an attempt to determine cause of death.* | autopsie |
| **autosomal** *Referring to an autosome.* | autosomique |
| **autotransfusion** *The reinfusion of one's own blood.* | autotransfusion |
| **availability** | disponibilité |
| **available** | disponible |
| **avascular** *An area with no blood supply.* | avasculaire |
| **avian flu** *A viral disease found in birds and fowl that can be transmitted to humans; it is exhibited by respiratory and gastrointestinal symptoms but can lead to encephalitis.* | grippe aviaire |
| **avian** *Referring to birds.* | aviaire |
| **avitaminosis** *A state of vitamin deficiency.* | avitaminose |
| **avoidable** | évitable |
| **awakening** | réveil |
| **away from** | éloigné de |
| **axilla** *The hollow beneath the arm.* | aisselle |
| **axillary** *Referring to the axilla.* | axillaire |
| **axis** *The second cervical vertebra.* | axe |
| **axon** *The structure along which nerve impulses are transmitted from the cell body to other cells.* | 1. axone 2. cylindraxe |
| **azoospermia** *The absence of spermatozoa in the semen.* | azoospermie |
| **azotemia** *Prerenal disease.* | azotémie |
| **azoturia** *An excess of urea in the urine.* | azoturie |
| **baby** | bébé |
| **baby-scale** | pèse-bébé |
| **bacillary** *Referring to bacilli.* | bacillaire |
| **bacillus** *A rod-shaped bacterium.* | bacille |
| **back pain** | dorsalgie |
| **bacteremia** *The presence of bacteria in the blood.* | bactériémie |
| **bacteria** *Plural for any organism of the order Eubacteriales.* | bactéries |
| **bacterial** *Referring to bacteria.* | bactérien |
| **bactericidal** *An agent that destroys bacteria.* | bactéricide |
| **bacteriostatic** *An agent that impedes bacterial growth.* | bactériostatique |
| **bacteriuria** *The presence of bacteria in the urine.* | bactérurie |
| **bagassosis** *A pulmonary disorder contracted from inhalation of the waste of sugar cane (bagasse dust).* | bagassose |
| **balanitis** *Inflammation of the glans of the penis.* | balanite |
| **ballottement** *Presence of movement of a floating object by palpation.* | ballottement |
| **balm** | baume |

| English | French |
|---|---|
| **balneology** *The "science" of baths.* | 1. balnéologie 2. thermalisme |
| **bandage** | bandage |
| **banding** *The process of encircling with a thin piece of material.* | cerclage |
| **barber's itch** *Ringworm that is transmitted by contaminated shaving equipment.* | sycosis trichophytique |
| **barium enema** *Administration of barium into the rectum followed by roentgenography to check for rectal or colon abnormalities.* | lavement baryté |
| **barium enema** *Roentgenography after administration of barium via a tube into the rectum.* | repas baryté |
| **basal ganglia** *Structures adjacent to the thalamus that are involved with coordination of movement.* | noyaux gris centraux |
| **basal** *Referring to the base.* | basal |
| **basilar** *Referring to the base or lower segment.* | basilaire |
| **basilic vein** *A vein in the hand that joins the brachial veins to form the axillary vein.* | veine basilique |
| **basin** | cuvette |
| **basophil** *A polymorphonuclear granulocyte.* | basophile |
| **bear, to** | donner naissance |
| **bearing down** *As in during labor.* | efforts expulsifs |
| **beat** | battement |
| **bed** | lit |
| **bed rest** | alitement |
| **bedbug** *Cimex lectularius. A small insect that is parasitic and hides in clothing or bedding.* | punaise de lit |
| **bedpan** | bassin de lit |
| **bedridden** | grabataire |
| **bee sting** | piqûre d'abeille |
| **beforehand** | préalable au |
| **behavior disorder** *An abnormal mental state.* | trouble du comportement |
| **below** | dessous |
| **belt; waist** | ceinture |
| **benign** *Not harmful.* | bénin |
| **berylliosis** *A lung exhibited by granulomas and caused by inhalation of beryllium.* | bérylliose |
| **best** | meilleur |
| **betablocker** *A substance that inhibits adrenergic stimulation. It is used to reduce pulse, blood pressure and to treat angina.* | bêta-bloquant |
| **beyond** | au-delà |
| **bezoar** *A concretion composed of either hair, vegetable/fruit fibers or hair and vegetable/fruit fibers that is found in the stomach.* | bézoard |
| **biased** *Prejudiced.* | biaisé |

| English | French |
|---------|--------|
| **biceps** *A muscle with two heads usually referring to the biceps brachii which is used for forearm flexion.* | biceps |
| **biceps reflex** *The biceps brachii tendon is hit with a reflex hammer and results in flexion of the forearm as a normal response. This assesses the C5-C6 region.* | réflexe bicipital |
| **bicuspid** *Having two points as in bicuspid valve or a premolar tooth.* | bicuspide |
| **bifid** *Presence of two branches.* | bifide |
| **bifurcate ligament** *A ligament on the dorsum of the foot that includes the calcaneonavicular and calcaneocuboid ligaments.* | ligament de Chopart |
| **bifurcate** *When one branch divides into two branches.* | bifurqué |
| **bilateral** | bilatéral |
| **bile** *An alkaline fluid secreted by the liver to aid digestion.* | bile |
| **bile duct** *The structure that is a conduit for passage of bile from the liver and gallbladder to the duodenum.* | canal biliaire |
| **bile pigment** *The golden brown or green-yellow color associated with bile.* | pigment biliaire |
| **bile salts** *Normally occurring salts of bile acids.* | sels biliares |
| **Bilharzia** *Historical name of a genus of flukes or nematodes now known as Schistosoma.* | Schistosoma |
| **biliary** *Referring to bile, bile ducts or gallbladder.* | biliaire |
| **bilious** *Something that contains bile.* | bilieux |
| **bilirubin** *A pigment found in bile that is responsible for the yellow color seen in patients with elevated serum levels of bilirubin.* | bilirubine |
| **biliuria** *The presence of bile in the urine.* | biliurie |
| **biliverdin** *A green pigment formed by oxidation of bilirubin.* | biliverdine |
| **bill** | facture |
| **bimanual** *Use of two hands, as in bimanual pelvic examination in which the right hand touches the cervix uteri and the left hand presses above the mons pubis.* | bimanuel |
| **binaural** *Referring to both ears.* | biauriculaire |
| **binocular** *Referring to both eyes.* | binoculaire |
| **binovular** *Derived from two different ova.* | biovulé |
| **bioassay** *A laboratory test determination as compared to normal.* | dosage biologique |
| **bioavailability** *The portion of a drug that is able to be utilized by the body after it is introduced to the body.* | biodisponibilité |
| **biochemistry** *The study of chemistry and physiochemical processes in living organisms.* | biochimie |
| **biology** *The study of living organisms.* | biologie |
| **biopsy** *The removal and examination of bodily tissues or fluids.* | biopsie |
| **biotin** *A vitamin involved in the synthesis of fatty acids and glucose.* | biotine |
| **birth** | naissance |
| **birth control** *Any method of limiting contraception.* | limitation des naissances |
| **birth defect** *A congenital anomaly.* | anomalie congénitale |

| English | French |
|---|---|
| **birth rate** *The number of live births per 1000 of a given population per year.* | taux de natalité |
| **bistoury; scalpel** *A surgical knife.* | bistouri |
| **bitemporal hemianopsia** *A visual defect seen commonly in pituitary tumors in which the visual defect is in the temporal portion of each eye.* | hémianopsie bitemporale |
| **bitter** | amer |
| **black** | noir |
| **black fly** *From the family Simuliidae that can cause disease in humans.* | simulie |
| **black stools** *Common term for melena.* | selles noires |
| **blackout** *Common term for loss of consciousness.* | voile noir |
| **blackwater fever** *A term used to describe the fever associated with malaria when the urine is reddish-black.* | fièvre bileuse hémoglobinurique |
| **blast injury** *Trauma from a wave of air pressure.* | lésion par souffle |
| **blastomycosis** *Infection caused by organisms of genus Blastomyces.* | blastomycose |
| **bleach** | eau de javel |
| **bleeding** | saignement |
| **bleeding time** *The time of bleeding after a controlled standardized puncture of the earlobe.* | temps de saignement |
| **blennorrhea** *Discharge from the mucous membranes, usually referring to gonorrhea.* | blennorrhée |
| **blepharitis** *Inflammation of the eyelids.* | blépharite |
| **blepharospasm** *A spasm of the orbicularis oculi muscle that causes closure of the eyelid.* | blépharospasme |
| **blind** | aveugle |
| **blind loop syndrome** *A condition in which there is a non-functional section of the bowel that is thought to be responsible for malabsorption and Vitamin B12 deficiency.* | syndrome de l'anse borgne |
| **blind spot** *An area of insensitivity to light located at the point of entry of the optic nerve on the retina.* | tache aveugle |
| **blindness** | cécité |
| **blinking** | clignement |
| **blister** *Common term for bulla.* | cloque |
| **bloating** *Sensation of having an abnormally large amount of air in the viscera.* | ballonnement |
| **blood** | sang |
| **blood alcohol level** *A quantitative measurement of the amount of alcohol in the blood.* | alcoolémie |
| **blood bank** | banque de sang |
| **blood brain barrier** *A matrix of capillaries that move blood between the blood and brain, as well as, limiting some substances from passing.* | barrière hématoméningée |
| **blood cell** | globule sanguin |
| **blood clot** | caillot sanguin |
| **blood grouping** *Testing blood to determine which type should be used for transfusion.* | groupage sanguin |

| English | French |
|---|---|
| **blood pressure** *Written as the measurement in mmHg at the time of systole of the left ventricle over the time of diastole.* | 1. tension artérielle 2. pression artérielle |
| **blood sedimentation rate (ESR)** *The settling time of erythrocytes in a prepared sample. This is a measure of the abnormal concentration of substances that are associated with pathological states.* | vitesse de sédimentation |
| **blood stream** *Common term or the arterial or venous systems.* | circulation sanguine |
| **blood tubing (used for infusion of blood)** | trousse de transfusion |
| **blood type** *Determined and listed in the ABO system.* | groupe sanguin |
| **blood volume** | 1. volémie 2. sanguin |
| **blue** | bleu |
| **blunt** | 1. contondant 2. émoussé |
| **blurred vision** | vision trouble |
| **blurt out, to** | lâcher |
| **blush, to** | rougir |
| **body surface area** *Dubois formula is: (weight in kilograms)to the 0.425th power x (height in centimeters) to the 0.725th power x 0.007184.* | surface corporelle |
| **body weight** | poids corporel |
| **bolus** *A fluid bolus is a phrase used for rapid infusion of fluid.* | bol |
| **bone** | os |
| **bone graft** *The transfer of bone to aid in the healing of a complex fracture.* | greffe osseuse |
| **bone marrow** *The soft material filling the cavity of bones.* | moelle osseuse |
| **bone marrow aplasia** *Suppression of bone marrow function leading to decreased production of erythrocytes, leukocytes and thrombocytes.* | aplasie médullaire |
| **bone marrow puncture** *The aspiration of marrow to look for pressure of disease.* | prélèvement de moelle osseuse |
| **bone scan** *Bone imaging using technetium 99m (99mTc) diphosphate.* | scintigraphie osseuse |
| **bonesetter** *A person who sets bones without being a physician.* | rebouteux |
| **border; margin** | bord |
| **born** | né |
| **bottle** | 1. bouteille 2. biberon |
| **bougienage** *Passage of a bougie through a body orifice with the goal of increasing the diameter of the orifice.* | bougirage |
| **brace** | appareil orthopédique |
| **brace; splint** | attelle |
| **brachial artery** *A continuation of the axillary artery and branches into the radial and ulnar among others.* | brachiale artère |
| **brachial plexus** *A cluster of nerves coming off the last four cervical and first thoracic spinal nerves form the nerve supply the the chest and arms.* | plexus brachial |
| **brachial** *Referring to the arm.* | brachial |
| **brachium cerebelli** *Synonym of pedunculus cerebellaris superior (upper portion the cerebellum).* | pédoncule cérébelleux |

| English | French |
|---|---|
| **brachycephaly** *The presence of a short broad skull.* | brachycéphalie |
| **bracing** | contention |
| **bradycardia** *Lower than normal cardiac rate measured in beats per minute.* | bradycardie |
| **bradykinin** *A peptide that causes contraction of smooth muscle and dilation of blood vessels.* | bradykinine |
| **brain** | encéphale |
| **brain** *A common term for cerebrum.* | cerveau |
| **brain death** *Cessation of cerebral functioning.* | 1. coma dépassé 2. mort cérébrale |
| **brain stem** *An organ that consists of the medulla oblongata, pons and midbrain.* | tronc cérébral |
| **branchial** *Referring to or resembling the gills of a fish.* | branchial |
| **break** | cassure |
| **breast** | sein |
| **breast feeding** | allaitement maternel |
| **breath** | haleine |
| **breath sound** *The noise heard upon auscultation with a stethoscope.* | murmure vésiculaire |
| **breath test (for alcohol)** | alcootest |
| **bregma** *Located at the convergence of the coronal and sagittal sutures.* | bregma |
| **bright** | brillant |
| **bring, to** | apporter |
| **brisk** | animé |
| **broad ligament of uterus** *Supports the uterus on both sides.* | ligament large de l'utérus |
| **broken** | cassé |
| **bromidrosis** *Foul smelling perspiration.* | bromhidrose |
| **bromism** *Poisoning caused by excessive intake of bromine.* | bromisme |
| **bronchial carcinoma** *A general term for a malignancy of the bronchi.* | cancer bronchique |
| **bronchial** *Referring to the bronchus.* | bronchique |
| **bronchiectasis** *The presence of abnormally wide bronchi or branches.* | bronchectasie |
| **bronchiole** *A small branch that a bronchus divides into.* | bronchiole |
| **bronchiolitis** *Inflammation of the pulmonary bronchioles.* | bronchiolite |
| **bronchitis** *Inflammation of the mucous membranes of the bronchioles that causes bronchospasm and cough.* | bronchite |
| **bronchogenic** *Referring to the bronchi.* | bronchogénique |
| **bronchography** *Roentgenography of the bronchi after administration of contrast media.* | bronchographie |
| **bronchopneumonia** *Pneumonia that starts in the distal bronchioles.* | bronchopneumonie |
| **bronchoscope** *The device used to visualize the bronchi.* | bronchoscope |
| **bronchoscopy** *The direct visualization of the bronchi with the aid of a scope.* | bronchoscopie |
| **bronchospasm** *Bronchial smooth muscle spasm.* | bronchospasme |

| English | French |
|---|---|
| **bronchus** *The major air channels that bifurcate from the distal trachea.* | bronche |
| **brow presentation** *The term used to describe which part of the body (forehead) is being delivered first in childbirth.* | présentation frontale |
| **brown** | brun |
| **brucellosis** *A gram-negative bacteria in cattle that causes persistent fever in humans.* | brucellose |
| **bruit** *An abnormal sound heard through a stethoscope indicating turbulent blood flow.* | bruit |
| **brush** | brosse |
| **bubo** *An inflamed, swollen lymph node in the axilla or inguinal region.* | bubon |
| **bubonic plague** *A form of plague exhibited by the formation of buboes.* | peste bubonique |
| **buccal** *Referring to the cheek.* | buccal |
| **buccinator** *A thin, flat muscle in the cheek wall.* | buccinateur |
| **bug** | hémiptère |
| **bulbar palsy** *Paralysis due to changes in the motor center of the medulla oblongata.* | paralysie bulbaire |
| **bulging** | 1. saillant 2. bombé |
| **bulimia** *Pathologic increase in hunger.* | boulimie |
| **bulky** | abondant |
| **bulla** *A large cutaneous serous filled vesicle.* | bulle |
| **bundle branch block** *A cardiac dysrhythmia produced by a blockage of a branch of the bundle of His.* | bloc de branche |
| **bundle of His** *The atrial contraction rhythm is facilitated by this bundle to the ventricles.* | faisceau de His |
| **bunion** *Swelling of the bursa of the metatarsal head of the first metatarsal.* | oignon |
| **burn** | brûlure |
| **burr** | fraise |
| **burr hole** *A treatment of subdural hematoma that involves drilling a hole into the cranium to release the hematoma.* | trou pratiqué avec une fraise |
| **bursitis** *Inflammation of the bursa.* | bursite |
| **burst, to** | éclater |
| **bush** | buisson |
| **buttock** | fesses |
| **button** *Synonym for pimple.* | bouton |
| **bypass** | pontage |
| **byssinosis** *A disease caused by inhalation of cotton dust; a type of pneumoconiosis.* | byssinose |
| **cachexia** *Generalized weakness and severe wasting.* | cachexie |
| **cadaver** *A dead body.* | cadavre |
| **caduceus** *An ancient herald's wand with two serpents twined around that is a symbol of the medical arts.* | caducée |
| **caesarian section** *Incision of the abdominal and uterine walls in order to deliver a fetus when natural delivery is not possible.* | césarienne |

| English | French |
|---|---|
| **caisson disease** *Decompression sickness.* | caissons, maladie des |
| **calcaneal spur** *A bony protrusion on the calcaneus.* | épine calcanéenne |
| **calcaneus** *Commonly called the heel bone.* | calcanéum |
| **calcareous** *Referring to something containing lime or calcium.* | calcaire |
| **calcemia** *The presence of an abundance of calcium in the blood.* | calcémie |
| **calciferol** *It is formed when egesterol is exposed to ultraviolet light; a D vitamin.* | calciférol |
| **calciferol** *It is formed when egesterol is exposed to ultraviolet light; a D vitamin.* | vitamine D |
| **calcification** *Deposition of calcium salts causing hardening of an organic tissue.* | calcification |
| **calcitonin** *A thyroid hormone that lowers serum calcium levels.* | calcitonine |
| **calcium** *A chemical element that is an essential component in teeth and bone.* | calcium |
| **calcium channel blocker** *A medication used to treat angina, supraventricular arrhythmias and hypertension; it works by blocking calcium influx into myocytes and vascular smooth muscle cells.* | inhibiteur calcique |
| **calculus** *A stone of minerals that can lead to the blockage of the bile duct or ureters.* | 1. calcul 2. lithiase |
| **calf** | mollet |
| **calibrate, to** *To adjust an instrument using a standard.* | calibrer |
| **calibration** *The process of calibrating an instrument.* | étalonnage |
| **callosity** *Callus; thickened hardened skin.* | callosité |
| **callus** *Thickened hardened skin.* | 1. cal 2. durillon |
| **calorie** *A unit of heat.* | calorie |
| **calvaria** *The portion of the skull that is composed of the superior aspects of the occipital, parietal and frontal bones.* | calotte crânienne |
| **calvaria** *The superior portions of the frontal, parietal and occipital bones.* | 1. voûte crânienne 2. calotte crânienne |
| **calyx** *A cup shaped organ or cavity.* | calice |
| **canaliculus** *A term for various small channels.* | canalicule |
| **cancel** | annuler |
| **cancellous** *A bony mesh-like structure with many pores.* | disposé en réseau |
| **cancellous bone** *Describing the cancellous interior of bone.* | spongieux os |
| **cancer; carcinoma** *A disease of uncontrolled abnormal cell growth.* | cancer |
| **cancroid** *A tumor occurring in the stomach, small or large bowel.* | cancroïde |
| **cancrum oris** *Gangrenous stomatitis.* | 1. noma 2, stomatite gangreneuse |
| **candle** | bougie |
| **canine teeth** *Located between the incisors and premolars.* | canine |
| **canker** *An ulceration, usually of the mouth or lips.* | ulcération |
| **cannabis** *A plant from the Cannibidaceae family that is known for its psychotropic effects.* | 1. cannabis 2. haschisch |
| **cannula** *A tube inserted into the body.* | canule |

27

| English | French |
|---|---|
| **cantering rhythm** *Gallop rhythm.* | rythme de galop |
| **capillary** *A vessel that connects arterioles to venules.* | capillaire |
| **capillary fragility test** *Application of a blood pressure cuff high enough to restrict venous return and after five minutes count the number or petechiae produced.* | signe du lacet |
| **capillary nevus** *A growth of skin that involves the capillaries.* | angiome plan |
| **capitate bone** *The bone at the base of the palm that articulates with the third metacarpal.* | carpe, grand os du |
| **capsule** | gélule |
| **capsulitis** *Inflammation of a capsule.* | capsulite |
| **capsulotomy** *Incision of a capsule as in with eye surgery.* | capsulotomie |
| **caput** *The head.* | chef d'un muscle |
| **caput succedaneum** *Edema that occurs in the scalp of an infant during child-birth.* | bosse sérosanguine |
| **carbohydrate** *A group of organic compounds including sugar and starch.* | glucide |
| **carbon dioxide gas** | 1. anhydride carbonique 2. gaz carbonique |
| **carbon monoxide poisoning** *This tasteless, odorless gas causes constitutional symptoms but can lead to death upon inhalation.* | intoxication par le monoxyde de carbone |
| **carboxyhemoglobin** *A compound formed from hemoglobin when it is exposed to carbon monoxide.* | carboxyhémoglobine |
| **carcinogenic** *That which causes cancer.* | carcinogène |
| **carcinoid** *A tumor occurring in the stomach, intestine and colon.* | carcinoïde |
| **carcinoma** *A malignant growth.* | carcinome |
| **carcinomatosis** *Dissemination of cancer throughout the body.* | carcinomatose |
| **cardia** *The superior aspect of the stomach at the opening of the esophagus.* | cardia |
| **cardiac** *Referring to the heart.* | cardiaque |
| **cardiac arrest** *Cessation of function of the heart.* | arrêt cardiaque |
| **cardiac failure** *Decreased cardiac output of the heart.* | insuffisance cardiaque |
| **cardiac output** *Amount of blood pumped by the heart in liters per minute.* | débit cardiaque |
| **cardiac pacing** *Electromechanical stimulation of the heart.* | entraînement électrosystolique |
| **cardiology** *A specialty of medical practice involve treatment and prevention of heart disease.* | cardiologie |
| **cardiomyopathy** *Chronic cardiac muscle disease.* | cardiomyopathie |
| **cardiorespiratory assistance** *Use of artificial means to support respiration and circulation.* | assistance cardiorespiratoire |
| **cardiovascular** *Referring to the heart or circulatory system.* | cardiovasculaire |
| **carditis** *Inflammation of the heart.* | cardite |
| **caregiver** | 1. aidant 2. soignant |

| English | French |
|---|---|
| **caries** *Referring to decay or death of a tooth.* | carie |
| **carina** *The protrusion of the lowest tracheal cartilage.* | carène |
| **carneous** *Synonym of fleshy.* | carné |
| **carotene** *A hydrocarbon that can be converted to vitamin A.* | carotène |
| **carotid body** *Carotid artery receptors that are sensitive to blood chemistry changes.* | glomus carotidien |
| **carotid bruit** *An abnormal noise heard over the carotid artery that may be a sign of stenosis or aortic valvular disease.* | souffle carotidien |
| **carotid sinus syncope** *Dizziness and syncope that results from hyperactivity of the carotid sinus reflex.* | syncope par hyperexitabilité du sinus carotidien |
| **carotid** *The large artery in the neck.* | carotide |
| **carpal tunnel syndrome** *Paresthesia that results from compression of the median nerve.* | canal carpien, syndrome du |
| **carpometacarpal** *Referring to the carpus and metacarpus.* | carpométacarpien |
| **carpopedal spasm** *A spasm of the carpus and the foot.* | spasme carpopédal |
| **carpus** *The joint between the hand and wrist.* | carpe |
| **caruncle** *A small fleshy protuberance.* | caroncule |
| **casein** *The principal protein in milk, a phospholipid.* | caséine |
| **Casoni's test** *Hydatid fluid is injected intradermally; subsequent formation of a larger papule indicates hydatid disease.* | Casoni, épreuve de |
| **cast** | moule |
| **casting gauze** *Gypsum impregnated gauze used to immobilize fractured extremities.* | bande plâtrée |
| **castor bean** *A bean that can yield the poisonous compound ricin.* | ricin |
| **castration** *Excision of the gonads.* | castration |
| **casualty** *A person killed or injured.* | accidenté |
| **cat cry syndrome** *A hereditary congenital disorder exhibited by microcephaly, hypertelorism, and cognitive deficits.* | cri du chat, maladie du |
| **cat scratch fever** *An infectious disease characterized by local inflammation a the site of the scratch, local lymph adenopathy and fever.* | 1. griffes du chat,maladie des 2. lymphoréticulose bénigne d'inoculation |
| **catabolism** *The reduction of complex molecules to more simple ones in living organisms.* | catabolisme |
| **catalepsy** *A condition exhibited by rigidity and the person maintains the same position if he is moved by another.* | catalepsie |
| **cataphoresis** *The use of an electric field to move charged particles in fluid.* | cataphorèse |
| **cataplexy** *A condition exhibited by rigidity and immobility.* | cataplexie |
| **cataract** *An opacity of an eye lens or the capsule.* | cataracte |
| **catarrh** *Inflammation of a mucous membrane.* | catarrhe |
| **catatonia** *Seen in schizophrenia, it is a state of stupor or excitability and abnormal movements.* | catatonie |
| **catch a cold** | enrhumer, s' |

| English | French |
|---|---|
| **catharsis** *The act of cleansing or purging, usually referring to thought.* | catharsis |
| **cathartic** *To be cleansed or evacuated, referring to thought or the cleansing of the bowels.* | cathartique |
| **catheter** *A flexible tube inserted into the body.* | cathéter |
| **cauda equina** *The roots of the lower spinal nerves.* | queue de cheval |
| **caudal** *Referring to a cauda.* | caudal |
| **caudate** *Referring to the caudate nucleus.* | caudé |
| **causative** | causal |
| **caustic** *Abrasive or corrosive.* | caustique |
| **cautery** *Application of an electric current to cut something.* | cautère |
| **cavernous hemangioma** *A tumor composed of connective tissue with blood filled areas.* | angiome caverneux |
| **cavernous sinus** *Large venous sinus located adjacent to the sphenoid bone and posterior to the petrosal sinuses.* | sinus caverneux |
| **cavity** *Pouch or chamber.* | caverne |
| **cecum** *The portion of the bowel between the ileum and and the ascending colon.* | cæcum |
| **celiac** *Referring to the abdominal cavity.* | cœliaque |
| **cell body** | corps cellulaire |
| **cell membrane** *The semipermeable structure surrounding the cytoplasm of a cell.* | membrane cellulaire |
| **cell** *The smallest functional unit of an organism.* | cellule |
| **cell wall** | paroi cellulaire |
| **cellulitis** *Infection characterized by diffuse, subcutaneous inflammation.* | cellulite |
| **cellulose** *A polysaccharide that occurs naturally in fibrous products.* | cellulose |
| **center** | centre |
| **centigrade** *A scale with 100 gradations, usually referring to a temperature scale.* | centigrade |
| **centimeter** *One hundredth of a meter.* | centimètre |
| **central nervous system (CNS)** *The brain and spinal cord.* | système nerveux central (SNC) |
| **centrifuge** *Machine used to separate substances of different weights.* | centrifugeuse |
| **centripetal** *The movement toward the center.* | centripète |
| **cephalic** *Towards the head.* | céphalique |
| **cercaria** *Larval trematode worm that live in a molluscan.* | cercaire |
| **cerebellum** *The part of the brain in the posterior portion of the skull that controls muscle coordination and movement.* | cervelet |
| **cerebral palsy** *A condition exhibited by motor incoordination and speech changes that is the result of brain injury occurring ante-, intra- or post- partum.* | infirme moteur cérébral |
| **cerebral** *Referring to the cerebrum.* | cérébral |
| **cerebration** *Operating activity of the cerebrum.* | cérébration |

| English | French |
|---|---|
| **cerebrospinal fluid (CSF)** *The fluid between the pia mater and arachnoid membrane.* | liquide céphalorachidien (LCR) |
| **cerebrovascular accident (stroke)** *A decrease in level of consciousness and paralysis caused by a cerebrovascular thrombosis, hemorrhage or vasospasm.* | accident vasculaire cérébral |
| **cerumen** *Waxy substance found normally in the external ear canals.* | cérumen |
| **Cervical insufficiency (formerly incompetent cervix)** *Painless changes in the cervix that result in recurrent second semester pregnancy loss.* | béance du col utérin |
| **cervical pleura** *The dome-like cap of the pleura.* | dôme pleural |
| **cervical** *Referring to the neck or the cervix.* | cervical |
| **cervicectomy** *Excision of the cervix uteri.* | cervicectomie |
| **cervicitis** *Inflammation of the cervix.* | cervicite |
| **cervix uteri** *The narrow end of the uterus.* | col de l'utérus |
| **cestode** *A class of parasitic flatworms.* | cestode |
| **chancre** *The initial ulcer that is the source of entry for a pathogen.* | chancre |
| **chancroid** *A sexually transmitted disease caused by Haemophilus ducreyi that is exhibited by ulcers without indurated margins.* | chancrelle |
| **check for, to** | vérifier |
| **cheek** | joue |
| **chelating agent** *A compound used to bind with metal typically used in the treatment of poisoning.* | chélateur |
| **chelilitis** *Inflammation of the lip.* | chéilite |
| **chemoreceptor** *A sense organ that responds to stimuli.* | chémorécepteur |
| **chemosis** *Swelling of conjunctival tissue adjacent to the cornea.* | chémosis |
| **chemotaxis** *The response of an organism to chemical agents.* | chimiotactisme |
| **chemotherapy** *Use of medication (chemical agents) in the treatment of disease. This term is commonly used to refer to the treatment of cancer patients with medication.* | chimiothérapie |
| **chest** | poitrine |
| **chest wall** | paroi thoracique |
| **chest x-ray** | cliché thoracique |
| **chew, to** | mâcher |
| **chiasma** *The optic chiasma is the area inferior to the hypothalamus where the optic nerves cross.* | chiasma |
| **chigger** *A parasitic mite of the genus Trombicula.* | aoûtat |
| **child** | enfant |
| **childbirth** | accouchement |
| **childhood** | enfance |
| **chill** | frisson |
| **chimera** *A mixture of genetically distinct tissues.* | chimère |
| **chin** | menton |
| **chiropodist** *A doctor trained in the treatment of feet.* | pédicure |

| English | French |
|---|---|
| **chiropractic** *Referring to the medical practice of adjusting malaligned joints.* | chiropraxie |
| **chiropractor** *A medical practitioner who is involved with the treatment of disease by manipulating malaligned joints.* | chiropracteur |
| **chlamydiosis** *A disease caused by the species Chlamydia.* | chlamydiase |
| **chloasma** *Brown or black macula that occur on the face during pregnancy or when there is ovarian dysfunction.* | chloasma |
| **chloroform** *A colorless, sweet smelling liquid formerly used as a general anesthetic.* | chloroforme |
| **chloroma** *A malignant tumor associated with myelogenous leukemia.* | chlorome |
| **choanae** *The two openings between the nasal cavity and the nasopharynx.* | choanes |
| **choice** | choix |
| **choke, to** | étouffer |
| **cholagogue** *A compound used to stimulate flow of bile from the liver.* | cholagogue |
| **cholangiogram** *Radiologic imaging of the gallbladder and bile ducts.* | cholangogramme |
| **cholangitis** *Inflammation of the bile ducts.* | cholangite |
| **cholangitis** *Inflammation of the bile ducts.* | angiocholite |
| **cholecystectomy** *Surgical excision of the gallbladder.* | cholécystectomie |
| **cholecystenterostomy** *Creation of a surgical anastomosis between the intestine and the gallbladder.* | cholécystenstérostomie |
| **cholecystitis** *Inflammation of the gallbladder.* | cholécystite |
| **cholecystolithiasis** *The presence of gallstones in the gallbladder.* | cholécystolithiase |
| **choledocholithotomy** *Creation of an incision in the bile duct for the purpose of removing a stone.* | cholédocholithotomie |
| **cholelithiasis** *Presence or creation of gallstones.* | cholélithiase |
| **cholemia** *Bile or bile products in the blood.* | cholémie |
| **cholera** *An infectious disease exhibited by vomiting and diarrhea and caused by Vibrio cholerae.* | choléra |
| **cholesteatoma** *A cystic mass that has a lining made of keratinizing material and cholesterol.* | cholestéatome |
| **cholesterol** *A compound or its derivatives are found in cell membranes and precursors to hormones but high levels can cause atherosclerosis.* | cholestérol |
| **cholinergic** *Referring to the stimulation, activation or transmission of acetylcholine.* | cholinergique |
| **cholinesterase** *An esterase used to cleave acetylcholine into choline and acetic acid.* | cholinestérase |
| **choluria** *Term indicating the presence of bile in the urine.* | cholurie |
| **chondralgia** *Cartilaginous pain.* | 1. chondralgie 2. chondrodynie |
| **chondritis** *Cartilaginous inflammation.* | chondrite |
| **chondroma** *Cartilaginous hyperplastic growth.* | chondrome |
| **chondromalacia** *Excessive softening of the cartilages.* | chondromalacie |
| **chondrosarcoma** *Cartilaginous tumor which exhibits rapid growth.* | chondrosarcome |

| English | French |
|---|---|
| **chorda** *A cord or sinew.* | corde |
| **chordee** *Downward bending of the penis.* | chordée |
| **chorditis** *Inflammation of a vocal or spermatic cord.* | 1. chordite 2. cordite |
| **chorea** *Involuntary, continuous rapid, jerking movements.* | chorée |
| **chorionic villus** *Cord-like projections of a fertilized ovum.* | villosité chorionique |
| **choroid** *Similar to the chorion (fertilized ovum or zygote)* | choroïde |
| **choroiditis** *Inflammation of the choroid.* | choroïdite |
| **choroidocyclitis** *Inflammation of the ciliary processes and choroid.* | choroïdocyclite |
| **chromatin** *A desocyribose nucleic acid that carries the genes of inheritance.* | chromatine |
| **chromosome** *A structure in the nucleus of living cells that carries genetic information.* | chromasome |
| **chronic** *When referring to an illness, it means recurring or persistent.* | chronique |
| **chyle** *A combination of lymph fluid and fat that enters the blood via the thoracic duct.* | chyle |
| **chylomicron** *A one micron particle of emulsified fat.* | chylomicron |
| **chylous** *Referring to chyle.* | chyleux |
| **chyme** *The gruel produced by gastric digestion.* | chyme |
| **cicatricial** *Referring to cicatrix.* | cicatriciel |
| **cicatrix (scar)** *New tissue in a healed wound.* | cicatrice |
| **cilia** *The hairs growing on the eyelid.* | cils |
| **ciliary body** *The connection between the iris and the choroid.* | corps ciliaire |
| **cinchonism** *The toxic effects induced by ingestion of cinchona bark; it is exhibited by tinnitus, deafness and cognitive changes.* | quinquinisme |
| **circadian** *Referring to a 24 hour period.* | circadien |
| **circadian rhythm** *Naturally recurring fluctuations in a 24 hour period.* | rythme circadien |
| **circumcision** *Surgical excision of the foreskin.* | circoncision |
| **circumference** *The distance around an object or part.* | circonférence |
| **circumflex nerve** *The axillary nerve that has an origin in the posterior branch of the brachial plexus.* | circonflexe nerf |
| **circumscribed** *Well defined borders.* | circonscrit |
| **cirrhosis** *A liver disease characterized by destruction of liver cells and increased connective tissue.* | cirrhose |
| **cirsoid** *Similar to a tortuous vein, artery or lymph vessel.* | cirsoïde |
| **cisternal puncture** *A trans-occipitoatlantoid ligament puncture of the cisterna magna so CSF can be obtained.* | ponction cisternale |
| **clasp** | agrafe |
| **clasp knife reflex** *The lengthening of the extensor muscles resulting in flexion.* | réflexe du canif |
| **claudication; limp** *Intermittent claudication is a phrase used to describe pain experienced in the leg from arterial insufficiency.* | claudication |
| **claustrophobia** *An unreasonable fear of being in an enclosed environment.* | claustrophobie |
| **clavicle** *A bone that articulates with the sternum and scapula.* | clavicule |

| English | French |
|---|---|
| **clavus** *A corn or horny protrusion.* | clou |
| **clavus** *A horny tubercle of the skin.* | cor |
| **clawhand** *A hand deformity caused by ulnar nerve palsy exhibited by the hyperextension of the metacarpophalangeal joints and flexion of the interphalangeal articulations.* | main en griffe |
| **clear** | clair |
| **clearance** | clearance |
| **clearing of throat** | raclement de gorge |
| **cleavage** *A sharp division or demarcation.* | segmentation |
| **cleft lip** | bec-de-lièvre |
| **cleft palate** *A congenital abnormal opening in the palate.* | fente palatine |
| **cleidocranial dysostosis** *A congenital condition exhibited by abnormal ossification of the cranial bones and absence of clavicles.* | 1. dysostose cléido-crânienne 2. Marie-Sainton, syndrome de |
| **cleidotomy** *A procedure used in difficult deliveries in which the clavicle is broken to facilitate childbirth.* | cléidotomie |
| **click** *A sound heard by the sudden closure of a heart valve.* | clic |
| **click; snap** | claquement |
| **clinic** | clinique |
| **clinical record** | dossier clinique |
| **clinical signs** *Physical assessment data.* | signes cliniques |
| **clitoris** *A small erectile body in the anterosuperior aspect of the vulva.* | clitoris |
| **clockwise** | sens des aiguilles d'une montre dans le |
| **clonic** *Referring to a spasm that alternates in rigidity and relaxation.* | clonique |
| **closed** | fermé |
| **clot** *A thrombus or embolus.* | caillot |
| **clubbing** *Increase in the mass of the soft tissue of the terminal phalanges.* | hippocrastisme digital |
| **cluster headache** *A unilateral, severe, recurrent headache.* | algie vasculaire de la face |
| **cnemial** *Referring to the shin.* | tibial |
| **coaching** | accompagnement |
| **coagulation** *The formation of a clot.* | coagulation |
| **coarctation** *A stricture, as in narrowing of the aorta with coarctation of the aorta.* | coarctation |
| **cobalt** *A metal that with causes polycythemia with increased ingestion.* | cobalt |
| **cocaine** *A highly addictive opiate derivative.* | cocaïne |
| **cocaine addiction** *Physical habituation to cocaine.* | cocaïnomanie |
| **coccus** *A spherical shaped bacterium.* | 1. coccus 2. coque |
| **coccydynia** *Coccygeal pain.* | coccygodynie |
| **coccyx** *The small bone formed by the natural fusion of rudimentary vertebrae.* | coccyx |
| **cochlea** *The essential organ of hearing which is in a spiral form.* | cochlée |

| English | French |
|---|---|
| **cock-up splint** *A splint used to maintain the wrist in dorsiflexion; used for carpal tunnel syndrome.* | attelle pour dorsiflexion du poignet |
| **cod** | morue |
| **codeine** *A morphine derived analgesic.* | codéine |
| **codon** *A series of three nucleotides that form a unit of genetic code.* | codon |
| **cog wheel** *As in cogwheel rigidity which is a jerky passive movement after there was increased tone.* | roue dentée |
| **cognition** *The process of acquiring thought or understanding.* | 1. cognition 2. connaissance |
| **cognitive disorders** *Any disease process that involves altered cognition.* | troubles cognitifs |
| **coitus** *Sexual intercourse between members of the opposite sex.* | coït |
| **cold** | froid |
| **cold sore** *A perioral blister caused by herpes simplex.* | bouton de fièvre |
| **colectomy** *Surgical removal of part of the colon.* | colectomie |
| **colic** *Acute abdominal pain.* | colique |
| **colitis** *Inflammation of the colon.* | colite |
| **collagen** *The principal supportive protein bone, skin, tendon and cartilage.* | collagène |
| **collapse** | collapsus |
| **collapsed** | collabé |
| **colloboma** *A congenital eye fissure.* | collobome |
| **collodion** *A product of the breakdown of colloid.* | collodion |
| **colloid** *A solution used for infusion, such as albumin or hetastarch, that are more likely to remain in the intravascular space than crystalloids.* | colloïde |
| **coloboma** *A congenital defect that involves a fissure of the eye.* | colobome |
| **colon** *The portion of the large intestine that goes from the cecum to the rectum.* | côlon |
| **color blindness** *The inability to distinguish colors.* | daltonisme |
| **color chart** | échelle colorimétrique |
| **color of conjunctiva** *A point of assessment to check for pallor.* | coloration conjonctive |
| **colostomy bag** *A pouch attached to the skin with a mild adhesive that collects stool emitted from a colostomy.* | sac de colostomie |
| **colostomy** *Surgically creating an opening in the colon that is extended to outside the abdominal wall.* | colostomie |
| **colostrum** *The fluid secreted by the mammary glands a few days around parturition.* | colostrum |
| **colpitis; vaginitis** *Inflammation of the vagina.* | 1. vaginite 2. colpite |
| **colpocele** *A hernia into the vagina.* | colpocèle |
| **colporrhaphy** *A surgical procedure that involves suturing the vagina.* | colporraphie |
| **colposcope** *A scope used to visualize the vagina.* | colposcope |
| **colposcopy** *Use of a scope to visualize the vagina and cervix.* | colposcopie |
| **coma** *A state of unconsciousness.* | coma |
| **comatose** *Referring to a coma.* | comateux |

| English | French |
|---|---|
| **comb** | peigne |
| **comedones** *The medical term for blackheads.* | comédons |
| **commensal** *Living in or on another organism without being a detriment.* | commensal |
| **comment** | commentaire |
| **common** *That which is usual.* | commun |
| **compatibility** *The existence without problems.* | compatibilité |
| **compendium** *A concise summary about a subject.* | recueil |
| **complaint** | 1. plainte 2. réclamation |
| **complement fixation test** *A laboratory test for the presence of an antibody in the serum that involves inactivation of the complement in the serum.* | test de fixation du complément |
| **complete blood count** *An assay that includes white blood cell, red blood cell, platelet count, hemoglobin, hematocrit and white blood cell differential.* | numération formule sanguine |
| **compliance** *The act of going along with a plan.* | 1. compliance 2. observance |
| **comply, to** | accepter |
| **compound** | composé |
| **compound fracture** *Open fracture.* | fracture ouverte |
| **comprehension** *Understanding.* | compréhension |
| **compression** | compression |
| **concavity** *The state of being concave.* | concavité |
| **concentration** | concentration |
| **concentric** *Referring to circles or arcs that share the same center.* | concentrique |
| **conception** *The act of an egg being fertilized by sperm.* | conception |
| **concha** *A part of the body that is spiral shaped. Nasal concha are the small bones in the sides of the nasal cavity.* | conque |
| **concretion** *A hard solid mass.* | concrétion |
| **concussion** *Head trauma resulting in temporary loss of consciousness.* | commotion |
| **condom** *A covering for the penis or the vagina (female condom) used during sexual intercourse that is meant to reduce the chance of pregnancy or infection.* | 1. condom 2. préservatif |
| **condyle** *A rounded protrusion of a bone.* | condyle |
| **condyloma** *A warty papule near the anus or vulva.* | condylome |
| **cone** | cône |
| **confabulation** *The fabrication of experiences to compensate for memory loss.* | confabulation |
| **confidence** | confiance |
| **confinement** | internement |
| **conflict** | conflit |
| **confusion** | confusion |
| **congenital** *A disease or anomaly present from birth.* | 1. congénital 2. inné |

| English | French |
|---|---|
| **congenital heart disease** *A cardiac disorder present prior to birth.* | cardiopathie congénitale |
| **congestive** | congestif |
| **congestive heart failure** *A diminished cardiac output leading to passive engorgement.* | insuffisance cardiaque congestive |
| **conjugate diameter** *A pelvic inlet measurement used to determine whether a woman is capable of delivering a fetus vaginally.* | diamètre promonto-rétropubien |
| **conjunctiva** *The membrane that lines the eyelid.* | conjonctif |
| **conjunctivitis** *Inflammation of the conjunctiva.* | conjonctivite |
| **consanguinity** *The relationship by blood.* | consanguinité |
| **conscious** *Being award and being able to respond to one's surroundings.* | conscient |
| **conservative** | conservateur |
| **consistent** | constant |
| **consolidation** *An area of fixed secretions in the lung.* | consolidation |
| **constipation** *A condition exhibited by difficulty in having a bowel movement due to hard stools.* | constipation |
| **constriction** | 1. constriction 2. étranglement |
| **contact** | contage |
| **contact lens** | lentille de contact |
| **contagious** *Description of a disease that can be spread by direct or indirect contact.* | contagieux |
| **contaminated** | contaminé |
| **content** | contenu |
| **contraceptive** *A device or medication used to prevent pregnancy.* | 1. anticonceptionnel 2. contraceptif |
| **contradictory** | contradictoire |
| **contraindication** | contre-indication |
| **contusion** *An area of broken capillaries in the skin causing discoloration; commonly called a bruise.* | contusion |
| **convenient** | adapté |
| **conversion** *When referring to a psychiatric condition it is the exhibition of physical symptoms as a manifestation of mental disease.* | conversion |
| **convex** *Having an exterior curved the outside of a sphere.* | convexe |
| **convulsion** *An involuntary series of tonic and clonic movements.* | convulsion |
| **cool** | frais |
| **cope, to** | faire face |
| **copper** | cuivre |
| **copulation** *Sexual relations.* | copulation |
| **cor pulmonale** *Heart disease that is secondary to lung disease.* | cœur pulmonaire |
| **coracoid** *A prominence on the scapula to which the biceps is attached.* | coracoïde |
| **cord compression** *Pressure being applied to the spinal cord.* | compression médullaire |

| English | French |
|---|---|
| core | partie centrale |
| cornea *The transparent segment located at the anterior part of the eye.* | cornée |
| corneal *Referring to the cornea.* | cornéen |
| corona dentis *The portion of the tooth covered by enamel.* | couronne dentaire |
| coronal suture *The line of intersection of the frontal bone and the two parietal bones.* | suture coronale |
| coronary angiography *Roentgenographic visualization of the coronary vessels after injection of dye.* | angiocardiographie |
| coronary vessel *Referring to a coronary artery.* | vaisseau coronaire |
| coroner *A person who investigates sudden or suspicious deaths.* | coroner |
| coronoid *Crown-shaped.* | coronoïde |
| corpulence *Fatness.* | corpulence |
| corpus callosum *A point of connection between the two cerebral hemispheres.* | corps calleux |
| corpus luteum *A structure that is discharged from an ovary; it degenerates if it is not impregnated.* | corps jaune |
| corpuscle *A red or white blood cell.* | corpuscule |
| cortex *An external layer.* | cortex |
| cortical *Referring to the cortex.* | cortical |
| corticosteroid *A hormone developed in the adrenal cortex.* | corticostéroïde |
| corticotrophic *That which exerts an effect on the adrenal cortex.* | corticotrope |
| cortisol *An adrenal cortical hormone, also called hydrocortisone.* | cortisol |
| cortisone *An adrenal cortical hormone responsible for carbohydrate regulation.* | cortisone |
| coryza *An acute condition exhibited by copious nasal discharge.* | coryza |
| cost | coût |
| costochondritis *Inflammation of the rib and or its cartiluge.* | costochondrite |
| cotton wool | ouate |
| cough | toux |
| coughing fit | quinte de toux |
| count | compte |
| counting | comptage |
| cowpox; vaccinia *A viral disease of cows that was used for an original smallpox vaccine.* | vaccine |
| cow's milk | lait de vache |
| coxalgia *Pain in the hip.* | coxalgie |
| crab louse *Phthirus pubis is formal name for a louse that infests pubic hair and causes intense itching.* | pou du pubis |
| crack | fêlure |
| crack one's knuckles | faire craquer ses doigts |
| cradle | 1. arceau 2. berceau |
| cramp | crampe |
| cranial *Referring to the skull.* | crânien |

| English | French |
|---|---|
| **cranioclast** *An instrument used to crush a fetal skull.* | cranioclaste |
| **craniopharyngioma** *A tumor that originates in the hypophyseal stalk.* | craniopharyngiome |
| **craniosynostosis** *Closure of the sutures of the skull that occurs prematurely.* | craniosynostose |
| **craniotabes** *Softening of the skull bones causing widened sutures; this occurs in rickets.* | craniotabès |
| **craniotomy** *Surgical creation of a hole in the skull.* | craniotomie |
| **cranium** *The skeleton of the head.* | crâne |
| **craving** | désir obsédant |
| **creatine** *A compound involved with muscle contraction.* | créatine |
| **creatinine** *A compound excreted in the urine that is produced by the metabolism of creatine.* | créatinine |
| **crenotherapy** *A form of treatment from mineral springs.* | crénothérapie |
| **crepitus** *A noise heard when one auscultates the lungs that is similar to the sound of rubbing hair between one's fingers. It is also considered the sound of two broken bones rubbing together.* | crépitation |
| **cretinism** *A chronic condition caused by diminished thyroid hormone secretion.* | crétinisme |
| **crevice** *A narrow opening.* | crevasse |
| **cribriform** *Like a sieve; the olfactory nerves pass through the cribriform plate of the ethmoid bone.* | cribriforme |
| **cricoid** *The ring-shaped cartilage of the larynx* | cricoïde |
| **cripple** | paralysé |
| **crisis** *Seizure.* | crise |
| **cross-immunity** *Attainment of immunity by receiving an inoculation of an organism similar to the one for which immunity is desired.* | immunité croisée |
| **cross-infection** *Transfer of infection between individuals, each with a different organism.* | contagion secondaire |
| **cross-matching (blood)** *Evaluation of blood to determine compatibility between the donor and recipient prior to transfusion.* | compatibilité sanguine, épreuve de |
| **cross-section** | coupe transversale |
| **croup** *An acute laryngeal condition that is accompanied by a hoarse, barking cough.* | croup |
| **cruciform** *Shaped like a cross.* | cruciforme |
| **crural; femoral** *Referring to the femur or leg.* | crural |
| **crush syndrome** *Rhabdomyolysis occurring as a result of muscle injury from mechanical stress.* | syndrome d'écrasement |
| **crust** | croûte |
| **crutches** | béquilles |
| **cryesthesia** *Abnormal sensitivity to cold.* | cryesthésie |
| **cryosurgery** *The application of extreme cold to destroy tissue.* | cryochirurgie |
| **cryotherapy** *The use of cold for therapeutic purposes.* | cryothérapie |
| **cryptorchism** *A condition characterized by the failure of the testes to descend into the scrotum.* | cryptorchidie |

| English | French |
|---|---|
| **crystalloid** *A substance that can pass through a semipermeable membrane; not a colloid.* | cristalloïde |
| **crystalluria** *The presence of crystals in the urine.* | cristallurie |
| **CSF** *Abbreviation for cerebrospinal fluid.* | LCR |
| **CT scan** *Computerized axial tomography.* | tomodensitométrie |
| **cubic millimeter** *A unit of volume.* | millimètre cube |
| **cubitus** *1. The bend at the elbow. 2. Ulna.* | cubitus |
| **cubitus** *Elbow.* | coude |
| **cuffed tube** *A cannula that has an balloon on the tip that can be inflated with air or fluid.* | sonde à ballonnet |
| **culdoscopy** *Examination of the female pelvic viscera with a scope inserted through the posterior vaginal fornix.* | culdoscopie |
| **culture** *The growth of bacteria in artificial medium.* | culture |
| **culture broth** *A medium used to grow bacteria.* | bouillon de culture |
| **cumulative effect** *A consequence of successive additions.* | effet cumulatif |
| **Cuneiform** *The three bones between the navicular bone and the metatarsals.* | cunéiforme |
| **curare** *A toxic botanical substance used at one time in poison darts in South America. Curare derivatives have been used in general anesthesia.* | curare |
| **curative** *A remedy capable of healing completely.* | curatif |
| **cure** | guérison |
| **curettage** *Removal of tissues from a cavity.* | curetage |
| **curette** *The instrument used during a curettage.* | curette |
| **current** | actuel |
| **current complaint (chief complaint)** | plainte actuelles |
| **currently** | actuellement |
| **cushion** | coussinet |
| **cut** | couper |
| **cutaneous** *Referring to the skin.* | cutané |
| **cuticle** *The dead skin at the base of the toenail or fingernail, also called the eponychium.* | cuticule |
| **cyanocobalamin** *Also called B12; used to treat pernicious and other macrocytic anemias.* | cyanocobalamine |
| **cyanosis** *Bluish discoloration of the skin and mucous membranes.* | cyanose |
| **cyclical vomiting** *Periods of recurrent vomiting with no apparent pathologic cause and the person has a normal state of health between the episodes.* | vomissement acétonémique |
| **cyclitis** *Inflammation of the ciliary body.* | cyclite |
| **cyclodialysis** *The surgical creation of a communication between the anterior chamber of the eye and the suprachorodial space for the purpose of treating glaucoma.* | cyclodialyse |
| **cycloplegia** *Paralysis of the ciliary muscle.* | cycloplégie |
| **cyclothymia** *Manic-depressive tendencies.* | cyclothymie |

| English | French |
|---|---|
| **cyclotomy** *Surgically creating an opening in the ciliary body.* | cyclotomie |
| **cystadenoma** *Adenoma associated with cysts of neoplastic origin.* | cystadénome |
| **cystectomy** *Surgical removal of a cyst or the bladder.* | 1. cystectomie 2. kystectomie |
| **cystic** *Referring to a cyst.* | cystique |
| **cystic duct** *The duct connecting the gallbladder to the common bile duct.* | canal cystique |
| **cystic fibrosis** *A congenital disorder exhibited by abnormal thick mucous which leads to problems in the intestines, pancreas and lungs.* | mucoviscidose |
| **cysticercosis** *The state of being infected with a type of tapeworm.* | cysticercose |
| **cystinosis** *A congenital disorder of increased cystine that leads to renal insufficiency, rickets and dwarfism.* | cystinose |
| **cystinuria** *The presence of cystine in the urine.* | cystinurie |
| **cystitis** *Inflammation of the urinary bladder.* | cystite |
| **cystocele** *Protrusion of the urinary bladder through the vaginal wall.* | cystocèle |
| **cystography** *Roentgenographic visualization of the urinary bladder after insertion of contrast media.* | cystographie |
| **cystolithiasis** *Presence of a calculus in the urinary bladder.* | 1. calcul vésical 2. cystolithiase |
| **cystoscope** *A device used to visualized the urinary bladder.* | cystocope |
| **cystoscopy** *Direct visualization of the urinary bladder with a cystoscope.* | cystoscopie |
| **cytology** *The study of cells, their function and structure.* | cytologie |
| **cytoplasm** *The protoplasm of the cell except for the nucleus.* | cytoplasme |
| **cytotoxic** *Referring to being harmful to cells.* | cytotoxique |
| **cytotoxin** *That which is harmful to cells.* | cytotoxine |
| **dacryoadenitis** *Inflammation of the lacrimal gland.* | dacryoadénite |
| **dacryocystitis** *Inflammation of a lacrimal sac.* | dacryocysitite |
| **dacryocystorhinostomy** *Surgical reaction of a communication between the lacrimal sac and nasal cavity.* | dacryocysto-rhinostomie |
| **dacryolith** *A stone in the lacrimal sac or duct.* | dacryolithe |
| **dandruff** *Dead skin found in the hair.* | pellicules |
| **dark adaptation** *Adjustment to low light by reflex dilation of the pupil.* | adaptation à l'obscurité |
| **date of admission** | date d'entrée |
| **date of birth** | date de naissance |
| **date of discharge (hospital discharge)** | date de sortie |
| **daughter** | fille |
| **dead space** *The area in the respiratory tract where air is not exchanged.* | espace mort |
| **deadline** | date limite |
| **deaf** | sourd |
| **deaf-mute** | sourd-muet |
| **deafness** | surdité |

| English | French |
|---|---|
| **death** | décès |
| **debility** *Physical weakness.* | débilité |
| **decade** | décennie |
| **decapitation** *The physical separation of the head from the body.* | décapitation |
| **decerebrate rigidity** *Rigid extension of the arms which is an abnormal posture associated with increased intracranial pressure.* | rigidité décérébration |
| **decerebrate** *The removal of the brain.* | décérébré |
| **decibel** *A unit used in the measurement of sound.* | décibel |
| **decidua** *The mucous membrane lining the uterus during pregnancy.* | 1. caduque 2. decidua |
| **deciduous teeth** *The first teeth.* | dents de lait |
| **decline** | 1. baisse 2. déclin |
| **decompensation** *The inability of an organ to respond to functional overload.* | décompensation |
| **decompression** *The surgical procedure relieving pressure on a part.* | décompression |
| **decrease** | diminution |
| **decubitus ulcer** *A wound caused by laying in one position for too long; also referred to as a pressure ulcer.* | escarre de décubitus |
| **decussation** *An area of intersection.* | décussation |
| **deep** | profond |
| **deep tendon reflex** *Reflexes exhibited by the stretching of a tendon.* | ostéo-tendineux réflexe |
| **defecation** *The discharge of feces from the rectum.* | 1. défécation 2. exonération |
| **defect** | défaut |
| **defibrillator** *A device used to convert an abnormal cardiac rhythm (ventricular fibrillation) into a normal rhythm with use of electrical stimulation.* | défibrillateur |
| **deficiency** | déficit |
| **deformity** | déformation |
| **deglutition** *The process of swallowing.* | déglutition |
| **dehydration** | déshydratation |
| **delirium** *An acute mental state exhibited by altered thought processes and restlessness.* | confusion mentale |
| **delirium tremens** *A condition seen when alcohol is withdrawn which is exhibited by restlessness, hallucinations and tremors.* | delirium tremens |
| **deliver, to** | livrer |
| **deltoid** *A term referring to "three". The deltoid muscle has its origin at three areas: clavicle, acromion, and spine of the scapula.* | deltoïde |
| **delusion** *A belief that is contradictory to rational thought.* | délire |
| **delusional** *Referring to a delusion.* | délirant |
| **demanding** | contraignant |
| **demarcation** *Having a fixed boundary.* | démarcation |
| **dementia** *A chronic brain disorder exhibited by memory loss, personality changes and faulty reasoning.* | démence |

| English | French |
|---|---|
| **demography** *The study of the structure of human populations.* | démographie |
| **demulcent** *Something that relieves irritation or inflammation.* | adoucissant |
| **demyelinating disease** *A condition characterized by the loss of myelin.* | affection démyélinisante |
| **dendrite** *Impulses are transmitted along a dendrite to a nerve cell body.* | dendrite |
| **denervated** *To remove nerve supply.* | dénervé |
| **dengue** *A mosquito-borne viral disease exhibited by fever and joint pain.* | dengue |
| **density** *The denseness of an object.* | densité |
| **dental** *Referring to teeth.* | dentaire |
| **dental calculus** *Calcium phosphate and carbonate adhered to the teeth.* | tartre dentaire |
| **dental caries** *Decay of teeth.* | carie dentaire |
| **dentatum** *Also referred to as nucleus dentatus.* | olive cérébelleuse |
| **dentist** *A professional capable of treating diseases of the teeth and gums.* | dentiste |
| **dentition** *The natural teeth.* | dentition |
| **denture** *A frame that holds artificial teeth.* | dentier |
| **deny, to** | nier |
| **deoxyribonucleic acid (DNA)** *The carrier of genetic information.* | désoxyribonucléique acide |
| **depilatory** *An agent used to remove hair.* | dépilatoire |
| **depressed** | déprimé |
| **depression** *A medical condition exhibited by profound despondency.* | dépression |
| **deprivation** *The lack of a necessity.* | privation |
| **dermatitis** *Non-specific inflammation of the skin.* | dermatite |
| **dermatography** *A description of the skin.* | dermatographie |
| **dermatologist** *A physician specializing in dermatology.* | dermatologiste |
| **dermatology** *The medical profession involving the treatment of skin conditions.* | dermatologie |
| **dermatome** *The area of sensation of the skin supplied by a single posterior spinal root.* | 1. dermatome 2. rhizomère |
| **dermatomycosis** *An infection of the skin by Trichophyton, Microsporum or Epidermophyton fungi.* | dermatoycose |
| **dermatomyositis** *Inflammation of the skin, subcutaneous tissue and adjacent muscle.* | dermatomyosite |
| **dermatophyte** *A fungal parasite living on the skin.* | 1. dermaphyte 2. dermatophyte |
| **dermatosis** *Any skin disease.* | dermatose |
| **dermis** *The "true skin" that lies beneath the epidermis.* | derme |
| **dermographia** *A raised, pale line with hyperemic borders is elicited upon scratching the skin with a dull instrument, in this condition.* | dermographie |
| **dermoid cyst** *An abnormal growth containing hair follicles, skin and sebaceous glands.* | kyste dermoïde |
| **descending** | descendant |

| English | French |
|---|---|
| **desensitization** *The gradual exposure of an offending agent to prevent an abnormal response upon a secondary exposure.* | désensibilisation |
| **desiccation** *The act of drying up.* | dessiccation |
| **desmoid** *A tumor typically found in the abdomen which contains. muscle and connective tissue.* | desmoïde |
| **despite** | malgré |
| **desquamation** *The shedding of skin in flakes or sheets.* | desquamation |
| **deterioration** | détérioration |
| **detoxication** *The process of removing toxins from the body.* | désintoxication |
| **detrimental** *Harmful.* | nocif |
| **detritus** *Particulate matter produced by the decomposition of an organic substance.* | détritus |
| **detrusor urinae** *Smooth muscle fibers that extend from the urinary bladder to the pubis.* | détrusor |
| **deuteranomaly** *Abnormal color vision sometimes called "green weakness".* | deutéranomalie |
| **deviation** *Away from the norm.* | déviation |
| **dexter;** *right;* **straight;** *erect* | droit |
| **dextran** *A high glucose polymer used as a plasma substitute.* | dextran |
| **dextrocardia** *Location of the heart in the right hemithorax.* | dextrocardie |
| **dhobie itch** *So called because the contact dermatitis is caused by the soap used by laundry workers in India who are called "dhobie".* | gale des blanchisseurs |
| **diabetes insipidus** *Caused by a deficiency in vasopressin, it is exhibited by great thirst and large volume urine output (and normal blood sugar).* | diabète insipide |
| **diabetes mellitus** *A disease exhibited by a deficiency of the pancreatic hormone insulin.* | diabète sucré |
| **diabetic** *A person who has diabetes mellitus.* | diabétique |
| **diagnostic** *A specific symptom or characteristic.* | diagnostique |
| **diapedesis** *The outward passage of blood elements through an intact vessel wall.* | diapédèse |
| **diaper** | couche de bébé |
| **diaper rash** | érythème fessier du nourrisson |
| **diaphoretic** *Exhibited by profuse perspiration.* | diaphorétique |
| **diaphragm** *The muscular separation between the thoracic and abdominal cavities.* | diaphragme |
| **diaphragmatic hernia** *Protrusion of visceral contents through the diaphragm.* | hernie diaphragmatique |
| **diaphysis** *The central part of a long bone.* | diaphyse |
| **diarrhea** *Increase in frequency and a loose consistency of the stools.* | diarrhée |
| **diarthrosis** *An articulation allowing free movement.* | diarthrose |
| **diastase** *Amylase.* | diastase |
| **diastole** *The period of dilatation of the heart; between the first and second heart sounds.* | diastole |

| English | French |
|---|---|
| **diathermy** *The use of heat produced from high-frequency electric currents to medically or surgically treat someone.* | diathermie |
| **diathesis** *A medical tendency to develop a specific condition.* | diasthèse |
| **die, to** | mourir |
| **diet** | 1. diète 2. régime alimentaire |
| **dietitian** *A professional who works with diet and nutrition.* | diététicien |
| **differential** *A term used to refer to the various options for diagnoses.* | différentiel |
| **differential diagnosis** *A list of possible alternative diagnoses for a patient who is ill.* | diagnostic differentiel |
| **differential leukocyte count** *The percentage of different types of leukocytes.* | formule leucocytaire |
| **digestion** *The process of enzymatic breakdown of food in the alimentary canal.* | digestion |
| **digit** *Finger.* | doigt |
| **digitalis** *Cardiac medication derived from the leaf of Digitalis purpurea.* | digitale |
| **dilatation** *The process of becoming wider or larger.* | dilatation |
| **dilator** *An instrument that dilates.* | dilatateur |
| **dilution** *The process of making a weaker solution.* | dilution |
| **dimercaprol** *A medication used as a binding agent for heavy metal poisoning.* | dimercaprol (BAL) |
| **dimmed** | obscurci |
| **dioptre** *Referring to refraction or transmitted and refracted light.* | dioptrie |
| **dioxide** *A compound containing two oxygen atoms.* | dioxyde |
| **diphtheria** *A contagious bacterial disease characterized by a grey membrane on the pharynx along with respiratory or cutaneous symptoms; caused by Corynebacterium diphtheriae.* | diphtérie |
| **diplegia** *The paralysis of both arms or both legs.* | diplégie |
| **diplococcus** *A bacterium that occurs in pairs including pneumococcus and Neisseria gonorrhoeae and Neisseria meningitidis.* | diplocoque |
| **diploid** *A nucleus containing two complete sets of chromosomes.* | diploïde |
| **diplopia** *Double vision.* | diplopie |
| **dipsomania** *Twins that are joined at some part of their bodies.* | dipsomanie |
| **dirty** | sale |
| **disability** | incapacité |
| **disaccharide** *A type of sugar that yields two monosaccharides upon hydrolysis.* | disaccharide |
| **disappearance** | disparition |
| **disarticulation** *The separation or amputation of a joint.* | désarticulation |
| **discomfort** | gêne |
| **discrete** | discret |
| **disease** | mal |
| **disease outcome** *The response obtained from treatment.* | évolution de la maladie |
| **disequilibrium** *The absence of stability.* | déséquilibre |

| English | French |
|---|---|
| **disinfectant** *A substance that kills bacteria.* | désinfectant |
| **dislocation** *The displacement of a bone when referring to an articulation.* | 1. déboîtement 2. dislocation 3. luxation |
| **disorder** *Impairment.* | atteinte |
| **disorientation** *Mental confusion.* | désorientation |
| **displacement** *Movement from normal position.* | déplacement |
| **disrobe** | déshabiller |
| **dissecting aneurysm** *A condition in which blood is present between the layers of an artery.* | anévrisme disséquant |
| **dissection** *To cut up in order to analyze or study.* | dissection |
| **dissemination** *To be spread or dispersed widely.* | dissémination |
| **dissolution** *Disintegration.* | dissolution |
| **distal** *Situated away from the center of the body.* | distal |
| **distended** *Swollen.* | distendu |
| **distichiasis** *Presence of two rows of eyelashes on one eyelid which are turned inward toward the globe.* | distichiase |
| **distribution** | distribution |
| **diuresis** *Increased excretion of urine.* | diurèse |
| **diuretic** *Medication which causes an increased excretion of urine.* | diurétique |
| **diurnal** *Occurring during the day.* | diurne |
| **diverticulitis** *Inflammation of the diverticulum.* | diverticulite |
| **diverticulosis** *Presence of diverticulum.* | diverticulose |
| **diverticulum** *A sac or pouch created by herniation of a mucous membrane in the alimentary canal.* | diverticule |
| **diving** | plongée |
| **dizygotic twins** *Twins from two separate zygotes (non-identicle twins).* | jumeaux hétérozygotes |
| **dizziness** *Sensation of losing one's balance.* | étourdissement |
| **DNA** *Deoxyribonucleic acid.* | ADN |
| **donor** *Referring to a person who gave an organ or part.* | donneur |
| **dopa reaction** *A dopa-oxidase reaction, changing dopa into melanin.* | dopa-réaction |
| **dopamine** *An intermediate product in the creation of norepinephrine.* | dopamine |
| **dorsal** *Referring to the back or back surface.* | dorsal |
| **dorsal root** *A description of the site of ganglion found on the dorsal root of each spinal nerve.* | racine dorsale |
| **dorsiflexion** *Backward bending of the foot or hand.* | dorsiflexion |
| **dorsum** *The back part.* | dos |
| **dosage** *The frequency and amount of a medication.* | dosage |
| **dose regimen** *The amount, frequency and length of treatment of a medication.* | posologie |
| **dose** *The quantity of a medication.* | dose |
| **dosing interval** *The number of times per unit a medication is given.* | intervalle entre les prises |
| **double** | double |

| English | French |
|---|---|
| **douche** *Cleansing of a canal; unless otherwise specified it refers to cleansing of the vaginal canal.* | lavage vaginal |
| **Douglas' pouch** *A recess in the peritoneum between the rectum and the uterus. Also called the rectouterine pouch.* | cul-de-sac de Douglas |
| **down** | vers le bas |
| **Down's syndrome** *A congenital chromosomal defect (trisomy 21) that caused diminished intellectual function, short stature and a broad face.* | Down, syndrome de |
| **drainage tube** *A cannula used to allow outflow of fluids.* | drain |
| **drape** *The fabric used as a sterile covering in the OR.* | champ opératoire |
| **drawing** | dessin |
| **drawsheet** *The topsheet of a bed.* | alèse |
| **dream** | rêve |
| **dressing** *The gauze applied to a wound.* | pansement |
| **dribble, to** | baver |
| **drill** | 1. foret 2. perceuse |
| **drink, to** | boire |
| **drinking water** | eau potable |
| **drop** | goutte |
| **drop by drop** | goutte-à-goutte |
| **drop foot gait** *A gait characterized by dragging the foot, as there is no ankle dorsiflexion.* | steppage |
| **drop foot** *The symptom in a person with a nerve injury causing impaired ankle dorsiflexion.* | pied tombant |
| **dropper** *A device used to administer medicines one drop at a time.* | compte-gouttes |
| **drops per minute** | gouttes par minute |
| **drowning** | noyade |
| **drowsiness** | assoupissement |
| **drug** | drogue |
| **drug dependence** *Addiction to a substance.* | pharmacodépendance |
| **drug eruption** *A diffuse rash caused by a medication.* | 1. dermatite médicamenteuse 2. toxidermie |
| **drug reaction** | réaction médicamenteuse |
| **drunkenness** *Inebriation.* | ébriété |
| **dry** | sec |
| **ductus arteriosus** *A fetal artery that communicates between the pulmonary artery and the descending aorta.* | canal artériel |
| **dumping syndrome** *Characterized by rapid bowel evacuation after eating in patients with prior gastric surgery.* | syndrome de chasse |
| **duodenal** *Referring to the duodenum.* | duodénal |
| **duplication** | dédoublement |
| **dura mater** *The outermost covering of the brain and spinal cord.* | dure-mère |
| **dust** | poussière |

| English | French |
|---|---|
| **dwarf** *Abnormally small person.* | nain |
| **dysarthria** *Difficulty in articulation of speech.* | dysarthrie |
| **dyschezia** *Pain experienced during defecation.* | dyschésie |
| **dyschondroplasia** *The formation of cartilaginous and bony tumors near the epiphyses.* | dyschondroplasie |
| **dyscoria** *A discordance in pupillary reaction.* | dyscorie |
| **dysdiadocokinesia** *The inability to arrest one motor response and substitute its opposite.* | dysdiadococinésie |
| **dysentery** *A severe form of diarrhea with blood and mucous in the stool.* | dysenterie |
| **dysesthesia** *1. Impairment of the sense of touch. 2. The presence of persistent pain upon receiving a light touch.* | dysesthésie |
| **dysfunction** | dysfonction |
| **dyskinesia** *Abnormal movement.* | dyskinésie |
| **dyslalia** *The absence of comprehensible speech articulation.* | dyslalie |
| **dyslexia** *Difficulty in learning or reading written language with no effect on intelligence.* | dyslexie |
| **dysmenorrhea** *Pain during menstruation.* | dysménorrhée |
| **dyspareunia** *Pain during sexual intercourse.* | dypareunie |
| **dyspepsia** *Indigestion.* | dyspepsie |
| **dysphagia** *Difficulty in swallowing.* | dysphagie |
| **dysplasia** *The increase in organ size due to an increase in the number of abnormal cell types.* | dysplasie |
| **dyspnea** *Difficult breathing.* | dyspnée |
| **dystocia** *Difficult birth caused by fetal position, narrow pelvis or lack of opening of the cervix.* | dystocie |
| **dysuria** *Painful urination.* | dysurie |
| **ear** | oreille |
| **eat, to** | manger |
| **eating disorder** *General term for pathologic eating habits.* | trouble de l'alimentation |
| **ecchondroma** *Hyperplastic growth of cartilage on the surface of other cartilage.* | ecchondrome |
| **ecchymosis** *Skin discoloration caused by bleeding beneath the epidermis.* | ecchymose |
| **Echinococcus** *A tapeworm of the family Taeniidae that can cause hydatid cysts.* | échinocoque |
| **echocardiographic** *Referring to echocardiography.* | échocardiographic |
| **echocardiography** *The use of ultrasound waves to visualize the heart and its structures.* | échocardiographie |
| **echolalia** *The meaningless repetition of the words spoken by another person.* | écholalie |
| **eclampsia** *A maternal condition characterized by convulsions and hypertension that can lead to maternal and fetal death.* | éclampsie |

| English | French |
|---|---|
| **ecmnesia** *Memory loss for recent events but retained memory of remote events.* | ecmnésie |
| **ectasia** *Expansion or distension.* | ectasie |
| **ectoderm** *The outermost layer of the three layers of the embryo.* | ectoderme |
| **ectopic** *Abnormal position.* | ectopique |
| **ectopic pregnancy** *A pregnancy that is not intrauterine.* | grossesse extra-utérine |
| **ectrodactylia** *A congenital anomaly exhibited by absence of one digit or part of a digit.* | ectrodactylie |
| **eczema** *A medical condition exhibited by pruritic, red, scaly patches on the scalp, cheeks and extensor surfaces.* | eczéma |
| **edema** *Extravascular fluid accumulation.* | œdème |
| **edematous** *Referring to the presence of edema.* | œdémateux |
| **education** | enseignement |
| **effector** *An organ that responds to a stimulus.* | effecteur |
| **efficacious** *Effective.* | efficace |
| **effleurage** *A form of massage involving circular stroking.* | effleurage |
| **effort** | effort |
| **effusion** *The accumulation of fluid in a body cavity.* | effusion |
| **egg** | œuf |
| **egocentric** *Thinking of self without considering the feelings or thoughts of others.* | égocentrique |
| **ejaculation** *The emission of semen at the moment of sexual climax in a male.* | éjaculation |
| **elastic bandage** *A stretch gauze used for compression of an extremity.* | bande élastique |
| **elastin** *A connective tissue-based glycoprotein.* | élastine |
| **elderly** | personnes âgées |
| **elective** *Non-urgent and not life-saving.* | électif |
| **electrocardiogram** *Display of a person's heart beat that can be used in the diagnosis of cardiac disorders.* | électrocardiogramme |
| **electroconvulsive therapy** *The electrical stimulation of the brain to treat mental disorders.* | électrochoc |
| **electrode** *A device used to facilitate conduction of electricity to or from a body.* | électrode |
| **electroencephalogram** *A display of brain waves used in the diagnosis of brain disorders, especially epilepsy.* | électroencéphalo-gramme |
| **electrolyte** *The ionized constituents including potassium, sodium, chloride and others.* | électrolyte |
| **electromyography** *The display of the electrical activity f muscle.* | électromyographie |
| **electron microscopy** *The use of electron beams and lenses to give high magnification.* | microscopie électronique |
| **electrophoresis** *The movement of charged particles in a fluid that is under the influence of an electric field. This is used in testing for various maladies in the form of serum protein electrophoresis.* | électrophorèse |

| English | French |
|---|---|
| **elephantiasis** *A condition caused by nematode parasites leading to lymphatic obstruction and limb or scrotal swelling.* | 1. éléphantiasis 2. lymphangite endémique tropicale |
| **elixir** *A medical solution.* | élixir |
| **emaciation** *Abnormally thin and weak.* | émaciation |
| **embolectomy** *The removal of an embolus.* | embolectomie |
| **embolus** *A blood clot, air bubble or fatty deposit that cause obstruction of a vessel.* | embole |
| **embryo** *The term used to describe a fertilized ovum in the first 8 weeks of development.* | embryon |
| **embryology** *The study of the embryo.* | embryologie |
| **emergence** *Coming into prominence.* | apparition |
| **emergency** *An urgent, life-threatening situation.* | urgence |
| **emesis** *Vomiting.* | vomissement |
| **emetic** *An agent that induces vomiting.* | émétique |
| **emmetropia** *The normal correlation between eye refraction and the axial length of the eyeball.* | emmétropie |
| **emollient** *Having softening or soothing qualities.* | émollient |
| **emotion** *An intense feeling.* | émotion |
| **empathy** *To be concerned for and share the feelings of another.* | empathie |
| **emphysema** *Abnormal enlargement of the airspaces distal to the terminal bronchioles.* | emphysème |
| **empty** | vide |
| **empyema** *A collection of purulent material in a body cavity, usually referring to a thoracic empyema.* | empyème |
| **emulsion** *The dispersion of one liquid into another, but it is not dissolved.* | émulsion |
| **enarthrosis** *The type of joint in which a spherical bone is set into the socket of another bone.* | énarthrose |
| **encephalic** *Referring to the brain.* | encéphalique |
| **encephalitis** *Inflammation of the brain.* | encéphalite |
| **encephalocele** *The protrusion of the brain through a defect in the skull.* | encéphalocèle |
| **encephalography** *Roentgenography of the brain.* | encéphalographie |
| **encephalomacia** *Abnormal softness of the brain.* | encéphalomacie |
| **encephalomyelitis** *Inflammation of the brain and spinal cord.* | encéphalomyélite |
| **encephalopathy** *Degeneration of cerebral function.* | encéphalopathie |
| **enchondroma** *An abnormal increase in cartilage growth on the inside of bone or of other cartilage.* | enchondrome |
| **encopresis** *Involuntary defecation.* | encoprésie |
| **end organ** *The encapsulated end of a sensory nerve.* | terminaison d'un nerf afférent |
| **end point** *The last stage of a process.* | aboutissement |
| **end stage** *Terminal stage. End stage cancer means there is no cure possible and death is imminent.* | étape terminale |

| English | French |
|---|---|
| **endarteritis** *Tunica intima inflammation.* | enartérite |
| **endemic** *When a disease is commonly found in a location or in a people group.* | endémique |
| **endocarditis** *Inflammation of the endocardium.* | endocardite |
| **endocervicitis** *Inflammation of the mucosal lining of the cervix.* | endocervicite |
| **endocrine gland** *A gland that secretes hormones and other substances into the blood.* | gland endocrine |
| **endocrine** *Referring to glands that secrete hormones and other chemicals into the blood.* | endocrine |
| **endocrinology** *The study of endocrine glands and hormones.* | endocrinologie |
| **endoderm** *The innermost layer of the embryonic germ cell layers.* | endoderme |
| **endogenous** *Originating from within.* | endogène |
| **endolymph** *The fluid collection the labyrinth of the ear.* | endolymphe |
| **endometrioma** *An isolated benign mass containing endometrial tissue.* | endométriome |
| **endometriosis** *Presence of uterine mucosal tissue in the pelvis in abnormal locations.* | endométriose |
| **endometritis** *Inflammation of the endometrium.* | endométrite |
| **endometrium** *The mucous membrane lining of the uterus.* | endomètre |
| **endoneurium** *The tissue in a peripheral nerve that separates the individual nerve fibers.* | endonèvre |
| **endoplasmic reticulum** *A framework of tubules within the cytoplasm of eukaryotic cells.* | réticulum endoplasmique |
| **endorphin** *Hormones secreted that activate the body's opiate receptors and act as analgesics.* | endorphine |
| **endoscope** *A device used to view the interior of a hollow organ (sigmoidoscope, gastroscope)* | endoscope |
| **endothelioma** *A mass that propagates from the endothelium of blood vessels, lymphatics or serous cavities.* | endothéliome |
| **endotracheal** *Within the trachea.* | endotrachéal |
| **endow** | doter |
| **enema** *A procedure involving insertion of fluid into the rectum.* | lavement |
| **enkephalin** *A peptide found in the brain that has similar effects as the endorphins.* | encéphaline |
| **enlargement** *Becoming bigger.* | 1. agrandissement 2. augmentation de volume |
| **enophthalmos** *Posterior displacement of the eyeball in the orbit.* | énophtalmie |
| **enormous** *Very large.* | énorme |
| **enostosis** *The abnormal bony growth inside a bone or on the cortex.* | énostose |
| **ensure, to** *To make certain of.* | assurer de, s' |
| **ENT** *Abbreviation for ears, nose and throat.* | ORL |
| **enteral feeding** *Nutrition supplied via the alimentary canal.* | alimentation parentérale |
| **enterectomy** *Surgical resection of part of the intestine.* | entérectomie |

| English | French |
|---|---|
| **enteric** *Referring to the intestines.* | entérique |
| **enteritis** *Inflammation of the intestines.* | entérite |
| **enterobiasis** *An infection caused by worms from the genus Enterobius.* | oxyurose |
| **enterococcus** *A gram positive cocci that occurs naturally in the intestine but is pathogenic elsewhere in the body.* | entérocoque |
| **enterolith** *A calculus of the intestine.* | entérolithe |
| **enteroptosis** *Inferior displacement of the intestines in the abdomen.* | entéroptose |
| **enterotomy** *A surgical opening of the intestines.* | entérotomie |
| **entrapment neuropathy** *Weakness or numbness caused by compression of a peripheral nerve.* | syndrome canalaire |
| **enucleation** *Surgical removal of a globe.* | énucléation |
| **enuresis** *Involuntary urination.* | énurésie |
| **enzyme** *A compound that acts as a catalyst for reactions within cells as assists with digestion outside of cells.* | enzyme |
| **eosinophil** *A cell with eosin stain used to designate a type of leukocyte that is elevated during allergic reactions.* | éosinophile |
| **eosinophilia** *An increased number of eosinophils in the blood.* | 1. acidophilie 2. éosinophilie |
| **eosphagectomy** *Surgical removal of the esophagus.* | œsophagectomie |
| **ependyma** *The glial lined covering of the cerebral ventricles and the central portion of the spinal cord.* | épendyme |
| **ependymoma** *A tumor composed of cells that line the ventricles of the brain.* | épendymome |
| **ephedrine** *A chemical used to treat asthma because it expands bronchial passages and used to control spinal anesthesia associated shock because it constricts blood vessels.* | éphédrine |
| **ephelis** *Medical term for the common freckle.* | tache de rousseur |
| **epiblepharon** *A condition exhibited by the eyelashes pressing against the eyeball.* | épiblépharon |
| **epicardium** *The serous membranous, innermost lining of the pericardium.* | épicarde |
| **epicondyle** *A protrusion at the distal end of the humerus.* | épicondyle |
| **epicondylitis** *Inflammation of the epicondyle.* | épicondylite |
| **epicranium** *The skin, fibrous layer (aponeurosis), and muscles lining the scalp.* | épicrâne |
| **epidemic** *Ubiquitous development of an infectious disease.* | épidémie |
| **epidemiology** *The study of the incidence, development and control of disease.* | épidémiologie |
| **epidermis** *The skin cells overlying the dermis.* | épiderme |
| **epidermophytosis** *A fungal skin infection caused by an organism from the genus Epidermophyton.* | épidermophytose |
| **epididymitis** *Inflammation of the duct that moves sperm from the testis to the vas deferens.* | épididymite |
| **epididymo-orchitis** *Inflammation of the epididymis and the testis.* | épididymo-orchite |
| **epidural** *The space around the dura of the spinal cord.* | épidural |

52

| English | French |
|---|---|
| **epidural analgesia** *Medication into this space produces analgesia for surgical procedures.* | anesthésie péridurale |
| **epidural hematoma** *Formation of a collection of blood outside the dural layer of the brain; usually caused by trauma.* | hématome extradural |
| **epigastrium** *The section of the abdomen that overlies the stomach.* | épigastre |
| **epiglottis** *Tissue at the base of the tongue that covers the trachea when one swallows.* | épiglotte |
| **epilation** *Removal of hair and the roots.* | épilation |
| **epilepsy** *A condition associated with abnormal brain activity and exhibited by sudden, recurrent convulsions, sensory disturbances and loss of consciousness.* | épilepsie |
| **epileptic seizure** *A convulsion related to abnormal brain activity (as opposed to being precipitated by hypoglycemia.)* | épileptique crise |
| **epileptiform** *Being similar to epilepsy.* | épileptiforme |
| **epileptogenic** *That which induces seizures.* | épileptogène |
| **epinephrine** *A hormone secreted by the adrenal gland.* | épinéphrine |
| **epiphysis cerebri** *A small structure situated on the mesencephalon between the two sections of the thalamus.* | gland pinéale |
| **epiphysitis** *Inflammation of the end of a long bone that is separated from the shaft by a cartilaginous disc.* | épiphysite |
| **episcleritis** *Inflammation of the tissue lying above the sclera.* | épisclérite |
| **episiotomy** *A surgical incision of the vagina used to aid childbirth.* | épisiotomie |
| **epistaxis** *Bleeding emanating from the nose.* | épistaxis |
| **epithelial** *Referring to the epithelium.* | épithélial |
| **epithelial cast** *Debris found in the urine composed of columnar renal epithelium.* | cylindre épithélial |
| **epithelioma** *A malignant tumor composed of epithelial cells.* | épithéliome |
| **epithelium** *The tissue lining the skin and the gastrointestinal tract that is derived from the embryonic ectoderm and endoderm..* | épithélium |
| **epitrochlea** *The medial condyle of the humerus.* | épitrochlée |
| **equal** | égal |
| **equilibrium** *When opposing forces are in balance.* | équilibre |
| **equipment** | matériel |
| **ergometer** *A device that measures energy expenditure.* | ergomètre |
| **ergonomics** *The study of workplace design that focuses on reducing work-related injuries.* | ergonomie |
| **ergosterol** *A compound converted to vitamin D2 upon exposure to ultraviolet light.* | ergostérol |
| **erosion** *The gradual destruction of surface tissue.* | érosion |
| **error** | erreur |
| **eructation** *A belch or burp.* | éructation |
| **erysipelas** *An acute infection caused by Streptococcus pyogenes that causes fever along with swelling and inflammation. The infection frequently effects the face or one leg.* | érysipèlas |

| English | French |
|---|---|
| **erythema mutliforme** *A skin condition exhibited by purpuric lesions and bullae usually on the distal parts of extremities but can affect the face and trunk.* | érythème polymorphe |
| **erythema nodosum** *The presence of red or purple nodules on the pretibial area.* | érythème noueux |
| **erythroblast** *A nucleus containing immature erythrocyte.* | érthyroblaste |
| **erythroblastosis fetalis** *A hemolytic disease of the newborn.* | érthyroblastose fœtale |
| **erythrocyanosis** *A condition exhibited by purple patches with asymmetric swelling, pruritis and burning.* | érthyrocyanose |
| **erythrocyte** *Called a red blood cell, it transports oxygen and carbon dioxide to and from the tissues.* | 1. érthyrocyte 2. globule rouge |
| **erythrocytopenia** *Low level of erythrocytes in the blood stream.* | érthyrocytopénie |
| **erythrocytosis** *A higher than normal level of erythrocytes in the blood stream.* | érthyrocytose |
| **erythropoiesis** *The production of red blood cells.* | érthyropoïèse |
| **eschar** *Dry, hard, dead tissue commonly seen with a chronic pressure ulcer or anthrax.* | escarre |
| **eserine** *Physostigmine.* | ésérine |
| **esophageal** *Referring to the esophagus.* | œsophagien |
| **esophagoscopy** *Visual inspection the esophagus utilizing a scope.* | œsophagoscopie |
| **esophagus** *The muscular tube that connects the throat to the stomach.* | œsophage |
| **esotropia** *Medial deviation of the eye at primary gaze.* | ésotropie |
| **essential** | essentiel |
| **estrogen** *A hormone involved with developing and maintaining female sexual characteristics.* | 1. estrogène 2. œstrogène |
| **ethanol** *Synonym for ethyl alcohol.* | alcool éthylique |
| **ethmoid** *A bone at the root of the nose which has perforations for the olfactory nerves to transit.* | ethmoïde |
| **etiology** | étiologie |
| **eunuch** *A man who has been castrated.* | eunuque |
| **euthanasia** *Killing someone painlessly who is thought to have a terminal condition.* | euthanasie |
| **evacuation** *The emptying of an organ of fluids or gas.* | évacuation |
| **evaluation** | évaluation |
| **eventration** *Protrusion of the intestines from the abdomen.* | éventration |
| **eversion** *To turn outward.* | éversion |
| **every** | chaque |
| **every day** | quotidien |
| **every other day** | tous les deux jours |
| **evident** *Obvious.* | évident |
| **evisceration** *The removal of bowels from the body.* | éviscération |
| **evoked potential** *Electrical impulses that can be noted after stimulation of sensory organs.* | potentiel évoqué |
| **evulsion** *Forcible extraction.* | évulsion |

| English | French |
|---|---|
| **exacerbation** *Worsening of an existing problem.* | exacerbation |
| **examination** | examen |
| **exanthema** *A rash that accompanies a disease or fever.* | exanthème |
| **excess** | excès |
| **exchange transfusion** *Treatment of hyperbilirubinemia in neonates.* | exsanguino-transfusion |
| **excipient** *An inactive substance used to deliver an active substance.* | excipient |
| **excisional biopsy** *Surgical removal of tissue for pathologic examination.* | biopsie-exérèse |
| **excoriation** *Superficial loss of skin.* | excoriation |
| **excrement** *Feces.* | excrément |
| **excrement (slang)** | caca |
| **excreta** *Fecal material.* | excreta |
| **exenteration** *Complete surgical removal of an organ.* | exentération |
| **exercise-induced dyspnea** | dyspnée d'effort |
| **exercised induce angina** | angor d'effort |
| **exfoliation** *The shedding of scales.* | exfoliation |
| **exhumation** *The process of removing a dead body from a grave.* | exhumation |
| **exogenous** *Referring to external factors.* | exogène |
| **exomphalos** *Umbilical hernia.* | exomphale |
| **exostosis** *A bony prominence growing from the surface of a bone.* | exostose |
| **exotoxin** *A toxin released from a living cell.* | exotoxine |
| **expansion** | ampliation |
| **expect** | attendre |
| **expectorant** *A substance that promotes the secretion of sputum.* | expectorant |
| **expectoration** *The presence of sputum that has been coughed out.* | expectoration |
| **expiration date** | date de péremption |
| **expiratory** *Referring to exhalation of air from the lungs.* | expiratoire |
| **expiratory flow rate** *Amount of air exhaled in liters per unit of time.* | débit expiratoire |
| **expiratory reserve volume** *Amount of air left in the lung after a maximal exhalation, in liters.* | 1. air de réserve 2. volume de réserve expiratoire |
| **expulsion** *Evacuation or elimination.* | expulsion |
| **expulsion of placenta** | délivrance |
| **extended** | prolongé |
| **extension** *Going from a bent to straight position.* | délai supplémentaire |
| **extensor plantar response** *Great toe extension indicating a positive Babinski sign.* | signe de Babinski positif |
| **extensor** *Referring to the extension of an extremity or part of an extremity.* | extenseur |
| **external ear** | oreille externe |
| **external** *Outside of the body.* | externe |
| **extirpate** *To totally destroy.* | exirper |
| **extracapsular** *Situated outside a capsule.* | extracapsulaire |
| **extracellular** *Outside the cell.* | extracellulaire |

| English | French |
|---|---|
| **extract** *A substance in a concentrated form.* | extrait |
| **extrapyramidal tract** *Motor nerves that are not part of the pyramidal tract.* | voie extrapyramidale |
| **extrasystole** | extrasystole |
| **extravasation** *Referring to a situation in which blood or fluid goes out of a vessel it is normally flowing into.* | 1. épanchement 2. extravasation |
| **extremity** | extrémité |
| **extrinsic** *Coming from outside or external sources.* | extrinsèque |
| **exudate** *The fluid, cells, and debris found in the tissues or a cavity (like pleural space) during inflammation.* | exsudat |
| **eye drops** | collyre |
| **eyebrow** *Supercilium.* | sourcil |
| **eyeground** *The fundus that is visualized with an ophthalmoscope.* | fond d'œil |
| **eyelash** | cil |
| **eyelid** *Palpebra.* | paupière |
| **face** | 1. face 2. figure |
| **face presentation** *Referring to the part of the body coming out of the cervix first during childbirth.* | présentation de la face |
| **facet** *A small flat surface of a bone.* | facette |
| **facial nerve** *Cranial nerve VII that supplies the face and tongue.* | facial nerf |
| **facial paralysis** *Lack of movement or sensation in the distribution of the facial nerve.* | paralysie faciale |
| **facies** *A facial expression that is typical for a particular disease.* | faciès |
| **faint** *Weak and dizzy.* | évanouissement |
| **fair** | juste |
| **falciform** *Referring to something that is curved. The falciform ligament attaches the liver to the diaphragm.* | falciforme |
| **falx cerebri** *A fold in the dura that separates the two cerebral hemispheres.* | faux du cerveau |
| **familial** *Referring to the family* | familial |
| **family** | famille |
| **family history** | antécédents familiaux |
| **family planning** *Birth control.* | planification familiale |
| **faradism** *The gradual increasing and decreasing of the amplitude of electricity.* | faradisation |
| **farmer's lung** *Coined because farmers are susceptible to this disease by inhaling fungi from hay; also called Aspergillosis.* | poumon du fermier |
| **fart** *Slang term for flatus.* | pet |
| **fascia** *The fibrous sheath enclosing a muscle or organ.* | fascia |
| **fascicle** *A bundle of nerve or muscle fibers.* | fascicule |
| **fasciculation** *Minute muscle contractions that are visible.* | fasciculation |
| **fasting** *Absence of caloric intake for a specified period.* | 1. jeun à 2. jeûne |
| **fat** | graisse |

| English | French |
|---|---|
| **fat embolism** *A deposit of fat that obstructs a vessel.* | embolie graisseuse |
| **fat soluble** *Referring to the ability of a substance to dissolve in fat.* | liposoluble |
| **fatal** | fatal |
| **fatness** | adiposité |
| **fatty** | gras |
| **fatty acid** *A carboxylic acid occurring as a an ester in fats and oils.* | acide gras |
| **favus** *Tinea capitis caused by Trichopyton schoenleini.* | favus |
| **fear** | crainte |
| **febrile** *Presence of an supraphysiologic temperature.* | fébrile |
| **fecal impaction** *The presence of hard excrement in the rectum that requires manual removal.* | fécalome |
| **feces** *Excrement.* | 1. fèces 2. selles |
| **fecundity** *The capability of producing offspring quickly and frequently.* | fécondité |
| **feeble minded** *A person unable to make seemingly simple decisions because of a cognitive impairment.* | arriéré |
| **feeding behavior** | comportement alimentaire |
| **female** | 1. femelle 2. femme |
| **feminine pad** *Gauze specially designed to absorb menstrual flow.* | serviette hygiénique |
| **femoral nerve** *Supplies the motor function of the quadriceps and the sensation over the anterior and medial thigh.* | 1. crural nerf 2. fémoral nerf |
| **femoral triangle** *An area that is bordered by the sartorius muscle, the adductor longus muscle and the inguinal ligament.* | triangle de Scarpa |
| **femur** *The long bone in the thigh.* | fémur |
| **fenestra** *Usually referring to a surgical window.* | fenêtre |
| **fertility** *The ability of a person to contribute to contraception.* | fertilité |
| **fertilization** *The melding of male and female gametes to form a zygote.* | fertilisation |
| **fester** *To become infected.* | suppurer |
| **festinating gait** *Walking with increased speed involuntarily; often seen in Parkinson's disease.* | démarche festinante |
| **fetal distress** *Term used to describe an abnormal heart rate or rhythm in a fetus indicating the need for urgent childbirth.* | souffrance fœtale |
| **fetal** *Referring to the fetus.* | fœtal |
| **fetichism** *The glorification of an inanimate object.* | fétichisme |
| **fetor** *A foul odor.* | puanteur |
| **fever** | fièvre |
| **fibrillation** *Uncoordinated, ineffective contraction as in atrial fibrillation.* | fibrillation |
| **fibrin** *An insoluble protein formed when fibrinogen is acted upon by thrombin.* | fibrine |
| **fibroadenoma** *A benign breast mass composed of fibrous and glandular tissue.* | fibroadénome |
| **fibroblast** *A collagen producing cell in connective tissue.* | fibroblaste |

57

| English | French |
|---|---|
| **fibrochondritis** *The inflammation of a structure composed of cartilage and fibrous tissue.* | fibrochondrite |
| **fibroelastosis** *The abnormal increase in growth of fibrous and elastic tissue.* | fibro-élastose |
| **fibroid** *A benign mass, typically uterine, composed of fibrous and muscle tissue.* | fibreux |
| **fibromyoma** *A mass containing fibrous and muscle tissue.* | fibromyome |
| **fibrosarcoma** *A sarcoma composed primarily of malignant fibroblasts.* | fibrosarcome |
| **fibrosis** *Connective tissue that is scarred and thickened after injury.* | fibrose |
| **fibrositis** *Fibrous connective tissue that is inflammed.* | fibrosite |
| **fibula** *The smaller of two bones in the lower leg.* | 1. fibula 2. péroné |
| **filaria** *A parasitic nematode worm that is transmitted by flies and mosquitos causing filariasis.* | filaire |
| **file** *Patient record or folder.* | dossier |
| **filiform** *Threadlike.* | filiforme |
| **filum terminale** *The thin structure at the end of the conus medullaris which connects the spinal cord with the coccyx.* | filum terminale |
| **fimbria** *A slender projection at the end of the fallopian tube near the ovary.* | 1. fimbria 2. frange |
| **finger cot** *A rubber or plastic covering for a finger that is used to enter an orifice.* | doigtier fingerstall |
| **fingerstick device** *A device used to project a lancet into the skin so a drop of blood can be obtained for analysis.* | appareil autopiqueur |
| **fingertip** | bout du doigt |
| **firm** | solide |
| **first aid** | premiers secours |
| **first line** | de première intention |
| **fish** | poisson |
| **fissure** *A general term for a cleft or deep groove. An anal fissure, for example, is a small ulcer adjacent to the anus.* | 1. fissure 2. scissure |
| **fist** | poing |
| **fistula** *An abnormal communication between two organs or an organ and the skin, as in rectovaginal fistula.* | fistule |
| **fixation** *1. An obsessive interest. 2. The securing of a body part.* | fixation |
| **flaccid** *Limp. A term applied to an extremity one cannot move actively.* | flasque |
| **flagellation** *1. The protrusion found on flagella. 2. Massage administered by tapping a body part with fingers.* | flagellation |
| **flagellum** *A slender appendage that allows protozoa to swim.* | flagelle |
| **flame photometer** *A device used to measure the intensity of light.* | photomètre à flamme |
| **flap** *A term used to describe a piece of tissue partially excised and placed over an adjacent surface.* | lambeau |
| **flare** *A sudden intensity or dilatation.* | poussée |
| **flask** | fiole |
| **flat** | plat |

| English | French |
|---------|--------|
| **flatten** | aplatir |
| **flatulence** *The gas expulsed from the anus.* | 1. flatulence 2. météorisme |
| **flatworm** *A class of worms that includes parasitic flukes and tapeworms.* | plathelminthe |
| **flea** | puce |
| **flesh** | chair |
| **flexor** *A muscle that bends an extremity or part of an extremity.* | fléchisseur |
| **flexure** *The action of bending.* | 1. angle 2. courbure |
| **floating** | flottant |
| **flow** | écoulement |
| **flow-volume loop** *A graph of inspiratory and expiratory flow against volume.* | boucle débit-volume |
| **fluid intake** *The amount of oral consumption plus the amount of intravenous fluids administered.* | apport hydrique |
| **fluke** *Parasitic nematode worm; an example is Schistosoma.* | douve |
| **fluoresceine** *A fluorane dye used to check for corneal ulcers.* | fluorescéine |
| **fluorescent antibody test (FTA test)** | réaction d'immuno-fluorenscence |
| **fluorescent screen** *A screen used to view x-rays.* | écran fluorescent |
| **fluoridation** *The addition of fluorine to something.* | fluoration |
| **fluorine** *A chemical that causes severe burns if exposed to the skin.* | fluor |
| **fluoroscopy** *The continuous viewing of roentgenographic images with a fluorescent screen.* | fluoroscopie |
| **flush, to** | rougeur |
| **flutter** *Used to describe a cardiac rhythm disturbance, as in atrial flutter.* | flutter |
| **foam** | 1. mousse 2. spume |
| **foley placement (urinary catheter)** | sondage vésicale |
| **folic acid** *Also called pteroylglutamic acid; a deficiency can cause megaloblastic anemia.* | folique acide |
| **follicle stimulating hormone (FSH)** *An anterior pituitary gland hormone responsible for production of sperm or ova.* | folliculostimulante hormone |
| **follicular** *Referring to a small secretory gland.* | folliculaire |
| **fontanelle** *The space between the bones in the skull that are separate at birth.* | fontanelle |
| **food** | aliment |
| **food intake** | apport alimentaire |
| **food poisoning** | 1. toxicose alimentaire 2. intoxication alimentaire |
| **foot and mouth disease** *A contagious viral disease exhibited by oral and digital vesicles.* | fièvre aphteuse |
| **foramen** *An opening in a bone.* | foramen |

| English | French |
|---|---|
| **foramen magnum** *The hole in the skull that the spinal cord passes through.* | trou occipital |
| **foramen ovale** *A hole in the atrial septal wall in a fetus.* | trou de Botal |
| **forced expiratory volume per second (FEV1)** *The amount of air exhaled with maximal effort, measured in liters, over one second.* | volume expiratoire maximal par seconde (VEMS) |
| **forceps** *A surgical instrument, commonly called tweezers.* | 1. forceps 2. pince 3. clamp |
| **forearm** | 1. antebrachium 2. avant-bras |
| **forearm crutch** *A long stick with a place for a hand-grip to aid in ambulation when there is lower extremity weakness.* | canne anglaise |
| **forebrain** *The part of the brain that includes the thalamus, hypothalamus and cerebral hemispheres.* | cerveau antérieur |
| **forehead** | front |
| **foreign body** *Term used to describe an object found in a body orifice that is not part of the body.* | corps étranger |
| **forensic** *Referring to the scientific method of studying crime.* | juridique |
| **foreskin** *Also called prepuce, the skin that naturally covers the glans but can be rolled back.* | prépuce |
| **former** | ancien |
| **formulary** *A list of medicines that are permissible to prescribe.* | formulaire |
| **fornix** *A vaulted structure.* | fornix |
| **forwards** | avant en |
| **fossa** *A shallow depression.* | fosse |
| **fovea** *The area on the retina where the visual acuity is optimal.* | fovea |
| **fracture** | fracture |
| **fragilitas ossium** *A condition exhibited by excessively brittle bones. Also called osteogenesis imperfecta.* | fragilité osseuse |
| **framboesia; yaws** *An endemic tropical disease caused by Treponema pertenue.* | pian |
| **free** | libre |
| **free of** | dépourvu de |
| **freedom** | liberté |
| **freezing** | congélation |
| **fremitus** *A vibration that is appreciated with palpation.* | frémissement |
| **frenulum** *The tissue that connects the inferior portion of the tongue to the base of the mouth.* | frein |
| **frequency** | fréquence |
| **friction** | friction |
| **friction rub** *A noise heard during cardiac auscultation in patients with pericarditis, for example.* | frottement |
| **frog** | grenouille |

| English | French |
|---|---|
| **frog in the throat, to have** | chat dans la gorge, avoir un |
| **frontal** *Referring to the anterior aspect, as in frontal lobe.* | frontal |
| **frostbite** | gelures |
| **frothy** | écumeux |
| **frozen** | gelé |
| **fructosuria** *The presence of fructose in the urine.* | lévulosurie |
| **FTA test** *Fluorescent treponemal antibody test for syphilis.* | anticorps tréponémiques fluorescents (test FTA) |
| **full-term** *A normal length pregnancy.* | terme à |
| **fulminating** *Sudden and severe.* | foudroyant |
| **function** | fonction |
| **fundus** *Referring to the upper part of the stomach or the part of the globe opposing the pupil.* | fundus |
| **fungicide** *An agent that destroys fungus.* | fongicide |
| **fungus** *A spore-producing organism that feeds on organic matter.* | champignon |
| **funiculi of the spinal cord** *The white matter of the spinal cord that is further defined by location.* | cordons de la moelle spinale |
| **funiculitis** *Inflammation of the funiculi.* | funiculite |
| **funnel chest** *Anterior thorax funnel shaped depression, also called pectus excavatum.* | thorax en entonnoir |
| **funny bone** *The area adjacent to the olecranon where the ulnar nerve passes; local trauma yields numbness distally.* | petit juif |
| **furuncle** *A painful erythematous nodule with a central core.* | furoncle |
| **furunculosis** *The presence of multiple furuncles.* | furonculose |
| **fusiform** *Spindle-shaped.* | fusiforme |
| **gag reflex** *Contraction of the pharynx muscles when the back of the pharynx is stimulated by touch.* | réflexe nauséeux |
| **gag** *To choke or wretch.* | ouvre-bouche |
| **gait** *The way one walks.* | démarche |
| **galactocele** *A milk-filled cyst in the mammary gland.* | galactocéle |
| **galactorrhea** *Excessive production of milk.* | galactorrhée |
| **galactose** *A sugar that is a constituent of lactose.* | galactose |
| **galactosemie** *1. Galactose in the blood. 2. A congenital condition exhibited by impaired carbohydrate metabolism.* | galactosémie |
| **gallbladder** *The organ adjacent to the liver that stores bile and secretes it into the duodenum.* | vésicule biliaire |
| **gallop** *An abnormal heart sound.* | galop (bruit ou rythme de) |
| **gallstone** *A calculus produced in the bile duct or gallbladder.* | calcul biliaire |
| **galvanism** *The use of electric currents for medical treatment.* | galvanisme |
| **galvanometer** *A device used to measure small electric currents.* | galvanomètre |

| English | French |
|---|---|
| **gamete** *A germ cell that is able to unite with another germ cell of the opposite gender to form a zygote.* | gamète |
| **gamma globulin** *A blood serum protein with little electrophoretic mobility.* | gammaglobuline |
| **gamma ray** *A type of electromagnetic radiation.* | rayon gamma |
| **ganglionectomie** *The removal of a benign swelling on a tendon sheath.* | gangliectomie |
| **gangrene** *Tissue death from either impaired blood flow or an infection.* | gangrène |
| **gaping** *Wide open.* | béant |
| **gargle** | gargarisme |
| **gargoylism** *A congenital anomaly exhibited by mental retardation, bone deformities and an abnormally large head.* | gargoylisme |
| **gas gangrene** *A life and limb threatening disorder caused associated with tissue death and caused by an anaerobic bacterium in the genus of Clostridium.* | gangrène gazeuse |
| **gastrectomy** *Complete or partial surgical resection of the stomach.* | gastrectomie |
| **gastric lavage** *Instillation and removal of large quantities of saline into the stomach in order to treat poisoning.* | lavage gastrique |
| **gastric** *Referring to the stomach.* | gastrique |
| **gastric secretions** | suc gastrique |
| **gastrin** *A hormone that stimulates gastric secretions.* | gastrine |
| **gastritis** *Inflammation of the stomach.* | gastrite |
| **gastrocele** *Protrusion of part of the stomach in the form of a hernia.* | gastrocèle |
| **gastrocnemius** *A large muscle in the lower leg, responsible for ankle plantar flexion, that is attached to the distal femur and achilles tendon.* | gastrocnemius muscle |
| **gastrocolic reflex** *Peristalsis of the colon produced by food entering the stomach.* | réflexe gastrocolique |
| **gastroduodenal ulcer** *A lesion in the mucosal lining of the stomach or duodenum.* | ulcère gastro-duodénal |
| **gastroenteritis** *A bacterial or viral infection that leads to vomiting and diarrhea.* | gastro-entérite |
| **gastroenterostomy** *A surgical opening in the stomach or intestine.* | gastro-entérostomie |
| **gastrointestinal tract** *The alimentary canal from the distal esophagus to the cecum.* | tube digestif |
| **gastrojejunostomy** *A surgical procedure that directly connects the stomach to the jejunum.* | gastrojéjunostomie |
| **gastropexy** *Securing the stomach to the abdominal wall.* | gastropexie |
| **gastroscope** *A device used to directly visualize the stomach.* | gastroscope |
| **gastrostomy** *A surgical creation of an opening in the stomach.* | gastrostomie |
| **gauge** *The size or thickness of something. An 18gauge needle.* | 1. calibre 2. jauge |
| **gauze** *A fabric used for dressing changes.* | gaze |
| **gavage syringe** | seringue gavage |
| **gavage** *The instillation of food into the stomach with use of a tube.* | gavage |
| **gavage tube** *A tube used for instillation of liquids into the stomach.* | sonde pour gavage |
| **gaze** | regard |

| English | French |
|---|---|
| **gel** | gel |
| **gene** *A unit of heredity that is passed on from parent to child.* | gène |
| **general** | général |
| **genetic** *Referring to genes or heredity.* | génétique |
| **geniculate** *Bent at a sharp angle.* | géniculé |
| **geniculate body** *Protrusions on the thalamus that relay visual and auditory signals to the brain.* | corps genouillé |
| **geniculate ganglion** *The sensory ganglion of the facial nerve.* | ganglion gèniculè |
| **genitalia** *Genitals.* | génitaux organes |
| **genome** *A full set of genetic information for an organism.* | génome |
| **gentian violet** *An antiseptic derived from rosaniline.* | violet de gentiane |
| **genu valgum** *A condition exhibited by the knees turning inward, commonly referred to as knock-knee.* | genu valgum |
| **genu varum** *A condition exhibited by the knees turning outward, commonly referred to as bowleg.* | genu varum |
| **geriatrics** *The study of the health of old people.* | gériatrie |
| **germ** | germe |
| **German measles (rubella)** *A contagious viral infection.* | rubéole |
| **gerontology** *The study of old persons.* | gérontologie |
| **gestation** *The development of a fetus from conception until birth.* | gestation |
| **gestation; pregnancy** | grossesse |
| **giant** | géant |
| **giardiasis** *A flagellate protozoa, Giardia lamblia, that causes diarrhea.* | giardiase |
| **gigantism** *Abnormally large size.* | gigantisme |
| **gingival** *Referring to the gums.* | gingival |
| **gingivitis** *Inflammation of the gums.* | gingivite |
| **ginglymus** *A joint that allows movement in one direction only.* | ginglyme |
| **glabella** *The area of the forehead above and between the eyebrows.* | 1. antinion 2. glabelle |
| **glance** | coup d'œil |
| **glans** *The distal aspect of the penis or clitoris.* | gland |
| **glare** | éblouissement |
| **glaucoma** *A condition characterized by increased intraocular pressure.* | glaucome |
| **glenoid** *Referring to the fossa that is a shallow depression, such as the hollow of the scapula where the humeral head sets.* | glénoïde |
| **glioma** *A neural malignant tumor of glial cells.* | gliome |
| **gliomyoma** *A mass with gliomatous and myomatous characteristics.* | gliomyome |
| **globus pallidus** *A portion of the lentiform nucleus in the brain.* | pallidum |
| **glomerulonephritis** *Inflammation of the renal glomeruli, usually from hemolytic streptococcus.* | glomérulonéphrite |
| **glomerulus** *A grouping of capillaries where waste is filtered from the blood.* | glomérule |
| **glomus tumor** *A reddish-blue painful papule that occurs on the distal aspects of the digits.* | 1. glomangiome 2. glomique tumeur |

| English | French |
|---|---|
| **glossal** *Referring to the tongue.* | lingual |
| **glossectomy** *Surgical resection of the whole or part of the tongue.* | glossectomie |
| **glossitis** *Inflammation of the tongue.* | glossite |
| **glossodynia** *Tongue pain.* | glossocynie |
| **glossopharyngeal** *The name for cranial nerve IX that supplies the tongue and pharynx.* | glossopharyngien |
| **glottis** *Essentially the vocal structure, including the true vocal cords and the opening between them.* | glotte |
| **glove** | gant |
| **glove anesthesia** *Absence of sensation of the hand and wrist.* | anesthésie en gant |
| **glucagon** *A pancreatic enzyme responsible for breakdown of glycogen to glucose.* | glucagon |
| **glucose tolerance test** *The oral administration of a carbohydrate load and then evaluation of the blood sugar at timed intervals.* | hyperglycémie provoquée, test d' |
| **glue** | colle |
| **glue ear** *Synonym for serous otitis media.* | otite moyenne adhésive |
| **glue sniffing addiction** | toxicomanie à la colle |
| **gluteal** *Referring to the gluteus.* | glutéal |
| **gluteal or gluteus muscle** *A paired set of three muscles, the gluteus maximus, medius and minimus, that all have origins in the ilium and insertions in the femur. (buttocks)* | fessier muscle 2. gluteus muscle |
| **glycemia** *The amount of glucose in the blood.* | glycémie |
| **glycerin** *A byproduct in the manufacture of soap that is used as a laxative.* | glycérine |
| **glycogen** *A compound that stores glucose and when it undergoes hydrolysis forms glucose.* | glycogène |
| **glycogenesis** *The production of glycogen from glucose.* | glycogenèse |
| **glycolysis** *The production of energy and pyruvic acid when glucose is broken down by enzymes.* | glycolyse |
| **glycoprotein** *A protein that has a carbohydrate attached to its polypeptide chain.* | glycoprotéine |
| **glycosuria** *Presence of glucose in the urine.* | glycosurie |
| **gnathic** *Referring to the jaws.* | 1. gnathique 2. mandibulaire |
| **goblet cells** *They aid in the secretion of respiratory and intestinal mucous.* | cellules caliciformes |
| **goggles** | lunettes de protection |
| **goiter** *Swelling of the thyroid gland.* | goitre |
| **gold** | or |
| **gonad** *A testis or an ovary.* | gonade |
| **gonadal dysgenesis** *The lack of complete development of the gonads.* | dysgénésie gonadique |
| **gonadotrophin** *Pituitary hormone that promotes gonadal activity.* | gonadotrophine |

| English | French |
| --- | --- |
| **gonococcus** *A diploccocal bacteria that is the causative agent in gonorrhea, formally Neisseria gonorrhoeae.* | gonocoque |
| **gonorrhea** *A sexually transmitted disease that is exhibited by purulent discharge from the vagina or penis.* | blénorragie |
| **goose bumps** | chair de poule |
| **gouge** *A chisel with a concave blade used in surgery.* | gouge |
| **gown** | 1. blouse 2. robe |
| **grade** | 1. degré 2. rang |
| **grading** | classement |
| **gram** | gramme |
| **granular layer** *A deep layer of the cerebellum.* | stratum granulosum |
| **granulation tissue** *The presence of fleshy, rounded areas of tissue in wounds.* | bourgeon charnu |
| **granulocyte** *A white blood cell with cytoplasmic secretory granules.* | granulocyte |
| **granuloma** *A mass of granulation tissue.* | granulome |
| **grasp reflex** *Flexion of the fingers or toes when stimulated.* | réflexe de préhension |
| **grasping** | agrippement |
| **Graves' disease** *A form of hyperthyroidism exhibited by a goiter and exophthalmos.* | Basedow-Graves, maladie de |
| **gravid** *Pregnant.* | 1. gravide 2. enceinte |
| **gray matter** *The section of the brain and spinal cord composed of branching dendrites and nerve cell bodies.* | substance grise |
| **greater than normal** | plus grand que la normale |
| **greenstick fracture** *Spiral fracture.* | fracture en bois vert |
| **grief** | chagrin |
| **grip strength** *Quantitative measurement of the force of a hand grip.* | force de préhension |
| **groan** | gémir |
| **groin** *The genital region.* | aine |
| **grommet** *A tube surgically placed in the tympanic membrane to drain the middle ear.* | yoyo |
| **gross** | brut |
| **ground** | broyé |
| **growth** | croissance |
| **growth factor** | facteur de croissance |
| **grunting** *A low guttural sound used to describe a person with profound respiratory difficulty.* | grognement |
| **guaiac** *A substance derived from guaiacum trees used to test for trace amounts of blood, in stool for instance.* | gaïac |
| **guarding** *A symptom used to describe a patient resisting an examination because of severe pain; often seen in patients with peritonitis.* | défense musculaire |
| **guinea worm** *A parasitic nematode worm that lives under the skin, formally called Dracunculus medinensis.* | 1. filaire de Médine 2. ver de Guinée |
| **gum** | gencive |

| English | French |
|---------|--------|
| **gumboil** *Swelling noted on the gingiva over a dental abscess.* | 1. abcès alvéolaire 2. abcès gingival |
| **gumma** *A soft granulomatous tumor of the skin or cardiovascular system seen in tertiary syphilis.* | gomme |
| **gurgling** | gargouillement |
| **gustatory** *Referring to sense of taste.* | gustatif |
| **gynecology** *The branch of medicine associated with the reproductive system of women.* | gynécologie |
| **gynecomastia** *Enlargement of the breasts.* | gynécomastie |
| **gyrus** *Convolutions of the brain where there is infolding.* | gyrus |
| **habit** | habitude |
| **hair** | 1. cheveu 2. poil |
| **hair cell** *Epithelial cells with hairlike projections.* | cellule ciliée |
| **hair follicle** | follicule pileux |
| **hairy** | pileux |
| **half** | 1. demi 2. moitié |
| **half-life** *The time required to reduce a chemical's activity in half.* | demi-vie |
| **halitosis** *Foul odor eminating from the mouth.* | halitose |
| **hallucination** *A perception that is not based on reality.* | hallucination |
| **hallucinogen** *A substance that elicits hallucinations.* | hallucinogène |
| **hallux** *Referring to the first toe.* | hallux 2. orteil |
| **hamartoma** *A nodule of superfluous tissue.* | hamartome |
| **hamate bone; uncinate bone** *The medial bone in the distal row of carpal bones adjacent to the fifth metacarpal.* | crochu du carpe |
| **hammer toe** *A condition characterized by extension of the proximal phalanx and flexion of the second and distal phalanges.* | orteil en marteau |
| **hamstrings** *Tendons of the posterior thigh.* | ischio-jambiers |
| **hand** | main |
| **hangnail** | envie de l'ongle |
| **haploid** *Either a single set of chromosomes or a set of nonhomologous chromosomes.* | haploïde |
| **hapten** *The molecular component that determines immunologic specificity.* | 1. haptène 2. partigène |
| **hard** | dur |
| **hard of hearing** | malentendant |
| **harmless** | anodin |
| **hay fever** *An allergy exhibited by pruritis of the eyes and nose, rhinorrhea and excessive lacrimal secretion.* | 1. coryza spasmodique 2. rhume des foins |
| **hazy** | flou |
| **head** | tête |
| **head trauma** *Any injury to the brain.* | traumatisme crânien |
| **headache** | 1. céphalée 2. mal de tête |

| English | French |
|---|---|
| healing | cicatrisation |
| health | santé |
| healthy | bien portant |
| hearing | 1. audition 2. ouïe |
| hearing aid | prothèse acoustique |
| heart | cœur |
| heart beat | battement cardiaque |
| heart block *An alteration in the cardiac electrical conduction system.* | bloc cardiaque |
| heart burn *Synonym of pyrosis.* | brûlures gastriques |
| heart lung machine *Device used during cardiac surgery to replace the function of the heart and lungs while surgery is performed.* | cœur-poumon artificiel |
| heart murmur | souffle cardiaque |
| heart rate | fréquence cardiaque |
| heat | chaleur |
| heat exhaustion *A condition that occurs secondary to prolonged exposure to high ambient temperature; it is exhibited by subnormal temperature, dizziness and nausea.* | épuisement par la chaleur |
| heat stroke *A condition caused by excessive exposure to high ambient temperature; it is exhibited by dry skin, thirst, vertigo, muscle cramps and nausea. The three forms are heat exhaustion, heat cramps and sunstroke.* | coup de chaleur |
| heavy | lourd |
| hebephrenia *A type of schizophrenia exhibited by hallucinations and inappropriate laughter.* | hébéphrénie |
| Heberden's node *Hard nodules formed at the distal interphalangeal joints in osteoarthritis.* | nodosité d'Heberden |
| hedonism *Devoting oneself to being happy.* | hédonisme |
| heel | talon |
| height | 1. hauteur 2. taille |
| heliotherapy *Treatment of disease with sunlight.* | héliothérapie |
| helium *An inert gas that is the lightest of the noble gases.* | hélium |
| helminth *A fluke, tapeworm or nematode.* | helminthe |
| helminthiasis *Being infected by a helminth.* | helminthiase |
| hemagglutinin *An antibody that facilitates the agglutination of blood.* | hémagglutinine |
| hemangioma *A benign tumor composed of blood vessels.* | hémangiome |
| hemarthrosis *Presence of intra-articular blood.* | hémarthrose |
| hematemesis *Vomiting blood.* | hématémèse |
| hematin *The insoluble iron protoporphyrin component of hemoglobin.* | hématine |
| hematinic *A substance that increases hemoglobin in the blood.* | hématinique |
| hematocele *A mass or area of swelling caused by the accumulation of blood.* | hématocèle |
| hematocrit *The measurement of the volume of red blood cells compared to the total volume of blood; recorded in percent.* | hématocrite |
| hematoma *A mass containing blood.* | hématome |

| English | French |
|---|---|
| **hematometra** *The accretion of blood in the uterus.* | hématomètre |
| **hematomyelia** *Accumulation of blood in the spinal cord.* | hématomyélie |
| **hematoporphyrin** *A derivative of heme that does not contain iron.* | hématoporphyrine |
| **hematosalpinx** *Presence of blood in the fallopian tube.* | hématosalpinx |
| **hematozoa** *Any organism living on blood.* | hématozoaire |
| **hematuria** *The presence of blood in the urine.* | hématurie |
| **heme** *A constituent of hemoglobin that is an insoluble iron protoporphyrin.* | hème |
| **hemeralopia** *Night blindness.* | héméralopie |
| **hemianopsia** *Blindness over half the field of vision.* | hémianopsie |
| **hemiballismus** *Severe motor restlessness unilaterally, usually from a subthalamic lesion.* | hémiballisme |
| **hemicolectomy** *Surgical removal of part of the colon.* | hémicolectomie |
| **hemicrania** *1. Pain on one side of the head. 2. Incomplete anencephaly.* | hémicrânie |
| **hemiparesis** *Unilateral muscle weakness (half the body).* | hémiparésie |
| **hemiplegia** *Paralysis of one side of the body.* | hémiplégie |
| **hemisphere** *Referring to either the right or left portion of the cerebrum.* | hémisphère |
| **hemizygote** *A cell with only one set of genes.* | hémizygote |
| **hemochromatosis** *A hereditary condition exhibited by iron deposition in the tissue and leading to liver disease, bronze discoloration of the skin and diabetes.* | hémochromatose |
| **hemoconcentration** *Decrease in the total fluid content of the blood, leading at times to a falsely elevated hematocrit.* | hémoconcentration |
| **hemocytometer** *A device used for counting cells from a blood sample.* | hémocytomètre |
| **hemodialysis** *The process of filtering blood outside the body to remove toxins normally excreted by functioning kidneys.* | hémodialyse |
| **hemoglobin** *An iron containing protein used for the transport of oxygen in blood.* | hémoglobine |
| **hemoglobinuria** *Presence of free hemoglobin in the urine.* | hémoglobinurie |
| **hemolysis** *Breakdown of hemoglobin.* | hémolyse |
| **hemolytic** *Something that causes hemolysis.* | hémolytique |
| **hemolytic anemia** *Reduced number of erythrocytes due to shortened survival and inability of the bone marrow to compensate.* | anémie hémolytique |
| **hemopericardium** *Abnormal presence of blood in the pericardium.* | hémopéricarde |
| **hemoperitoneum** *Abnormal presence of blood in the peritoneum.* | hémopéritoine |
| **hemophilia** *A hereditary bleeding disorder characterized by hemarthroses and deep tissue bleeding as a result of absence of a coagulation factor such as factor VIII.* | hémophilie |
| **hemophiliac** *A person with hemophilia.* | hémophile |
| **hemophilic arthropathy** | arthropathie des hémophiles |
| **hemophthalmia** *Bleeding within the eye.* | hémophtalmie |
| **hemopoiesis** *The production of blood cells from stem cells.* | hémopoïèse |

| English | French |
|---|---|
| **hemopoietin** *A hormone secreted by the kidneys that stimulates the bone marrow to produce erythrocytes.* | hémopoïétine |
| **hemoptysis** *Expectoration of blood.* | hémoptysie |
| **hemorrhage** *Bleeding from a damaged blood vessel.* | hémorragie |
| **hemorrhoidectomy** *Surgical excision of a hemorrhoid.* | hémorroïdectomie |
| **hemorrhoids** *Engorgement of the veins in the anus or rectum.* | hémorroïdes |
| **hemostasis** *The control of bleeding.* | hémostase |
| **hemothrorax** *The abnormal presence of blood in the pleural cavity.* | hémothorax |
| **hence** | d'où |
| **Henoch purpura** *Exhibited by vomiting, diarrhea, abdominal pain and hematuria; a non-thrombocytopenic purpura.* | purpura rhumatoïde |
| **Henri, syndrome of** *Congenital anomaly exhibited by different sized external orifices of the nostrils.* | Henri, syndrome d' |
| **heparin** *A polysaccharide that occurs naturally in the liver and is used as a medication to induce a hypocoagulable state.* | héparine |
| **hepatectomy** *Partial or complete surgical resection of the liver.* | hépatectomie |
| **hepatic ducts** *The right and left hepatic ducts join the cystic duct to form the common bile duct.* | voies biliaires |
| **hepatic flexure of the colon** | angle droit du côlon |
| **hepatic** *Referring to the liver.* | hépatique |
| **hepatitis** *Inflammation of the liver.* | hépatite |
| **hepatocyte** *A liver cell.* | hépatocyte |
| **hepatoma** *A tumor of the liver.* | hépatome |
| **hepatomegaly** *Enlargement of the liver.* | hépatomegaly |
| **hepatosplenomegaly** *Enlargement of the spleen and the liver.* | hépatosplénomégalie |
| **hereditary spherocytosis** *A familial hemolytic disease exhibited by abnormally thick erythrocytes.* | 1. microsphérocytose héréditaire 2. Minkkowski=Chauffard, maladie de |
| **hereditary** *That which is transmitted genetically* | héréditaire |
| **hermaphrodite** *A person possessing gonadal characteristics of both sexes.* | hermaphrodite |
| **herniated disc** *Prolapse of the nucleus pulposus into the spinal cord.* | hernia discale |
| **herniorrhaphy** *The surgical repair of a hernia.* | herniorraphie |
| **heroin** *A morphine derivative that is highly addictive.* | héroïne |
| **herpangina** *An infectious disease caused by Coxsackie virus exhibited by vesicular lesion on the soft palate.* | 1. angine herpétiforme 2. herpangine |
| **herpes** *A skin condition exhibited by formation of clustered vesicular lesions; herpes simplex is at times referred to, albeit incompletely, as herpes.* | herpès |
| **herpes zoster; shingles** *A unilateral vesicular rash along one dermatome and caused by inflammation of a posterior nerve root by "the chicken pox virus".* | zona |
| **herpetic** *Referring to herpes.* | herpétique |

| English | French |
|---|---|
| **herpetiform** *Something that is characteristic of herpes.* | herpétiforme |
| **heterochromia iridis or syndrome of Eric** *Congenital anomaly in which the iris of each eye is of a different color.* | hétérochromie (iris), Syndrome d'Eric |
| **heterogenous** *That which originates outside the organism.* | hétérogène |
| **heterotropia** *Synonym of strabismus.* | hétérotropie |
| **heterozygous** *Having different alleles concerning a certain trait.* | hétérozygote |
| **hiatus hernia** *Protrusion of part of the stomach through the esophageal hiatus of the diaphragm.* | hernia hiatale |
| **hiccup** | hoquet |
| **hidradenitis** *Inflammation of a sweat gland. When there is purulent discharge it is called hidradenitis suppurativa.* | hidradénite |
| **hidrosis** *The production and secretion of sweat.* | hidrose |
| **high** | élevé |
| **hilar** *Referring to a hilus.* | hilaire |
| **hilum or hilus** *A depression where blood vessels and nerve fibers enter an organ.* | hile |
| **hindbrain** *The brainstem which includes the pons, medulla oblongata and cerebellum.* | cerveau postérieur |
| **hip** | hanche |
| **hip girdle** *The bony supporting structure for the legs.* | ceinture pelvienne |
| **hip girth** *The measurement around a person's waist.* | tour de hanches |
| **hip joint** | articulation cox-fémorale |
| **hippocampus** *The area at the base of the cerebral ventricles thought to be the center of memory and emotion.* | hippocampe |
| **Hippocratic oath** *An vow taken by doctors, indicating they will treat people properly.* | serment d'Hippocrate |
| **hirsutism** *Abnormal growth on hair on a person's face and body.* | hirsutisme |
| **hissing** | chuintement |
| **histamine** *A chemical responsible for the reaction exhibited when a person has an allergic reaction.* | histamine |
| **histidine** *An amino acid precursor to histamine.* | histidine |
| **histiocyte** *A phagocytic cell found in connective tissue.* | histiocyte |
| **histochemistry** | histochimie |
| **histology** *The study of the structure and composition of minute structures.* | histologie |
| **histoplasmosis** *A fungal pulmonary infection from bat and bird excrement.* | histoplasmose |
| **history taking** | interrogatoire |
| **hit** | frapper |
| **HIV** *Abbreviation for human immunodeficiency virus.* | VIH |
| **hoarse** *A rough, harsh sounding voice.* | 1. enroué 2. rauque |
| **hold one's breath** | retenir son souffle |
| **hollow** | creux |

| English | French |
|---|---|
| homeless | sans-abri |
| homeopathy *A treatment of disease by use of minute doses of toxic substances that would normally be harmful.* | homéopathie |
| homeostasis *The tendency of an organism to maintain a stable and uniform state.* | homéostasie |
| homicide *When one person kills another.* | homicide |
| homograft *A graft of tissue from the same species as the recipient.* | homogreffe |
| homolateral *Ipsilateral.* | dimidié |
| homologous *Referring to something derived from the same species but different genotype.* | homologue |
| homosexuality *Being sexually attracted to someone of the same gender.* | homosexualité |
| homozygous *Having identical alleles for a particular trait.* | homozygote |
| hookworm *A parasitic infection of the family Strongylidae that can cause anemia.* | ankylostome |
| hordeolum *Inflammation of the sebaceous gland of the eye.* | orgelet |
| hormone *A substance produced in the body that effects a specific organ.* | hormone |
| horn *A keratinized outgrowth.* | corne |
| horseshoe kidney *Anomalous renal development.* | rein en fer à cheval |
| hospital | hôpital |
| hot | chaud |
| hot flash *A symptom of menopause manifested as a sudden sensation of fever.* | bouffée de chaleur |
| human | humain |
| humerus *The long bone in the upper arm.* | humérus |
| hunchback *Synonym of kyphosis.* | gibbosité |
| hunger | faim |
| hyaline *Having a glassy, transparent appearance.* | hyalin |
| hyaloid *Transparent.* | hyaloïde |
| hybrid *An animal or plant produced from two different species.* | hybride |
| hydarthrosis *An accumulation of water-like fluid in a joint cavity.* | hydarthrose |
| hydatid cyst *A cyst produced by and containing tapeworm larvae.* | kyste hydatique |
| hydatiform *Referring to a hydatid cyst.* | hydatiforme |
| hydration *Used to describe fluid balance.* | hydratation |
| hydrocele *The accumulation of fluid in a body sac.* | hydrocèle |
| hydrocephalus *The excessive accumulation of cerebral spinal fluid in the brain causing enlargement of the head.* | hydrocéphalie |
| hydrochloric acid *A solution with a low pH formed by dissolving hydrogen chloride in water.* | chlorhydrique acide |
| hydrochloride | chlorhydrate |
| hydrocortisone *A natural steroid hormone secreted by the adrenal cortex and used in a synthetic formulation for treatment of various medical conditions.* | hydrocortisone |
| hydrolysis *A reaction with water causing a compound to breakdown.* | hydrolyse |

| English | French |
|---|---|
| **hydronephrosis** *Enlargement of a kidney due to interruption of outflow of urine from that kidney.* | hydronéphrose |
| **hydrophobia** *Abnormal fear of water.* | hydrophobie |
| **hydropneumothorax** *Abnormal accumulation of fluid and air in the pleural space.* | hydropneumothorax |
| **hydrops** *The abnormal collection of fluid in a cavity.* | hydropisie |
| **hydrops fetalis** *The total body accumulation of fluid in a fetus; the result of a hemolytic reaction in a Rh neg mother.* | anasarque fœtoplacentaire |
| **hydrosalpinx** *Collection of fluid in a fallopian tube.* | hydrosalpinx |
| **hydrothorax** *Accumulation of fluid within the thoracic cavity.* | hydrothorax |
| **hygroma** *A cyst or bursa filled with fluid.* | hygroma |
| **hygroscopic** *The tendency to absorb moisture from the air.* | hygroscopique |
| **hymen** *A membrane in the vagina.* | hymen |
| **hymenotomy** *Surgically creating an opening in the hymen.* | hyménotomie |
| **hyperacidity** *An abnormally high acid level.* | hyperacidité |
| **hyperactivity** *Abnormal increase in activity.* | hyperactivité |
| **hyperalgesia** *Greater than normal sensitivity to pain.* | hyperalgésie |
| **hyperbaric** *Use of gas at a higher than normal pressure.* | hyperbare |
| **hyperbaric chamber** *A device used to treat decompression illness.* | caisson hyperbare |
| **hyperbilirubinemia** *Higher than normal level of bilirubin in the blood.* | hyperbilirubinémie |
| **hypercalcemia** *Higher than normal level of calcium in the blood.* | hypercalcémie |
| **hypercapnia** *Higher than normal level of carbon dioxide in the blood stream.* | hypercapnie |
| **hypercholesterolemia** *Higher than normal level of cholesterol in the blood.* | hypercholestérolémie |
| **hyperchromia** *An excessive level of hemoglobin in erythrocytes.* | hyperchromie |
| **hyperemia** *An increase in blood for the area of concern.* | hyperémie |
| **hyperesthesia** *Higher than normal skin sensitivity.* | hyperesthésie |
| **hyperextension** *Extension of an articulation beyond the normal range.* | hyperextension |
| **hyperflexion** *Flexion of an articulation beyond the normal range.* | hyperflexion |
| **hyperglycemia** *Higher than normal level of glucose in the blood.* | hyperglycémie |
| **hypergonadism** *A condition of excessive gonadal activity and subsequently precocious sexual development.* | hypergonadisme |
| **hyperhidrosis** *Excessive perspiration.* | hyperéphidrose |
| **hyperkalemia** *Higher than normal level of potassium in the blood stream.* | hyperkaliémie |
| **hyperkeratosis** *Excessive thickening of the outer layer of skin.* | hyperkératose |
| **hyperkinesis** *Excessive activity and inability to concentrate.* | hyperkinésie |
| **hyperlipidemia** *Higher than normal level of lipids in the blood stream.* | hyperlipémie |
| **hypermetropia** *Farsightedness.* | hypermétropie |
| **hypermnesia** *Unusually good memory.* | hypermnésie |
| **hypermyotonia** *Excessive muscle tone.* | hypermyotonie |
| **hypernephroma** *A renal tumor that mimic adrenal cortical tissue.* | hypernéphrome |

| English | French |
|---|---|
| **hyperonychia** *Hypertrophic nails.* | hyperonychose |
| **hyperparathyroidism** *Excessive level of parathyroid hormones in the blood stream causing weak bones and hypocalcemia.* | hyperparathyroïdie |
| **hyperphagia** *Excessive food ingestion.* | hyperphagie |
| **hyperphoria** *Upward deviation of the visual axis of the eye.* | hyperphorie |
| **hyperpituitarism** *Excessive eosinophilic hormone resulting in acromegaly or excessive basophilic hormone resulting in pituitary compression and ultimately hypopituitarism.* | hyperpituitarisme |
| **hyperplasia** *Excessive growth of normal cells.* | hyperplasie |
| **hyperpnea** *Abnormal increase in rate and depth of respiration.* | hyperpnée |
| **hyperpyrexia** *Fever.* | hyperpyrexie |
| **hypersensitivity** *Abnormal increase in sensitivity.* | hypersensibilité |
| **hypersplenism** *Excessive splenic activity resulting in decreased peripheral blood elements and sometimes splenomegaly.* | hypersplénisme |
| **hypertension** *Higher than normal blood pressure.* | hypertension |
| **hyperthermia** *Fever.* | hyperthermie |
| **hyperthyroidism** *Increased thyroid activity resulting in exophthalmos and increased metabolic rate.* | hyperthyroïdie |
| **hypertonia** *Excessive tone or tension.* | hypertonie |
| **hypertonic** *Increased osmotic pressure.* | hypertonique |
| **hypertrichosis** *Excessive hair growth.* | hypertrichose |
| **hypertrophy** *Pathologic organ enlargement.* | hypertrophie |
| **hyperventilation** *Increase in the rate and depth of ventilation causing reduced blood carbon dioxide level.* | hyperventilation |
| **hypervolemia** *Abnormally large amount of fluid in the blood stream.* | hypervolémie |
| **hypnotic** *Sleep inducing agent.* | 1. hypnotique 2. somnifère |
| **hypocalcemia** *Lower than normal level of calcium in the blood.* | hypocalcémie |
| **hypochondriac** *A person suffering from hypochondriasis.* | hypocondriaque |
| **hypochondriasis** *Abnormal increase in concern about one's own health.* | hypocondrie |
| **hypochondrium** *The upper abdomen lateral to the epigastrium.* | hypocondre |
| **hypochromic** *Referring to the abnormal decrease in hemoglobin content of erythrocytes.* | hypochrome |
| **hypodermic needle** | aiguille hypodermique |
| **hypoesthesia** *Abnormally decreased skin sensitivity.* | hypoesthésie |
| **hypofibrinogenemia** *Diminished blood fibrinogen level.* | hypofibrinogénémie |
| **hypogastric** *Referring to the hypogastrium.* | hypogastrique |
| **hypogastrium** *The area of the central abdomen located below the stomach.* | hypogastre |
| **hypoglossal nerve** *Twelfth cranial nerve pair.* | nerf hypoglosse |
| **hypoglossal triangle** *The area in the subhyoid region, bordered by the hypoglossal nerve, the mylohyoid muscle and the tendon of the digastric muscle.* | aile blanche interne |
| **hypoglycemia** *Abnormally low blood sugar.* | hypoglycémie |

| English | French |
|---|---|
| **hypogonadism** *Abnormal decrease in gonadal function with associated diminished growth and sexual development.* | hypogonadisme |
| **hypokalemia** *Diminished level of potassium in the blood stream.* | hypokaliémie |
| **hypomania** *A moderate form of mania.* | hypomanie |
| **hyponatremia** *Diminished level of sodium in the blood stream.* | hyponatrémie |
| **hypoparathyroidism** *Abnormal decrease in parathyroid function.* | hypoparathyroïdie |
| **hypophoria** *Downward deviation of the visual axis of the eye.* | hypophorie |
| **hypophosphatasia** *A genetic defect of diminished alkaline phosphatase in the cells leading to bone demineralization.* | hypophosphatasie |
| **hypophysectomy** *Surgical removal of the pituitary gland.* | hypophysectomie |
| **hypophysis** *Pituitary gland.* | hypophyse |
| **hypopituitarism** *Diminished pituitary activity exhibited by obesity and persistence of adolescent characteristics.* | hypotituiarisme |
| **hypoplasia** *Incomplete development.* | hypoplasie |
| **hypopyon** *The presence of purulent fluid in the anterior chamber of the eye.* | hypopion |
| **hyposecretion** *Secretion below the normal rate.* | hyposécrétion |
| **hypospadias** *Congenital condition exhibited by development of the urethral meatus on the inferior aspect of the penis.* | hypospadias |
| **hypostasis** *The formation of a deposit.* | hypostase |
| **hypotension** *Abnormally low blood pressure.* | hypotension |
| **hypothalamus** *Located inferior to the thalamus it controls visceral activities, water balance, temperature and sleep.* | hypothalamus |
| **hypothenar eminence** *The prominence on the palm at the base of the fingers adjacent to the ulna.* | éminence hypothénar |
| **hypothermia** *Lower than normal temperature.* | hypothermie |
| **hypothyroidism** *Reduced functioning of the thyroid.* | hypothyroïdie |
| **hypotonia** *Reduced tone or activity.* | hypotonie |
| **hypoxia** *Diminished oxygen content.* | hypoxie |
| **hysterectomy** *Surgical removal of the uterus.* | hystérectomie |
| **hysteria** *A psychological condition exhibited by uncontrolled emotion or exaggerated manifestations.* | hystérie |
| **hysterography** *1. Recording of uterine contractions. 2. Roentgenography of the uterus after administration of contrast media.* | hystérographie |
| **hysteromyomectomy** *Surgical removal of a uterine myoma.* | hystéromyomectomie |
| **hysteropexy** *Surgical fixation of the uterus by shortening of the round ligaments or by other means.* | hystéropexie |
| **hysterosalpingography** *Roentgenography of the uterus and fallopian tubes after instillation of contrast media.* | hystérosalpinographie |
| **hysterotomy** *Surgical opening of the uterus.* | hystérotomie |
| **i.e.** *A latin derived abbreviation for "that is to say"(In latin: id est)* | c.à.d. (c'est-à-dire) |
| **iatrogenic** *A problem caused by medical treatment.* | iatrogène |
| **ichthyosis** *A congenital anomaly exhibited by excessively dry, thick skin.* | ichtyose |
| **icterus** *Yellowing of the skin and sclerae because of excess bilirubin.* | ictère |

| English | French |
|---------|--------|
| **identical twins** *Twins from the same zygote.* | jumeaux homozygotes |
| **idiopathic** *Relating to a disease with an unknown cause.* | idiopathique |
| **ileitis** *Inflammation of the ileum.* | iléite |
| **ileocecal valve** *The membranous folds between the ileum and cecum.* | valvule iléo-cæcale |
| **ileocolitis** *Inflammation of the ileum and cecum.* | iléocolite |
| **ileocolostomy** *Creating a surgical opening between the ileum and colon.* | iléocolostomie |
| **ileoproctostomy** *Creating a surgical opening between the ileum and the rectum.* | iléorectostomie |
| **ileorectal** *Referring to the ileum and rectal.* | iléorectal |
| **ileostomy** *Surgical creation of an opening in the ileum that is placed at the skin surface.* | iléostomie |
| **ileum** *The portion of the small bowel from the jejunum to the cecum.* | iléon |
| **ileus** *A temporary obstruction in the intestine.* | iléus |
| **iliac crest** *The upper border of the ilium.* | crête iliaque |
| **iliococcygeal** *Referring to the ilium and coccyx.* | ilio-coccygien |
| **ilium** *The large bone at the superior aspect of the pelvis which is present bilaterally.* | ilion |
| **immediate-acting** *In reference to a drug, one that has no delay in its action.* | action immédiate |
| **immune** *Being resistant to an infection.* | immun |
| **immune response** *The body's reaction to what is perceived as a foreign substance.* | réponse immunologique |
| **immunization** *A medication given to provide immunity.* | immunisation |
| **immunochemistry** *The study of immune response and biochemistry.* | immunochimie |
| **immunodeficiency** *An inadequate immune response.* | 1. déficit immunitaire 2. immunodéficience |
| **immunoelectrophoresis** *A means of differentiating proteins and other compounds by comparing their mobility and antigenic specificities.* | immuno-électrophorèse |
| **immunoglobulin** *Serum and cellular proteins of the immune system.* | immunoglobuline |
| **immunosuppression** *The inhibition of the immune response.* | immunosuppression |
| **impacted tooth** *A tooth that does not erupt because adjacent teeth prevent it.* | dent incluse |
| **impaired** | altéré |
| **impairment** | altération |
| **imperforate** *Lack of an opening. An infant with an imperforate anus has a congenital defect with no anal opening.* | imperforé |
| **impervious** *Not affected by.* | étanche |
| **impingement syndrome** *Tendinitis of the rotator cuff causing decreased range of motion a the shoulder.* | tendinite de la coiffe des rotateurs |
| **implant** | implant |
| **implementation** | mise en œuvre |
| **impotence** *Absence of power. A term used to describe erectile dysfunction.* | impuissance |
| **in conformity with** | en conformité avec |

| English | French |
|---|---|
| **inanition** *Generalized weakness from lack of nutrition.* | inanition |
| **inarticulate** *Indistinct speech.* | inarticulé |
| **incest** *Sexual relations between related people.* | inceste |
| **incipient** *Starting to happen.* | incipiens |
| **incision** | incision |
| **incisor** *Sharp-edged tooth; humans have four incisors.* | incisive |
| **incisura** *A notch or indentation usually on the edge of a bone.* | échancrure |
| **incisure** *A notch or incision.* | incisure |
| **inclusion body** *Variably shaped bodies in the nuclei of cells found in infections such as rabies and herpes.* | inclusion cellulaire |
| **incoherent** *Absence of intelligible speech.* | incohérent |
| **incontinence** *Inability to control urination.* | incontinence |
| **incoordination** *Absence of smooth, efficient body movement.* | incoordination |
| **increment** | accroissement |
| **incubator** *A warming device for infants.* | 1. couveuse 2. étuve 3. incubateur |
| **incus** *The middle ear bone between the stapes and malleus.* | enclume |
| **indeed** | en effet |
| **indigenous** *Naturally occurring.* | autochtone |
| **indigestion** *Inadequate digestion for various reasons.* | indigestion |
| **indolent** *1. Causing little pain. 2. Slow healing ulcer.* | 1. indolent 2. torpide |
| **induced** *Facilitated. When referring to labor, it means medication was given to assist in delivery of the fetus.* | induit |
| **induced abortion** *Surgical or medical evacuation of the fetus.* | avortement provoqué |
| **induration** *An area that is abnormally hard.* | induration |
| **indwelling catheter** *Continuous use tube usually referring to a tube in the urinary bladder.* | sonde à demeure |
| **indwelling foley** *A catheter inserted into the urinary bladder with an inflatable ballon on the tip.* | sonde vésicale le à demeure |
| **inebriation** *Intoxication with drugs or alcohol.* | ivresse |
| **ineffective** | inefficace |
| **inertia** *The tendency to remain unchanged.* | inertie |
| **inevitable** *Not preventable.* | inévitable |
| **infancy** | petite enfance |
| **infant** | nourrisson (jusqu' à 12 mois) |
| **infantile** *Referring to babies or young children.* | infantile |
| **infarcted** *Referring to dead tissue.* | infarci |
| **infarction** *Dead tissue, for example, myocardial infarction.* | infarcissement |
| **infectious** | infectieux |
| **inferior** | inférieur |
| **inferior pelvis strait** *The pelvic outlet.* | détroit inférieur du bassin |

| English | French |
|---|---|
| **infestation** *The presence of large numbers, as in lice infestation.* | infestation |
| **inflammation** *Localized redness, excessive warmth and swelling.* | inflammation |
| **influenza** *Viral infection causing fever, muscle aches and catarrh.* | grippe |
| **infraspinous** *Below the scapular spine.* | 1. infra-épineux 2. sous-épineux |
| **infundibulum** *The connection between the hypothalamus and the posterior pituitary gland.* | infundibulum |
| **infusion** *The injection of fluid into tissue or a vein.* | infusion |
| **ingestion** *The intake of food or liquid orally.* | ingestion |
| **inguinal** *Referring to the groin.* | inguinal |
| **inhalation** *The act of breathing in.* | inhalation |
| **injection** *The act of a needle being inserted into a body.* | 1. injection 2. piqûre |
| **injure, to** | blesser |
| **injured person** | blessé |
| **injury** | blessure |
| **inner ear** | oreille interne |
| **innervation** *The presence of a nerve supply.* | innervation |
| **innominate artery** *The first branch off the aortic arch that branches into the right common carotid and right subclavian arteries.* | tronc artériel brachiocéphalique |
| **innominate** *Referring to the innominate artery.* | innominé |
| **inoculation** *Injection with a vaccine to provide immunity.* | inoculation |
| **inorganic** *Not coming from natural growth.* | anorganique |
| **insane** *A term not used in formal medical evaluations that when used by a layperson means a serious mental illness.* | 1. aliéné 2. fou |
| **insanity** *Referring to a serious mental illness.* | aliénation mentale |
| **insensible** *Unable to perceive a stimulus.* | insensible |
| **insertion** | insertion |
| **inside** | intérieur |
| **insidious** *A slow, gradual and harmful advancement.* | insidieux |
| **insomnia** *Sleeplessness.* | insomnie |
| **inspiration** *Drawing in a breath.* | inspiration |
| **inspiratory reserve volume** *The amount of air that can be inhaled after a normal inhalation.* | 1. air complémentaire 2. volume de réserve inspiratoire |
| **inspissated** *Thickened or congealed.* | épaissi |
| **instep** *The medial aspect of the foot between the ankle and the ball of the foot.* | cou-de-pied |
| **insulin** *A hormone produced by the pancreas and synthetically to control blood glucose levels.* | insuline |
| **insulinoma** *An islet cell tumor that causes abnormally high insulin secretion and thus hypoglycemia.* | insulinome |
| **intake** | ration |
| **integument** *Outer protective layer.* | tégument |

| English | French |
|---|---|
| **intelligence quotient (IQ)** *A number representing a person's ability to problem solve compared to a matched-control.* | quotient intellectuel |
| **intensive** | intensif |
| **intensive care** | soins intensif |
| **intensive care unit** | unité de soins intensifs |
| **intention tremor** *The tremulous movement noted when a person is beginning to perform a task but not seen at rest.* | tremblement intentionnel |
| **interarticular** *Between the articular surfaces of a joint.* | interarticulaire |
| **intercellular** *Between cells.* | intercellulaire |
| **intermittent** | intermittent |
| **internal** | interne |
| **interosseous** *Referring to something between bones, like the interosseous muscles of the hand.* | interosseux |
| **interstitial** *Referring to the interstices of tissue.* | interstitiel |
| **intertrigo** *Irritation present because adjacent surfaces rub together.* | intertrigo |
| **intertrochanteric** *Referring to the space within the trochanter.* | intertrochantérien |
| **interval** | écart |
| **interventricular** *Between the ventricles.* | interventriculaire |
| **intestinal obstruction** *Blockage of the intestine by mass or volvulus.* | occlusion intestinale |
| **intestinal** *Referring to the intestines.* | intestinal |
| **intestine** *A general term used for the section of bowel from the stomach to the anus.* | intestin |
| **intraabdominal** *Within the abdominal cavity.* | intra-abdominal |
| **intraarticular** *Within a joint space.* | intra-articulaire |
| **intracellular** *Within a cell.* | intracellulaire |
| **intracerebral** *Within the cerebrum.* | intracérébral |
| **intracranial** *Within the cranial vault.* | intracrânien |
| **intradermal** *Within the dermis.* | intradermique |
| **intradural** *Within the dural space.* | intradural |
| **intramedullary** *1. Within the medulla oblongata. 2. Within the bone marrow.* | intramédullaire |
| **intramuscular** *Within a muscle.* | intramusculaire |
| **intraocular fluid** | liquide intra-oculaire |
| **intraosseous** *Within a bone.* | intra-osseux |
| **intraperitoneal** *Within the peritoneal cavity.* | intrapéritonéal |
| **intrathecal** *Technically means within a sheath but this term is used when medication is instilled in the dura mater spinalis.* | intrathécal |
| **intrauterine contraceptive device** *A device used to physically prevent the implantation of a fertilized ovum.* | 1. dispositif intra-utérin 2. stérilet |
| **intrauterine** *Within the uterus.* | intra-utérin |
| **intravenous infusion** *Administration of fluid into a vein.* | perfusion intraveineuse |
| **intravenous tubing** | trousse de perfusion |
| **intravenous** *Within a vein.* | intraveineux |

| English | French |
|---|---|
| **intubation** *Placement of a tube; commonly used to refer to endotracheal intubation.* | 1. intubation 2. tubage |
| **intussusception** *The inversion of one portion of the bowel into another.* | invagination |
| **inulin** *A polysaccharide used in the testing of renal function.* | inuline |
| **inunction** *The application of lotion with friction.* | onction |
| **involucrum** *A wrap or covering (referring to a sequestrum).* | involucre |
| **involutional** *The shrinkage of an organ when it is not in use, as in the uterus after childbirth.* | d'involution |
| **involved** | impliqué |
| **iodine** *A chemical used as an antiseptic and a deficiency of it can lead to goiter.* | iode |
| **iodism** *A condition caused by excessive iodine intake resulting in diarrhea, weakness, and convulsions.* | iodisme |
| **ion channel** *A selectively permeable cell membrane to certain ions.* | canal ionique |
| **ionizing radiation** *High energy radiation that produces ion pairs in matter.* | rayonnement ionisant |
| **ipsilateral** *On the same side.* | 1. homolatéral 2. ipsilatéral |
| **iridectomy** *Surgical removal of part of the iris.* | iridectomie |
| **iridocyclitis** *Inflammation of the ciliary body and the iris.* | iridocyclite |
| **iridoplegia** *Paralysis of part of the iris with subsequent lack of contraction or dilation of the pupil.* | iridoplégie |
| **iridotomy** *A surgical opening of the iris.* | iridotomie |
| **iris** *The colored membrane posterior to the cornea.* | iris |
| **iron** *An element found in hemoglobin.* | fer |
| **iron-deficiency anemia** *A microcytic anemia.* | anémie ferriprive |
| **irradiation** *The process of being irradiated.* | irradiation |
| **irrelevant** *Not pertinent.* | sans objet |
| **irritable bowel syndrome** *A condition exhibited by chronic diarrhea or constipation and abdominal pain; it is sometimes associated with a labile emotional state.* | côlon irritable |
| **ischemia contracture** *A muscle's resistance to passive stretch that is related to a decrease in arterial flow from any reason.* | contracture ischémique |
| **ischemia** *Inadequate blood supply to a part of the body.* | ischémie |
| **ischemic heart disease** *Inadequate blood supply to the heart.* | cardiopathie ischémique |
| **ischium** *The inferoposterior portion of the pelvis.* | ischion |
| **islet** *Tissue that is structurally separate from adjacent tissues.* | ilot |
| **isoantibody** *A situation in which an antibody of person A reacts with an antigen of person B.* | isoanticorps |
| **isolation** *A ward where patients with infectious disease are housed.* | isolement |
| **isthmus** *A narrow piece of tissue connecting two larger body parts.* | isthme |
| **itch** | démangeaison |

| English | French |
|---|---|
| **jaundice** *Yellowing of the sclerae and skin because of excessive bilirubin in the blood.* | jaunisse |
| **jaw** | mâchoire |
| **jejunectomy** *Surgical removal of the jejunum.* | jéjunectomie |
| **jejunostomy** *Surgical creation of an opening in the jejunum.* | jéjunostomie |
| **joint space narrowing** *Decrease in the space between the two bones in an articulation.* | pincement articulaire |
| **jugular notch** *The notch on the upper border of the sternum.* | échancrure jugulaire |
| **jugular** *Referring to the neck, as in jugular vein.* | jugulaire |
| **juxta-articular** *Positioned near a joint.* | juxta-articulaire |
| **juxtaglomerular apparatus** *Cells located in the tunica media of the afferent glomerular arterioles.* | appareil juxtaglomérulaire |
| **kala-azar** *A disease caused by Leishmania donovani that is exhibited by weight loss, fever, anemia and hepatosplenomegaly.* | kala-azar |
| **karyokinesis** *A part of mitosis involving the cell nucleus division.* | caryocinèse |
| **karyotype** *The arrangement of chromosomes in a single cell.* | caryotype |
| **keloid** *Hypertrophic scar tissue that forms after a minor cut or surgical procedure.* | chéloïde |
| **keratectasia** *Obtrusion of the cornea.* | kératectasie |
| **keratectomy** *Excision of a portion of the cornea.* | kératectomie |
| **keratic** *Referring to the cornea.* | corné |
| **keratin** *A protein found in the skin, hair, nails and enamel of the teeth.* | kératine |
| **keratoma** *A protuberance of horny tissue.* | kératome |
| **keratomalacia** *Softening of the cornea.* | kératomalacie |
| **keratosis** *A growth of keratin such as a wart or callosity.* | kératose |
| **kernicterus** *A condition associated with high bilirubin levels that causes yellow staining of cerebral tissues and subsequent neurologic dysfunction.* | ictère nucléaire |
| **ketone** *A ketone containing a carbonyl group.* | cétone |
| **ketonemia** *Presence of ketone in the blood.* | cétonémie |
| **ketonuria** *Presence of ketone in the urine.* | cétonurie |
| **ketosis** *The presence of an abnormally high level of ketones in the blood and body tissues.* | cétose |
| **kick** | coup de pied |
| **kidney** *One of two glandular organs that form urine.* | rein |
| **kinase** *An enzyme that facilitates movement of phosphate from ATP to another molecule.* | kinase |
| **kineplasty** *An amputation done in a fashion to facilitate ambulation.* | 1. amputation orthopédique 2. cinéplastie |
| **kinesis** *Movement of a part in response to a stimulus.* | cinésie |
| **knee** | genou |
| **knee elbow position** *Knees and elbows are on the table and the chest is in the air.* | position genupectorale |

| English | French |
|---|---|
| **knee jerk reflex** *Contraction of the quadriceps, yielding leg extension when the quadriceps tendon is tapped.* | réflexe rotulien |
| **kneeling** | agenouillé |
| **knock knees** *Common term for genu valgum.* | genoux cagneux |
| **knot** | nœud |
| **known** | connu |
| **koilonychia** *Thin and concave fingernails.* | koïlonychie |
| **Koplik's spots** *Red buccal macules with a blue center; seen in measles.* | Koplik, taches de |
| **Köhler's disease** *Malformation of the navicular bone.* | 1. Köhler, maladie de 2. scaphoïdite tarsienne |
| **kraurosis vulvae** *Dryness and shrinkage of the vulva.* | atrophie sclérosante de la vulve |
| **Krebs cycle** *The process of aerobic respiration by which living cells generate energy.* | Krebs, cycle de |
| **Kussmaul respiration** *The slow, deep breathing noted in patients with acidosis.* | respiration de Kussmaul |
| **kwashiorkor** *A form of malnutrition from inadequate protein intake.* | kwashiorkor |
| **kyphoscoliosis** *An abnormal outward and lateral curvature of the spine.* | cyphoscoliose |
| **kyphosis** *Abnormal outward curvature of the spine.* | cyphose |
| **lab result** | résultat de laboratoire |
| **labial** *Referring to the lip.* | labial |
| **labile** *Easily altered; emotionally unstable.* | labile |
| **labium** *The lip.* | lèvre |
| **laboratory** | laboratoire |
| **labrum** *An edge or lip. The labrum acetabular is the fibrocartilagous rim attached to the acetabulum.* | 1. bourrelet 2. labrum |
| **labyrinth** *Inner ear structure concerned with balance.* | labyrinthe |
| **labyrinthitis** *Inflammation of the labyrinth.* | labyrinthite |
| **laceration** *An injury that produced a cut in the skin or tissue such as a tear during childbirth.* | déchirure |
| **lacrimal** *Referring to the secretion of tears.* | lacrymal |
| **lacrimation** *The secretion of tears.* | larmoiement |
| **lactalbumin** *Proteins found in milk.* | lactalbumine |
| **lactase** *An enzyme that facilitates the breakdown of lactose to glucose and galactose.* | lactase |
| **lactation** *The secretion of milk from mammary glands.* | lactation |
| **lactic** *Referring to milk.* | lactique |
| **lactiferous duct** *A canal that carries milk.* | 1. canal galactophore 2. conduit lactifère |
| **lactose** *A disaccharide present in milk.* | lactose |
| **lambdoid** *The suture connecting the parietal bones with the occipital bone.* | lambdoïde |
| **lamella** *A thin layer of bone.* | lamelle |

81

| English | French |
|---|---|
| **laminectomy** *The surgical removal of part of a vertebrae.* | laminectomie |
| **lancet** *A small sharp instrument used to obtain a drop of blood for testing.* | lancette |
| **laparoscope** *A fiber-optic instrument used to visualize the peritoneal contents.* | 1. cœlioscope 2. laparoscope |
| **laparoscopy** *A procedure utilizing a laparoscope.* | cœlioscopie |
| **laparotomy** *A surgical incision of the abdomen.* | laparotomie |
| **laryngeal** *Referring to the larynx.* | laryngé |
| **laryngectomy** *Surgical removal of the larynx.* | laryngectomie |
| **laryngismus stridulus** *Sudden, severe laryngeal spasm.* | laryngite striduleuse |
| **laryngitis** *Inflammation of the larynx.* | laryngite |
| **laryngology** *The study of the larynx and related diseases.* | laryngologie |
| **laryngopharynx** *The pharyngeal space between the superior aspect of the glottis and the opening of the larynx.* | laryngopharynx |
| **laryngospasm** *Sudden, involuntary muscle contraction of the larynx.* | laryngospasme |
| **laryngostenosis** *Abnormal narrowing of the larynx.* | laryngosténose |
| **laryngotomy** *Surgical creation of an opening in the larynx.* | laryngotomie |
| **larynx** *A hollow muscular structure that contains the vocal cords.* | larynx |
| **last** | dernier |
| **late** | tardif |
| **lateral** *Referring to the side of the body.* | latéral |
| **laugh, to** | rire |
| **laxity** *A description of a joint that is loose.* | laxité |
| **layer** | feuillet |
| **lead** | plomb |
| **lead poisoning** *The ingestion of lead, exhibited in severe cases by paralysis, encephalopathy, purple gingiva, and colic.* | saturnisme |
| **leaflet** *Cusp.* | dépliant |
| **leakage** | fuite |
| **learning** | apprentissage |
| **lecithin** *A compound widely used by tissues, derived from egg yolks and it consists of phospholipids linked to choline.* | lécithine |
| **leech** *An annelid used in some tropical regions for drawing out blood; they have an anticoagulant effect locally and have been attached to digits of persons with acute peripheral ischemia.* | sangsue |
| **left** | gauche |
| **left handed** | gaucher |
| **leg** | jambe |
| **legionnaires' disease** *The name was derived after an outbreak at a convention of the American Legion; it is manifested by fever, chills, dyspnea, and cough.* | légionnaires, maladie des |
| **leishmaniasis** *A condition caused by a flagellate protozoan parasite that is exhibited by visceral or dermatologic manifestations.* | leishmaniose |
| **length** | longueur |

| English | French |
|---|---|
| **lengthening** | allongement |
| **lens** *The transparent chamber between the posterior chamber and the vitreous body.* | 1. cristallin 2. lentille |
| **lenticular** *Referring to the lens of the eye.* | 1. cristallinien 2. lenticulaire |
| **lentigo** *A benign condition exhibited by flat brown patches on the skin.* | lentigo |
| **leontiasis ossea** *Bilateral hypertrophy of the bones of the face and cranium.* | leontiasis ossea |
| **leproma** *A superficial granulatomous papule that is seen in leprosy.* | léprome |
| **leprosy** *A contagious disease caused by Mycobacterium leprae that causes insensate papules and disfiguration.* | lèpre |
| **leptomeningitis** *A general term used to describe meningitis of the pia and arachnoid of the brain.* | leptoméningite |
| **leptospirosis** *A zoonosis caused by the spirochete Leptospira interrogans transmitted by rats and contaminated water.* | leptospirose |
| **lesbian** | lesbienne |
| **less** | moins |
| **lethal** | létal |
| **lethal dose** *The amount of a drug required to cause death.* | dose mortelle |
| **lethargy** *Absence of energy.* | léthargie |
| **leucinosis; maple syrup urine disease** *A condition characterized by an enzyme defect causing an increase in leucine in the urine.* | leucinose |
| **leukemia** *A malignant disease causing an increase in the number of abnormal and immature leukocytes.* | leucémie |
| **leukine (or leucine)** *An amino acid obtained from hydrolysis of some proteins.* | leucine |
| **leukocyte** *A white blood cell.* | leucocyte |
| **leukocythemia** *Synonym of leukemia.* | leucocythémie |
| **leukocytolysis** *Destruction of white blood cells.* | leucocytolyse |
| **leukocytosis** *An increase in the number of leukocytes.* | leucocytose |
| **leukodermia** *A localized loss of skin pigment.* | leucodermia |
| **leukonychia** *A whitish discoloration of the fingernails and toenails.* | leuconychie |
| **leukopenia** *A decreased number of leukocytes in the blood.* | leucopénie |
| **leukopoiesis** *Production of white blood cells.* | leucopoïèse |
| **leukorrhea** *Thick white vaginal discharge.* | 1. leucorrhée 2. pertes blanches |
| **levator** *A muscle that raises part of the body; the levator labii superioris raised the upper lip.* | releveur |
| **levulose** *Synonym for fructose.* | lévulose |
| **libido** *Sexual desire.* | libido |
| **library** | bibliothèque |
| **lice** *Plural for louse, a small parasite that lives on the skin. Pediculus humanus capitis is a head house.* | poux |

| English | French |
|---|---|
| **lichen** *A term used to describe a variety of papular skin diseases. Lichen planus is a shiny, flat, violaceous eruption of the mucous membranes, skin and genitalia.* | lichen |
| **life expectancy** | espérance de vie |
| **life-threatening** | menaçant la vie du patient |
| **lifetime** | durée de vie |
| **lift, to** | soulever |
| **ligature** *A thread used to tie a vessel.* | ligature |
| **light** | lumière |
| **light adaptation** *The pupillary adjustment after going from a dark environment to one of bright light.* | adaptation à la lumière |
| **likelihood** | vraisemblance |
| **limbus** *The margin of a structure, for example, of the cornea and sclera.* | limbe |
| **liminal** *Referring to a threshold.* | liminaire |
| **lincture** *A medicine mixed with a sweet substance.* | électuaire |
| **linea alba** *The tendinous portion of the anterior abdomen between the two rectus muscles.* | ligne blanche |
| **lingua nigra** *A condition characterized by a dark fur-like covering on the dorsum of the tongue.* | langue noire |
| **lipase** *A pancreatic enzyme that facilitates the breakdown of fats.* | lipase |
| **lipemia** *Abnormally high fat content in the blood.* | lipémie |
| **lipid** *A compound that is a fatty acid which is insoluble in water but soluble in organic solvents.* | lipide |
| **lipid-lowering agent** *A medication used to treat hyperlipidemia.* | hypolipémiant |
| **lipoatrophy** *Fatty tissue atrophy.* | lipo-atrophie |
| **lipochondrodystrophy** *A congenital condition exhibited by short stature, kyphosis, mental deficiency and short fingers.* | lipochondrodystrophie |
| **lipocyte** *A fat cell.* | lipocyte |
| **lipodystrophy** *Abnormal fat metabolism.* | lipodystrophie |
| **lipoid** *Referring to fat.* | lipoïdique |
| **lipoidosis** *Abnormal lipid metabolism.* | lipoïdose |
| **lipoma** *A benign tumor consisting of fat cells.* | lipome |
| **lipoprotein** *A soluble protein used to transport fat or lipids.* | lipoprotéine |
| **lipotrophic substance** *A compound which causes an increase in body fat.* | lipotrope substance |
| **lisping** *A speech problem in which "s" and "z" are pronounced "th".* | zézaiement |
| **liter** | litre |
| **lithagogue** *A treatment of a calculus.* | lithagogue |
| **litholapaxy** *The crushing and then removal of a calculus.* | litholapaxie |
| **lithotomy** *Surgical removal of a calculus.* | lithotomie |
| **lithotritor** *An instrument used to crush a calculus.* | lithotriteur |
| **litmus** *A dye that turns red with low pH and blue with high pH.* | tournesol |

| English | French |
|---|---|
| **liver** *A large glandular organ in the right upper quadrant that functions in digestive processes, as well as, neutralizing toxins.* | foie |
| **liver abscess** | abcès du foie |
| **lobar** *Referring to a lobe.* | lobaire |
| **lobe** *A body part divided by a fissure.* | lobe |
| **lobectomy** *Surgical removal of a lobe (generally lung or liver).* | lobectomie |
| **lobotomy** *Surgical incision into the prefrontal lobe; historically a treatment of mental illness.* | lobotomie |
| **Lobo's disease** *A condition exhibited by small, red, hard papules in the sacral region.* | 1. blastomycose chéloïdienne 2. Lobo, maladie de |
| **lobule** *A small lobe.* | lobule |
| **localization** *Establishment of a site of a disease process.* | localisation |
| **localized** *Toward one point or area.* | localisé |
| **lochia** *Vaginal secretions noted within two weeks of childbirth.* | lochies |
| **locked-in syndrome** *A neurologic condition characterized by a person by conscious of their surroundings but being unable to verbally communicate that understanding.* | verouillage, syndrome de |
| **loculated** *Divided into small cavities.* | loculaire |
| **long acting** | action prolongée |
| **long-standing** | longue date de |
| **longsighted** *Synonym of hyperopia.* | hypermétrope |
| **loose** | lâche |
| **looseness** | relâchement |
| **lordosis** *An abnormal depth of the inward curvature of the spine.* | lordose |
| **loss of consciousness** *Unresponsive to verbal and tactile stimuli.* | perte de connaissance |
| **lost to follow-up** *This describes a situation in which a patient has a chronic medical problem but has not been seen regularly.* | perdu de vue |
| **lots of** | beaucoup de |
| **low back pain** | lombalgie |
| **low-fat diet** | régime pauvre en graisses |
| **lower extremity edema** | œdema des membres inférieurs |
| **lowering** | abaissement |
| **lubricant** | lubrifiant |
| **lumbago** *Pain in the region of the lumbar spine.* | lumbago |
| **lumbar puncture** *Insertion of a needle into the spinal canal in the region of L3-4 to obtain a sample of CSF.* | ponction lombaire |
| **lumbar** *Referring to the spinal region inferior to the thoracic spine.* | lombaire |
| **lumen** *A hollow cavity.* | lumen |
| **lump** | 1. bosse 2. grosseur |
| **lunate bone** *A carpal bone that articulates with the wrist.* | 1. lunatum 2. semi-lunaire os |

85

| English | French |
|---|---|
| lung | poumon |
| lung capacity *The amount of air in the lungs after a maximal inhalation.* | capacité respiratoire |
| lunula *The pale area at the base of a fingernail.* | lunule |
| lupus erythematosous *An autoimmune inflammatory disease exhibited by a butterfly shaped rash on the face along with visceral and connective tissue abnormalities.* | lupus érythémateux |
| luteinizing hormone (LH) *A pituitary hormone that stimulates ovulation in females and androgen in males.* | lutéinisante hormone |
| luteotropic *Synonym of prolactin.* | lutéotrope |
| lymph *A transparent and sometimes opalescent fluid that flows in the lymph channels.* | lymphe |
| lymph node *An area of organized lymphatic tissue.* | ganglion lymphatique |
| lymphadenitis *Inflammation of a lymph node.* | lymphadénite |
| lymphangiectasis *Distention of the lymph channels.* | lymphangiectasie |
| lymphangioma *A mass composed of newly formed lymph tissue.* | lymphangiome |
| lymphangitis *Inflammation of the lymph vessels.* | lymphangite |
| lymphatic *Referring to the lymph system.* | lymphatique |
| lymphocyte *A white blood cell produced by the lymph tissue.* | lymphocyte |
| lymphocytemia *Abnormally high number of lymphocytes in the blood.* | lymphocythémie |
| lymphocytic leukemia *Chronic accumulation of functionally incompetent lymphocytes.* | leucémie lymphoïde |
| lymphocytopenia *Decrease in the usual number of lymphocytes in the blood.* | 1. lymphocytopénie 2. lymphopénie |
| lymphocytosis *The organization of cysts containing lymph.* | lymphoctyose |
| lymphoid *Similar to lymph.* | lymphoïde |
| lymphoma *A malignant disease of the lymph system, Hodgkin's lymphoma for example.* | lymphome |
| lymphosarcoma *A malignant disease of the lymph system that does not include Hodgkin's lymphoma.* | lymphosarcome |
| lysine *An amino acid found in most proteins.* | lysine |
| lysis *The rupture of a cell wall or membrane.* | lyse |
| lysosomal *Referring to an organelle contained in the cytoplasm of eukaryotic cells.* | lysosomial |
| lysozyme *An enzyme in tears that facilitates destruction of certain bacterial cell walls.* | lysozyme |
| lytic *Referring to lysis.* | lytique |
| macrocephalus *Having an abnormally large head.* | macrocéphale |
| macrocheilia *Abnormally large lips.* | macrochéilie |
| macrocyte *A large red blood cell.* | macrocyte |
| macrocytic *Referring to the status of an increased number of large erythrocytes as seen in Vitamin B12 deficiency.* | macrocytaire |
| macrodactyly *Abnormally large digits.* | macrodactylie |
| macroglobulinemia *A condition exhibited by an increase number of macroglobulins in the blood.* | macroglobulinémie |

| English | French |
|---------|--------|
| **macroglossia** *Abnormally large tongue.* | macroglossie |
| **macromastia** *Abnormally large breasts.* | macromastie |
| **macromelia** *Abnormally large head or extremity.* | macromélie |
| **macrophage** *A phagocytic cell that originates in the tissues.* | macrophage |
| **macrostomia** *Abnormal increase in the width of the mouth.* | macrostomie |
| **macula** *1. The area of the eye of greatest visual acuity that surrounds the fovea. 2. A small flat discoloration of the skin (synonym for macule).* | 1. macula 2. tache |
| **macula solaris** *Formal medical term describing a freckle.* | éphélide |
| **maculopapular** *A skin lesion that is similar to both a macule and a papule.* | maculopapulaire |
| **mad cow disease** *Bovine spongiform encephalopathy, a disease that cause cerebral degeneration exhibited by ataxia.* | vache folle, maladie de la |
| **madness** | folie |
| **magnet** | aimant |
| **magnetic** | magnétique |
| **magnetic resonance imaging (MRI)** *Images are produced by evaluating the response of body tissue. nuclei to radio waves in a magnetic field.* | imagerie par résonance magnétique |
| **maiden name** | nom de jeune fille |
| **maintenance** | entretien |
| **malacia** *The abnormal softening of a body part or tissue.* | 1. malacie 2. ramollissement |
| **maladjustment** | inadaptation |
| **malalignment (dental)** *Displacement of the teeth from their normal position.* | alignement dentaire défectueux |
| **malaria** *A condition caused by a protozoan of the genus Plasmodium. It is transmitted by mosquitos and is exhibited by fever, chills, headache. In the severe form it can lead to convulsions, increased ICP and death.* | malaria |
| **malignant** | malin |
| **malignant hypertension** *Sudden, severe hypertension associated with neuroretinitis.* | hypertension maligne |
| **malingering** *Feigning illness.* | simulation |
| **malleolus** *A bony protrusion on medial and lateral aspect of each ankle.* | malléole |
| **mallet finger** *Flexion contracture of the distal phalanx.* | doigt en marteau |
| **malleus** *Small bone in the inner ear that articulates with the incus.* | 1. malleus 2. marteau |
| **malnutrition** *Lack of appropriate nutrition.* | 1. malnutrition 2. sous-alimentation |
| **malpractice** *Negligent professional activity.* | 1. incurie 2. malversation |
| **maltose** *A disaccharide hydrolyzed by amylase.* | maltose |
| **malunion** *The union of a fracture in a faulty position.* | cal vicieux |
| **mammaplasty** *Plastic surgery of the breast.* | mammoplastie |
| **mammary** *Referring to the breast.* | mammaire |

| English | French |
|---------|--------|
| **mammary gland** *The mass of tissue posterior to the nipples which has the essential task of milk production.* | gland mammaire |
| **mammillary** *Referring to a nipple.* | mamillaire |
| **mammography** *Roentgenography of the breasts, used as a screening test for cancer.* | mammographie |
| **man** | homme |
| **management** | prise en charge |
| **mandatory** | obligatoire |
| **mandible** *The lower jaw.* | 1. mandibule 2. maxillaire inférieur |
| **mania** *A mental disorder exhibited by hyperexcitability, delusions and euphoria.* | manie |
| **manic-depressive psychosis** *A mental disorder exhibited by alternating periods of depression and mania.* | psychose maniacodépressive |
| **mankind** | humanité |
| **manometer** *Device used for pressure monitoring.* | manomètre |
| **manubrium sterni** *The superior segment of the sternum which articulates with the clavicle and first rib.* | manubrium sternal |
| **maple syrup urine disease** *A condition characterized by an enzyme defect causing an increase in leucine in the urine.* | urines à odeur de sirop d'érable, maladie des |
| **mapping** | cartographie |
| **marasmus** *Progressive weight loss and emaciation.* | 1. maigreur extrême 2. marasme |
| **marijuana** *Cannabis.* | marijuana |
| **marital counseling** | conseil conjugal |
| **marital status** | situation matrimoniale |
| **marsupialization** *Creation of a surgical pouch.* | marsupialisation |
| **mass** *Tumor.* | masse |
| **mast cell** *A cell containing basophilic granules that releases histamine and other substances during allergic reactions.* | mastocyte |
| **mastectomy** *Surgical resection of one or both breasts.* | 1. mammectomie 2. mastectomie |
| **mastication** *Chewing.* | mastication |
| **mastitis** *Inflammation of the breast.* | mastite |
| **mastodynia** *Breast pain.* | mastodynie |
| **mastoid** *Referring to the mastoid process.* | mastoïde |
| **mastoid process** *The posterior part of the temporal bone bordered by the parietal bone superiorly and the occipital bone posteriorly.* | apophyse mastoïde |
| **mastoidectomy** *Surgical removal of the mastoid.* | mastoïdectomie |
| **mastoiditis** *Inflammation of the mastoid process.* | mastoïdite |
| **matching** | appariement |
| **mattress** | matelas |
| **maxilla** *The upper jaw that also forms the inferior portion of the orbit and part of the nose.* | maxillaire supérieur |

| English | French |
|---|---|
| meaningless | sans signification |
| measles *A childhood viral, infectious disease exhibited by rash and fever.* | rougeole |
| meatus *Opening to the body, such as urethral meatus.* | méat |
| meconium *The first newborn feces which are green. Presence of meconium on the newborn is a sign there was fetal distress in utero.* | méconium |
| medial *Situated toward the midline.* | médial |
| median lethal dose (LD 50) *The average dose of a substance it takes to kill 50% of the subjects.* | dose létale médiane (DL 50) |
| medianoscopy *Visual inspection of the mediastinum with a scope.* | médianoscopie |
| mediastinum *The thoracic area between the lungs.* | médiastin |
| medical record | dossier médical |
| medication | médicament |
| medicine | médecine |
| medicosurgical *Referring to medicine and surgery.* | médicochirurgical |
| medulla oblongata *The inferior portion of the brainstem.* | bulbe rachidien |
| medullary *1. The inner part of an organ. 2. Referring to the medulla oblongata.* | médullaire |
| medulloblastoma *A malignant tumor of the cerebellum found mostly in children.* | médulloblastome |
| megacephaly *Having a larger than normal cranial capacity.* | mégacéphalie |
| megacolon *Profound dilation of the large bowel.* | mégacôlon |
| megakaryocyte *A cell found in the bone marrow that is a source of platelet production.* | mégacaryocyte |
| megaloblast *A large red blood cell noted primarily in pernicious anemia.* | mégaloblaste |
| megalomania *A mental disorder characterized by abnormal feelings of self-importance.* | mégalomanie |
| meibomian cyst *An enclosed fluid collection along a sebaceous gland of the eyelid.* | chalazion |
| meiosis *Cell division creating two daughter cells each with half the number of cells as the parent cell.* | méiose |
| melancholia *Profound sadness.* | mélancolie |
| melanin *A dark pigment found on the skin, hair or iris.* | mélanine |
| melanoma *Malignant cancer, typically found in the skin.* | mélanome |
| memory | mémoire |
| menarche *The time of the initial menstrual period.* | ménarche |
| meningeal *Referring to the dura mater, arachnoid and the pia mater.* | méningé |
| meningioma *A tumor of the meningeal tissue; generally benign.* | méningiome |
| meningism *Signs and symptoms of meningitis without infection of the meninges.* | 1. méningisme 2. pseudo-méningite |
| meningitis *Inflammation of the meninges exhibited by fever, photophobia, nuchal rigidity and in severe cases coma and convulsions.* | méningite |

| English | French |
|---|---|
| **meningocele** *A congenital defect exhibited by protrusion of the meninges through a defect in the spinal column.* | méningocèle |
| **meningococcemia** | méningococcémie |
| **meniscectomy** *Surgical excision of a meniscus.* | méniscectomie |
| **meniscus** *A thin cartilage between joint surfaces.* | ménisque |
| **menopause** *The time when menstruation ceases.* | ménopause |
| **menorrhagia** *Abnormally large amount of menstrual blood.* | ménorragie |
| **menses** *The blood and other material expelled from the uterus during menstruation.* | règles |
| **menstruation** | menstruation |
| **mental** | mental |
| **mention, to** | citer |
| **mesarteritis** *Inflammation of the middle layer of an artery.* | mésartéritie |
| **mesencephalon** *Midbrain.* | mésencéphale |
| **mesenchyme** *Organized mesodermal cells that produce connective tissue, lymphatics and bone.* | mésenchyme |
| **mesentery** *The fold of peritoneum that connects the small bowel, pancrease and spleen to the posterior portion of the abdominal wall.* | mésentère |
| **mesoappendix** *The portion of the mesentery vermiform appendix.* | méso-appendice |
| **mesocolon** *The mesentery connecting the colon to the posterior abdominal wall.* | mésocôlon |
| **mesoderm** *The middle germ layer in an embryo that is the source of bone, muscle and skin.* | mésoderme |
| **mesonephroma** *Usually a tumor of the female genital tract that is thought to stem from the mesonephros.* | mésonéphrome |
| **mesosalpinx** *A portion of the broad ligament supporting the fallopian tubes.* | mésosalpinx |
| **mesothelioma** *A tumor that stems from mesothelial tissue; a known cause is asbestos exposure.* | mésothéliome |
| **mesovarium** *The portion of the mesentery connecting the ovary with the abdominal wall.* | mésovarium |
| **metabolic** *Referring to the physical and chemical reactions involved with keeping an organism functioning.* | métabolique |
| **metacarpal** *The name for any of the five hand bones.* | métacarpe |
| **metacarpophalangeal** *Referring to the metacarpus and the phalanges.* | métacarpophalangien |
| **metaphysis** *The region between the diaphysis and the epiphysis.* | métaphyse |
| **metaplasia** *Abnormal change in the nature or character of tissue.* | métaplasie |
| **metatarsal** *Any of the bones of the foot.* | métatarsien |
| **metatarsalgia** *Foot pain.* | métatarsalgie |
| **meter** | mètre |
| **methemoglobin** *A substance formed with the oxidation of hemoglobin.* | méthémoglobine |
| **methionine** *A sulfur-containing amino acid used in the biosynthesis of cysteine.* | méthionine |
| **metric system** | système métrique |

| English | French |
|---|---|
| **metrorrhagia** *Uterine bleeding in normal amounts but at irregular intervals.* | métrorragie |
| **microbe** *A microorganism.* | microbe |
| **microbiology** *The study of microorganisms.* | microbiologie |
| **microcephalic** *A congenital deformity exhibited by an abnormally small head.* | microcéphale |
| **microcyte** *An unusually small erythrocyte associated with anemias, such as iron deficiency anemia.* | microcyte |
| **micrognathia** *Abnormally small maxilla or mandible.* | micrognathie |
| **microgram** *One millionth of one gram.* | microgramme |
| **micrometer** *One millionth of one meter.* | micromètre |
| **microorganism** *An organism only seen with a microscope.* | micro-organisme |
| **microphthalmos** *A congenital condition characterized by smallness of the eyes.* | microphtalmie |
| **microscope** | microscope |
| **micturition** *Synonym of urination.* | miction |
| **middle ear** | oreille moyenne |
| **midline** | ligne médiane |
| **midstream urine** *A specimen of urine that is collected after the initial stream of urine is initiated and before one finishes urinating.* | urines du milieu du jet |
| **midwife** *A person trained to assist in childbirth.* | sage-femme |
| **midwifery** *The occupation of assisting in childbirth.* | obstétrique |
| **migraine** *An episodic, unilateral headache accompanied by nausea.* | migraine |
| **mild** | doux |
| **milestone** *An event indicative of a certain stage of development.* | jalon |
| **miliary** *Referring to a disease that is exhibited by small seed-like lesions (millet), such as miliary tuberculosis.* | miliaire |
| **milligram** | milligramme |
| **milliliter** | millilitre |
| **millimeter** | millimètre |
| **Milroy's disease** *Hereditary disease exhibited by leg edema.* | 1. éléphantiasis familial 2. Milroy, maladie de |
| **minute** | minuscule |
| **mirror** | miroir |
| **miscarriage** *Spontaneous abortion.* | fausse-couche |
| **misspelling** | faute d'orthographe |
| **mite fever** *Synonym of typhus fever.* | typhus exanthématique |
| **mitochondria** *Organelle found in cells responsible for energy production.* | mitochondrie |
| **mitosis** *Cell division in which two daughter cells are formed that have the same number of chromosomes as the parent cell.* | mitose |
| **mitral** *Referring to the mitral valve.* | mitral |

| English | French |
|---|---|
| **mitral regurgitation** *Backflow of blood from the left ventricle to the left atrium because of dysfunctional valve.* | insuffisance mitrale |
| **mitral stenosis** *Narrowing of the left atrioventricular orifice.* | rétrécissement mitral |
| **mitral valve** *The valve with two cusps between the left atrium and ventricle.* | valve mitrale |
| **modiolus** *A column located in the cochlea.* | 1. columelle 2. modiolus |
| **moist** | humide |
| **molality** *The number of moles of a solution per kilogram of pure solvent.* | molalité |
| **molar teeth** *The most posterior teeth bilaterally which includes 8 deciduous and usually 12 permanent teeth.* | molaires |
| **molecule** *A combination of at least two atoms.* | molécule |
| **monitoring** | monitorage |
| **monoamine oxidase inhibitor (MAOI)** *A drug used to treat depression that allows accumulation of serotonin and norepinephrine.* | inhibiteur de la monoamine oxydase |
| **monoclonal** *Asexual formation of a clone from a single cell.* | monoclonal |
| **monocyte** *A leukocyte with an oval nucleus and grey cytoplasm.* | monocyte |
| **monocytosis** *An abnormal increase in the number of monocytes in the blood.* | 1. leucocytose monocytaire 2. monocytose |
| **monomania** *A psychotic obsession about a single subject.* | idée fixe |
| **mononeuritis** *Inflammation of a single nerve.* | mononévrite |
| **mononuclear** *A cell having only one nucleus.* | mononucléaire |
| **mononucleosis** *An infectious disease exhibited by malaise and lymphadenopathy.* | mononucléose |
| **monoplegia** *Paralysis of a single limb.* | monoplégie |
| **monopolar** *This refers to an electrosurgery device in which the power flows through only one electrode.* | unipolaire |
| **mons pubis** *The fleshy protuberance over the symphysis pubis.* | mont de Vénus |
| **mood** | thymie |
| **morbid** | morbide |
| **morgue** | morgue |
| **moribund** *Near death.* | moribond |
| **morning sickness** *Nausea associated with pregnancy.* | état nauséeux gravidique |
| **morphea** *A condition exhibited by an elevated or depressed patch of pink skin with a purple border.* | sclérodermie circonscrite |
| **morphine** *An opioid analgesic.* | morphine |
| **morphology** *The study of living organisms and the correlation between their structure.* | morphologie |
| **morula** *A solid mass created by the splitting of an ovum.* | morula |
| **mosquito net** | moustiquaire |
| **mossy fiber** *Nerve fibers that surround the nerve cells of the cerebellar cortex.* | fibre moussue |

| English | French |
|---|---|
| **motion sickness** *Nausea associated with travel.* | transports, mal des |
| **motor** | moteur |
| **motor end plate** *The expansions on a motor nerve where the branches terminate on muscle fiber.* | plaque motrice |
| **motor unit** *The complex of one motor cell and its attached muscle fibers.* | unité motrice |
| **mottling** *An irregular arrangement of patches of color.* | tacheture |
| **mourning** *A period of grieving.* | deuil |
| **mouth** | bouche |
| **mouth piece** | embout buccal |
| **mouth to mouth** *A manner of artificial respiration.* | bouche-à-bouche |
| **mouth to mouth resuscitation** *A form of emergency management of respiratory failure.* | souffle de vie |
| **mouthful** | bouchée |
| **mucilage** *1. A viscous bodily fluid. 2. A polysaccharide used in medicines and glue.* | mucilage |
| **mucin** *A glycoprotein that is the primary constituent in mucous.* | mucine |
| **mucocele** *An accumulation of mucous in a dilated cavity.* | mucocèle |
| **mucoid** *Referring to mucous.* | mucoïde |
| **mucolytic** *A substance that breaks down mucous.* | 1. fluidifiant 2. mucolytique |
| **mucopurulent** *That which contains both mucous and pus.* | mucopurulent |
| **mucosa** *A mucous membrane like the buccal mucosa.* | muqueuse |
| **mucus** *A substance secreted by mucous membranes.* | mucus |
| **multigravida** *A woman who has been pregnant more than once.* | multigeste |
| **multilocular** *The presence of more than one cells within a cavity.* | multiloculaire |
| **multipara** *A woman with more than one live births.* | multipare |
| **multiple sclerosis** *A chronic neurologic disease exhibited by numbness, vision and speech problems, and motor incoordination.* | sclérose en plaques |
| **mumble, to** | marmonner |
| **mumps** *A contagious viral disease that is exhibited by parotid swelling and puts males at risk for sterility.* | 1. oreillons 2. ourlien |
| **murmur** *An abnormal heart sound heard with a stethoscope.* | murmure |
| **muscle** | muscle |
| **muscle weakness** | déficit musculaire |
| **muscular** | musculaire |
| **muscular dystrophy** *A hereditary condition exhibited by progressive muscular weakness and muscle atrophy.* | dystrophie musculaire progressive |
| **mutation** *A gene alteration that can be passed to the next generation.* | mutation |
| **mute** | muet |
| **mutism** *Inability to speak.* | mutisme |
| **myalgia** *Muscle pain.* | myalgie |

| English | French |
|---|---|
| **myasthenia gravis** *An autoimmune disease characterized by fluctuating weakness of the ocular, limb and respiratory muscles.* | myasthénie |
| **mycetoma** *Persistent inflammation of the tissues caused by an infection.* | mycétome |
| **mycosis** *A disease caused by a fungal infection.* | mycose |
| **mycotoxin** *A substance toxic to fungus.* | mycotoxine |
| **mydriasis** *Pupillary dilation.* | mydriase |
| **myelin** *The substance that forms a sheath around some nerve fibers.* | myéline |
| **myelitis** *Inflammation of the spinal cord.* | myélite |
| **myelocele** *Protrusion of the spinal cord through a defect in the bony structure.* | myélocèle |
| **myelogram** *CT scan or roentgenography of the spinal canal after injection of contrast media.* | myélogramme |
| **myeloid** *Referring to the bone marrow or spinal cord.* | myéloïde |
| **myeloma** *Malignant tumor of the bone marrow.* | myélome |
| **myelomatosis** *A leukemic disease in which there is an abnormally high amount of myeloblasts in the blood.* | myélomatose |
| **myelomeningocele** *A protrusion of the spinal cord and its meninges through a defect in the vertebral canal.* | myéloméningocèle |
| **myelopathy** *A condition of the spinal cord.* | myélopathie |
| **myocardial** *Referring to the muscular tissue of the heart.* | myocardique |
| **myocardial infarction** *The death of myocardial tissue as a result of an interruption in flow to the region supplied by a coronary vessel.* | infarctus myocardique |
| **myocarditis** *An inflammation of the heart.* | myocardite |
| **myocardium** *The middle layer of the heart wall.* | myocarde |
| **myoglobin** *A heme protein that carries and stores oxygen in muscle tissue.* | myoglobine |
| **myoma** *A tumor composed partly of muscle.* | myome |
| **myomectomy** *Surgical resection of a myoma.* | myomectomie |
| **myometrium** *The smooth muscle layer of the uterus.* | myomètre |
| **myopathy** *Muscle disease.* | myopathie |
| **myope** *A person who is nearsighted.* | myope |
| **myopia** *Nearsightedness.* | myopie |
| **myosarcoma** *A mass with myoma and sarcoma characteristics.* | myocarcome |
| **myosin** *A protein that when coupled with actin form the contractile complex of a muscle cells.* | myosine |
| **myosis** *Profound pupillary constriction.* | myosis |
| **myositis** *Inflammation of muscle tissue.* | myosite |
| **myositis ossificans** *Inflammation of muscle tissue with presence of bony deposits.* | myosite ossifiante |
| **myotic** *Referring to miosis.* | myotique |
| **myotomy** *The surgical removal of muscle tissue.* | myotomie |
| **myotonia dystrophica; Steinert's disease** *A condition exhibited initially by hypertonic muscles followed by atrophy of the facial and neck muscles.* | 1. maladie de Steinert<br>2. myotonie atrophique |

| English | French |
|---|---|
| **myringitis** *Inflammation of the tympanic membrane.* | 1. myringite 2. tympanite |
| **myringoplasty** *Surgical repair of tympanic membrane defects.* | myringoplastie |
| **myringotomy** *Surgical opening of the tympanic membrane.* | 1. myringotomie 2. paracentèse tympanique |
| **myxedema** *Diffuse edema with a wax-like appearance of the skin; this condition is associated with hypothyroidism.* | myxœdème |
| **myxoma** *A tumor composed of mucous tissue.* | myxome |
| **myxosarcoma** *A sarcoma that alos has mucous tissue.* | myxosarcome |
| **nail** | ongle |
| **nailing** *Referring to placement of an intramedullary rod in a long bone in order to treat a fracture.* | enclouage |
| **name** | nom |
| **nap** | sieste |
| **narcissism** *Abnormally excessive self-interest.* | narcissisme |
| **narcolepsy** *A condition exhibited by a strong desire to sleep and by sudden onset of sleep at increased intervals.* | narcolepsie |
| **narcosis** *A reversible medication-induced condition of excessive drowsiness or unconsciousness.* | narcose |
| **narcotic** *A medication that produces narcosis.* | 1. narcotique 2. stupéfiant |
| **nasal** *Referring to the nose.* | nasal |
| **nasogastric tube** *A tube that is inserted into the nose with the distal tip in the stomach; it is used for irrigation or drainage of gastric contents.* | sonde naso-œsophagienne |
| **nasogastric tube placement** | sondage nasogastrique |
| **nasolacrimal** *Referring to the nose and tear apparatus.* | nasolacrymal |
| **nasopharyngeal** *Referring to the nose and pharynx.* | rhinopharyngien |
| **nasopharynx** *The part of the pharynx which lies superior to the soft palate.* | nasopharynx |
| **nausea** | nausée |
| **navicular** *1. boat shaped 2. Referring to the navicular bone of the hand or foot.* | naviculaire |
| **navicular bone** *The most lateral bone in the proximal row of carpal bones.* | os scaphoïde |
| **near** | proche |
| **nebula** *An opaque spot on the cornea causing impaired vision.* | néphélion |
| **nebulizer** *A device used for transforming a liquid into a fine mist for inhalation as in nebulized albuterol for an acute exacerbation of asthma.* | 1. nébuliseur 2. vaporisateur |
| **nebulizer treatment** *Administration of medication such as albuterol via a fine mist using a nebulizer.* | nébulisation |
| **neck** | 1. col 2. cou 3. nuque |
| **necropsy** *Synonym of autopsy.* | nécropsie |
| **necrosis** *The death of most of the cells of the affected part.* | nécrose |

| English | French |
|---|---|
| **necrotic** *Referring to necrosis.* | nécrotique |
| **need** | besoin |
| **needle** | 1. agacer 2. aiguille |
| **needle biopsy** *Use of a needle to aspirate body contents for microscopic or pathologic examination.* | 1. biopsie à l'aiguille 2. ponction-biopsie |
| **needle for lumbar puncture** | aiguille à ponction lombaire |
| **needle holder** *A surgical instrument used to grasp a needle during suturing.* | porte-aiguille |
| **negation** | dénégation |
| **nematode** *An endoparasite belonging to the class of the Nemathelminthes including roundworms and threadworms.* | nématode |
| **neonatal** *Referring to the first four weeks after birth.* | néonatal |
| **neonate** *The term for a newborn infant for the first four weeks.* | nouveau-né |
| **neoplasm** *A new and abnormal growth.* | néoplasme |
| **nephrectomy** *Surgical removal of a kidney.* | néphrectomie |
| **nephritis** *A general term meaning inflammation of a kidney that is further categorized depending on the associated pathology.* | néphrite |
| **nephroblastoma** *Congenital tumor of the kidney, also called Wilms' tumor.* | néphroblastome |
| **nephrocalcinosis** *A condition exhibited by calcium phosphate deposition in the renal tubules; a cause of renal insufficiency.* | néphrocalcinose |
| **nephrolithiasis** *A calculus in the kidney.* | lithiase rénale |
| **nephrolithotomy** *Surgical removal of a renal calculus.* | néphrolithotomie |
| **nephroma** *A renal tumor.* | néphrome |
| **nephron** *A functional unit of the kidney that consists of the glomerulus, the proximal and distal convoluted tubules, the loop of Henle and the collecting tubule.* | néphron |
| **nephropathy** *Renal disease.* | néphropathie |
| **nephropexy** *The surgical fixation of a kidney that was previously floating.* | néphropexie |
| **nephroptosis** *Inferior displacement of the kidney.* | néphroptose |
| **nephrosclerosis** *Hardening of the kidney.* | néphrosclérose |
| **nephrosis** *A kidney disease exhibited by edema and proteinuria; also called nephrotic syndrome.* | néphrose |
| **nephrostomy** *Surgical creation of an opening between the renal pelvis and an opening in the skin.* | néphrostomie |
| **nephrotic** *Referring to nephrosis.* | néphrotique |
| **nephrotomy** *Surgical incision of the kidney.* | néphrotomie |
| **nerve** | nerf |
| **nerve impulse** *A signal transmitted along a nerve fiber.* | influx nerveux |
| **nerve-block anesthesia** *Injection of an anesthetic agent near a nerve, thus blocking the sensation distal to the injection.* | anesthésie par bloc nerveux |
| **neural** *Referring to a nerve or nerve impulse.* | neural |

| English | French |
|---|---|
| **neuralgia** *Severe pain along the course of a nerve.* | névralgie |
| **neurapraxia** *Paralysis from nerve injury but no degeneration of the nerve.* | neurapraxie |
| **neurasthenia** *A psychoneurosis exhibited by severe fatigue.* | neurasthénie |
| **neurectomy** *Excision of a section of a nerve.* | neurectomie |
| **neurectomy** *Excision of a section of a nerve.* | névrectomie |
| **neurilemma** *The membrane covering a myelinated nerve fiber or the axon of an unmyelinated nerve fiber.* | 1. neurilemme 2. Schwann, gaine de |
| **neuritis** *Inflammation of a nerve.* | névrite |
| **neuroblastoma** *A nervous system malignant tumor composed of neuroblasts.* | neuroblastome |
| **neurodermatitis** *A pruritic, thickened eruption in the axillary and inguinal thought to be exacerbated by emotions.* | névrodermite |
| **neuroepithelium** *Cells specialized to serve as sensory cells such as cells of the cochlea and tongue.* | neuro-épithélium |
| **neurofibroma** *A tumor formed by excessive growth of perineurium and endoneurium.* | neurofibrome |
| **neurofibromatosis** *A hereditary condition exhibited by formation of multiple soft tumors scattered throughout the skin surface.* | neurofibromatose |
| **neuroglia** *A type of connective tissue of the nervous system.* | névroglie |
| **neuroleptic** *A drug that causes neurologic symptoms.* | neuroleptique |
| **neurologist** *A physician who specializes in the study of the nervous system.* | neurologue |
| **neurology** *The study of the nervous system.* | neurologie |
| **neuroma** *A mass composed of nerve cells and fibers.* | névrome |
| **neuron** *A nerve cell.* | neurone |
| **neuropathic** *Referring to neuropathy.* | neuropathique |
| **neuropathy** *Structural of pathologic changes of the peripheral nervous system.* | neuropathie |
| **neurosis** *A mental disorder.* | névrose |
| **neurosurgery** *Surgery of the brain or spinal cord.* | neurochirurgie |
| **neurosyphilis** *Infection of the central nervous system with Treponema pallidum.* | neurosyphilis |
| **neurotmesis** *The severing of a nerve.* | neurotmésis |
| **neurotomy** *Surgical incision into a nerve.* | neurotomie |
| **neurotransmitter** *A substance released at the end of a nerve fiber that facilitates transmission of an impulse.* | neurotransmetteur |
| **neutropenia** *Diminished number of neutrophils in the blood.* | neutropénie |
| **neutrophil** *A polymorphonuclear leukocyte.* | neutrophile |
| **nevus** *A benign, well-circumscribed growth of tissue of congenital origin.* | nævus |
| **next** | prochain |
| **nick** | entaille |
| **nicotinic acid** *A deficiency of this substance results in pellagra.* | acide nicotinique |

| English | French |
|---|---|
| **night shift** | garde ne nuit |
| **night terror** *Sensation of profound fear upon wakening.* | terreur nocturne |
| **nightmare** | cauchemar |
| **nipple** | mamelon |
| **nitrogen** *A colorless, odorless gas used as a coolant in the liquid form.* | azote |
| **nitrous oxide** *An inhalant gas used as an anesthetic agent.* | protoxyde d'azote |
| **nocturia** *Urination at night.* | 1. hypnurie 2. nycturie |
| **nocturnal** *Referring to events that happen at night.* | nocturne |
| **node** *A swelling or prominence.* | ganglion |
| **nodule** *A rounded collection of cells that is palpable.* | nodosité |
| **non-resorbable suture (nylon)** | fil non-résorbable (nylon) |
| **noon** | midi |
| **norepinephrine** *A hormone secreted by the adrenal medulla and a synthetic drug used as a pressor agent.* | noradrénaline |
| **normoblast** *A precursor cell for erythrocytes.* | normoblaste |
| **normocyte** *A normal erythrocyte.* | normocyte |
| **nose** | nez |
| **nosocomial infection** *An infection occurring after admission to a hospital.* | infection nosocomiale |
| **nosology** *The medical science of disease classification.* | nosologie |
| **nosophobia** *Unwarranted, excessive fear of any disease.* | nosophobie |
| **nostril** | narine |
| **noxious** *Harmful or poisonous.* | nuisible |
| **nuclear magnetic resonance (NMR)** *A type a diagnostic body imaging utilizing electromagnetic radiation in a magnetic field.* | résonance magnétique nucléaire |
| **nuclear medicine** *The branch of medicine associated with the use of radioactive material in the evaluation and treatment of disease.* | médecine nucléaire |
| **nuclear** *Referring to a nucleus.* | nucléaire |
| **nucleic acid** *An organic compound found in living cells; its molecules contain nucleotides linked in long chains.* | nucléique acide |
| **nucleoprotein** *A substance composed of a nucleic acid and a protein.* | nucléoprotéine |
| **nullipara** *A woman who has never given birth.* | nullipare |
| **numbness** | engourdissement |
| **nummulated** *Formed as round, flat discs.* | nummulaire |
| **nursing care** | soins infirmiers |
| **nutation** *Referring to nodding of the head.* | nutation |
| **nutrient** | nutriment |
| **nutrient foramen** *A conduit for passage of nutrient vessels in the marrow of bone.* | trou nourricier |
| **nutrition** | nutrition |
| **nutritional status** | statut nutritionnel |

| English | French |
|---|---|
| **nystagmus** *Rapid involuntary movement of the eyes; it can be horizontal, vertical or rotary.* | nystagmus |
| **obesity** | obésité |
| **obsession** *A pathologic preoccupation.* | obsession |
| **obsolete** | désuet |
| **obstetric** *Referring to The management of pregnancy, labor and the peuperium.* | obstétrical |
| **obstetrician** *A physician who specializes in the management of pregnancy, labor and the peuperium.* | 1. accoucheur 2. obstétricien |
| **obstructed** *To be blocked or halted.* | obstrué |
| **obturator** *A device used to close an artificial or natural opening.* | obturateur |
| **occipital** *Referring to the back part of the head.* | occipital |
| **occlusive dressing** *A synthetic covering for a wound that has a semipermeable membrane.* | pansement occlusif |
| **occult bleeding** *Loss of blood from an unknown source.* | hémorragie occulte |
| **occupational therapy** *Rehabilitation focusing on activities of daily living.* | erthothérapie |
| **ocular** *Referring to the eye.* | oculaire |
| **oculogyric** *Referring to movement of the eye around the anteroposterior axis.* | oculogyre |
| **oculomotor nerve** *Referring to cranial nerve III which is one of the nerves responsible for extraocular movements.* | moteur oculomoteur commun nerf |
| **odontalgia** *Tooth pain.* | odontalgie |
| **odontoid** *A prominence on the second cervical vertebra on which the first cervical vertebra pivots.* | 1. dentiforme 2. odontoïde |
| **odontology** *Synonym of dentistry.* | 1. médecine dentaire 2. odontologie |
| **odor** | odeur |
| **offspring** | progéniture |
| **ointment** | 1. onguent 2. pommade |
| **old age** | vieillesse |
| **older** | plus vieux |
| **olecranon** *The bony protrusion at the proximal ulna at the elbow.* | olécrâne |
| **olfactory** *Referring to the sense of smell.* | olfactif |
| **oligodendroglia** *The ectodermal cells forming part of the central nervous system.* | oligodendroglie |
| **oligomenorrhea** *Infrequent menstruation or low volume menstrual flow.* | oligoménorrhée |
| **oligospermia** *Abnormally low sperm count.* | oligospermie |
| **oligotrophia** *Inadequate nutritional state.* | oligotrophie |
| **oliguria** *Abnormally low urine output.* | oligurie |
| **omentocele** *A herniated protrusion of omentum.* | épiplocèle |
| **omentopexy** *Surgically fastening the omentum to an adjacent tissue it was not previously attached to.* | 1. épiploopexie 2. omentopexie |

| English | French |
|---|---|
| **omentum** *A fold of peritoneum fastening the stomach to other organs in the viscera.* | 1. épiploon 2. omentum |
| **omphalitis** *Inflammation of the umbilicus.* | omphalite |
| **omphalocele** *A large congenital, umbilical hernia with only a thin membranous covering.* | omphalocèle |
| **on all fours** | quatre pattes à |
| **on going** | cours en |
| **on hold** | attente en |
| **one year survival rate** *The number of patients out of 100 who are alive a year after they received treatment.* | taux de survie à un an |
| **onset** | début |
| **onychia** *Inflammation of the toenail or fingernail matrix.* | 1. onychie 2. onyxis |
| **onychocryptosis** *Ingrown toenail.* | ongle incarné |
| **onychogryphosis** *A deformed nail that is incurved or hooked.* | onychogryphose |
| **onychomycosis** *Fungal disease of the toenails or fingernails.* | onychomycose |
| **oocyte** *An ovarian cell that needs to undergo meiotic division to become an ovum.* | 1. oocyte 2. ovocyte |
| **oogenesis** *The initiation and development of an ovum.* | 1. oogenèse 2. ovogenèse |
| **oophorectomy** *Surgical removal of an ovary.* | 1. oophorectomie 2. ovariectomie |
| **oophoritis** *Inflammation of an ovary.* | oophorite |
| **oophoron** *Synonym for ovary.* | ovaire |
| **oophorosalpingectomy** *Surgical removal of an ovary and fallopian tube.* | 1. ovariosalping-ectomie 2. oophoro-salpingectomie |
| **oozing** *Slow leakage.* | suintement |
| **operative note** *A detailed description of a surgical procedure performed on a specific patient.* | protocole opératoire |
| **ophthalmia** *Profound inflammation of the eye or its structures.* | ophtalmie |
| **ophthalmic** *Referring to the eye.* | ophtalmique |
| **ophthalmologist** *A physician specializing in diseases of the eye.* | ophtalmologiste |
| **ophthalmology** *The study of diseases of the eye.* | ophtalmologie |
| **ophthalmoplegia** *Paralysis of the eye muscles.* | ophtalmoplégie |
| **ophthalmoscope** *A device used to visually inspect the interior eye.* | ophtalmoscope |
| **opiate** *Referring to opium.* | opiacé |
| **opioid** *A substance similar to opium that binds to at least one of the opium receptors in the body.* | opioïde |
| **opisthotonos** *A profound spasm in which the head/neck is hyperextended, the feet are touching the bed and with the patient supine the body arched upward.* | opisthotonos |
| **opium** *An addictive drug derived from opium poppy; synthetic versions are used as analgesics.* | opium |
| **opponens** *Synonym for opponent muscle.* | opposant |

| English | French |
|---|---|
| **opsonin** *An antibody used to facilitate phagocytosis of a bacterium.* | opsonine |
| **optic** *Referring to the eye.* | optique |
| **optic disk** *The area of the retina where the optic nerve enters.* | 1. disque optique 2. papille optique |
| **optician** *A person who makes eyeglasses.* | opticien |
| **optometry** *The profession of examination of the eyes for disease (not a medical doctor).* | optométrie |
| **oral** | oral |
| **oral contraceptive** *Tablet taken by mouth to prevent pregnancy.* | contraceptif oral |
| **oral intake** *Amount of liquid taken by mouth.* | ration alimentaire |
| **orally** | voie orale |
| **orbicular** *Rounded or circular.* | orbiculaire |
| **orbit** *The bony structure enclosing the eyeball.* | orbite |
| **orbital** *Referring to the orbit.* | orbitaire |
| **orchidectomy** *Synonym of orchiectomy; removal of one or both testes.* | orchidectomie |
| **orchidopexy** *Surgical repair of an undescended testis.* | orchidopexie |
| **orchiepididymitis** *Inflammation of the testis and epididymis.* | orchi-épididymite |
| **orchitis** *Inflammation of one or both testes.* | orchite |
| **organ** | organe |
| **oriental sore** *Cutaneous leishmaniasis.* | bouton d'Alep |
| **orifice** *Synonym of foramen.* | orifice |
| **ornithosis** *A viral infection transmitted by birds that is manifested by chills, headache, photophobia, fever, nausea and vomiting.* | ornithose |
| **oropharynx** *The portion of the pharynx between the soft palate and the superior aspect of the epiglottis.* | oropharynx |
| **orthodontics** *A subspecialty of dentistry concerned with treatment of dental irregularities and malocclusion, including the use of braces.* | orthodontie |
| **orthopedics** *A surgical specialty concerned with treatment of skeletal problems.* | orthopédie |
| **orthopnea** *The inability to breath comfortably except in the upright position.* | orthopnée |
| **orthosis** *Straightening of a malaligned part with the use of braces and other supportive devices.* | orthèse |
| **orthostatic** *Referring to the standing position. Orthostatic hypotension is low blood pressure in the standing position.* | orthostatique |
| **oscillating nystagmus** *Abnormal movement of the eyes in a wave-like pattern.* | nystagmus pendulaire |
| **osmolality** *The concentration expressed in total number of solute particles per kilogram.* | osmolalité |
| **osmole** *The recognized unit of osmotic pressure.* | osmole |
| **osmosis** *The movement of a solvent from a solution of greater concentration to one of lower concentration through a semi-permeable membrane until the two solutions have equal concentration.* | osmose |
| **osmotic** *Referring to osmosis.* | osmotique |

| English | French |
|---|---|
| **osmotic fragility test** *Detects hemolysis at progressively less concentrated salt solutions.* | résistance globulaire, épreuve de la |
| **osseous** *Possessing the quality of bone.* | osseux |
| **ossicle** *A small bone. The stapes is an auditory ossicle.* | osselet |
| **ossification** *The formation of bone.* | ossification |
| **osteitis** *Inflammation of the bone.* | ostéite |
| **ostensibly** *Synonym of apparently and seemingly.* | en apparence |
| **osteoarthritis** *A long term, progressive degenerative joint disease.* | arthrose |
| **osteoarthrosis** *Arthritis without inflammation.* | ostéo-arthrose |
| **osteoblast** *A cell that matures from a fibroblast and produces bone.* | ostéoblaste |
| **osteochondral** *Referring to bone and cartilage.* | ostéocartilagineux |
| **osteochondritis** *Inflammation of bone and cartilage.* | ostéochondrite |
| **osteochondroma** *A tumor with bony and cartilaginous characteristics.* | ostéochondrome |
| **osteoclasis** *The surgical fracture of a bone usually in order to restore proper alignment.* | ostéoclasie |
| **osteoclast** *A large bone cell that is associated with bone reabsorption and removal.* | 1. myéloplaxe 2. ostéoclaste |
| **osteoclastoma** *A tumor composed of giant cells or osteoclasts.* | 1. ostéoclastome 2. tumeur à myéloplaxes |
| **osteocyte** *An osteoblast within the bone matrix.* | ostéocyte |
| **osteodystrophy** *Abnormal bone formation.* | ostéodystrophie |
| **osteogenesis** *Development of new bones.* | ostéogenèsis |
| **osteolytic** *Referring to the removal or loss of calcium from the bone.* | ostéolytique |
| **osteomalacia** *Softening of the bones because of a deficiency of vitamin D, calcium or phosphorus.* | ostéomalacie |
| **osteomyelitis** *Inflammation of the bone or bone marrow because of a microorganism.* | ostéomyélite |
| **osteopathy** *1. Any disease of the bone. 2. Medical practice concerning treatment of disease by manipulation and massage of bones, joints, and muscles.* | ostéopathie |
| **osteopetrosis** *Increased bone density with no change in modeling.* | ostéopétrose |
| **osteophony** *The sound conduction of bone.* | 1. conduction osseuse 2. ostéophonie |
| **osteophyte** *Abnormal growth of a bone protuberance.* | ostéophyte |
| **osteoporosis** *Loss of bone substance because the osteoblasts fail to produce bone matrix.* | ostéoporose |
| **osteosarcoma** *A tumor composed of a sarcoma and osseous material.* | ostéosarcome |
| **osteosclerosis** *Abnormal hardening of bone.* | ostéosclérose |
| **osteotomy** *Creation of a surgical opening in bone.* | ostéotomie |
| **ostium** *A vessel or body cavity opening.* | ostium |
| **ostoarthropathy** *Any disease of the joints and bones.* | ostéo-arthropathie |
| **otalgia** *Ear pain.* | otalgie |
| **otitis** *Inflammation of the ear. (otitis media or otitis externa)* | otite |

| English | French |
|---|---|
| **otolaryngologist** *Surgical specialist concerned with organs of the ears, nose and throat.* | otorhinolaryngologie (ORL) |
| **otolith** *A calcium based calculus in the inner ear.* | otolithe |
| **otology** *Study of conditions and anatomy of the ear.* | otologie |
| **otomycosis** *Fungal infection of the ear.* | otomycose |
| **otosclerosis** *A hereditary condition exhibited by progressive hearing loss because of bone overgrowth in the inner ear.* | otosclérose |
| **otoscope** *A device used for inspection of the tympanic membrane.* | otoscope |
| **ototoxic** *A substance harmful to the ear or its nerve supply.* | ototoxique |
| **outbreak** | 1. éclosion 2. flambée |
| **outdated** | périmé |
| **ovaritis** *Synonym for oophoritis.* | ovarite |
| **overdose** *An above normal dose of a medication.* | surdose |
| **overring suture** *The overlapping of cranial sutures noted on vaginal exam when the head is descended.* | chevauchement |
| **overt** *Not hidden.* | manifeste |
| **overweight** | surcharge pondérale |
| **oviduct** *The channel which an ovum passes from the ovary.* | oviducte |
| **ovulation** *The release of an ova from the ovary.* | ovulation |
| **ovule** *An immature ovum.* | ovule |
| **owing to** | en raison de |
| **oxaluria** *Existence of oxalates in the urine.* | oxalurie |
| **oxidation** *The process of a chemical combining with oxygen.* | oxydation |
| **oximeter** *A medical device used to measure the percent of oxygen that is saturated in the blood (oxygen saturation).* | oxymètre |
| **oxycephaly** *The deformation of the skull so that it appears pointed.* | oxycéphalie |
| **oxygen** | oxygène |
| **oxygen consumption** *The body's utilization of oxygen per unit of time.* | consommation d'oxygène |
| **oxygen tent** *A manner of giving supplement oxygen to a neonate.* | tente à oxygène |
| **oxygen therapy** *Utilization of supplemental oxygen.* | oxygénothérapie |
| **oxygenation** *Saturated with oxygen.* | oxygénation |
| **oxyhemoglobin** *The combination of oxygen and hemoglobin using a covalent bond.* | oxyhémoglobine |
| **oxytocic** *Referring to rapid parturition.* | ocytocique |
| **oxytocin** *A natural hormone released by the pituitary or a synthetic hormone that facilitates uterine contraction.* | ocytocine |
| **ozena** *Various nasal conditions, all of which include fetid discharge.* | ozène |
| **ozone** *A toxic chemical that has profound oxidizing properties. It has three atoms in its molecule compared with oxygen which has two.* | ozone |
| **pace** | allure |
| **pacemaker** *An electrical device used to stimulate the heart used for bradyarrhythmias.* | 1. stimulateur cardiaque 2. entraîneur |

| English | French |
|---|---|
| **pachydermia** *An abnormally thick skin.* | pachydermie |
| **pachymeningitis** *Inflammation of the dura mater.* | pachyméningite |
| **pad** | compresse |
| **pain** | douleur |
| **pain relief** | soulagement de la douleur |
| **painful** | douloureux |
| **palate** *The roof of the mouth.* | palais |
| **palatoplegia** *Paralysis of the palate.* | palatoplégie |
| **palliative** *A treatment used to reduce pain when cure is not possible.* | palliatif |
| **pallidectomy** *Surgical resection of all or part of the palate.* | pallidectomie |
| **pallor** *Unusually pale appearance.* | pâleur |
| **palm** *The anterior aspect of the hand.* | 1. palmier 2. paume |
| **palmar** *Referring to the palm.* | palmaire |
| **palpation** *The assessment of the body with the use of one's hands.* | palpation |
| **palpitation** *Sensation of a forceful, rapid, irregular heartbeat present after exercise or with anxiety.* | palpitation |
| **paludism** *Synonym of malaria.* | paludisme |
| **pamper, to** | dorloter |
| **panarthritis** *Inflammation of the joints.* | panarthrite |
| **pancarditis** *Inflammation of pericardium, myocardium and endocardium.* | pancardite |
| **pancreas** *A gland that secretes digestive enzymes into the duodenum and insulin and glucagon into the blood.* | pancréas |
| **pancreatectomy** *Surgical excision of part or all of the pancreas.* | pancréatectomie |
| **pancreatitis** *Inflammation of the pancreas.* | pancréatite |
| **pancreozymin** *A duodenal mucosal enzyme that facilitates the secretion of amylase and other enzymes from the pancreas.* | pancréozymine |
| **pandemic** *When a disease is present over an entire region.* | pandémique |
| **panhypopituitarism** *Insufficiency of the anterior pituitary.* | panhypopituitarisme |
| **panic attack** *Sudden, profound anxiety.* | panique, attaque de |
| **panniculitis** *Inflammation of a section of subcutaneous tissue containing large amounts of fat.* | 1. hypodermite 2. panniculite |
| **panophthalmia** *Inflammation of the eye and all its structures.* | panophtalmie |
| **panotitis** *Inflammation of each part of a bone.* | panotite |
| **papilledema** *Swelling of the optic disc.* | œdème papillaire |
| **papillitits** *Swelling of a papilla.* | papillite |
| **papilloma** *A benign, lobulated tumor coming from epithelium.* | papillome |
| **papule** *A small, well-circumscribed elevation of the skin.* | papule |
| **para-aminobenzoic acid** *A natural product (not FDA approved) reportedly beneficial for Peyronie's disease and scleroderma. It is a component of folic acid.* | para-aminobenzoïque acide (PABA) |

| English | French |
|---|---|
| **para-aminohippuric acid (PAH)** *A chemical used for calculation of renal plasma flow.* | para-aminohippurique acide |
| **paracentesis** *A procedure involving aspiration of fluid from the abdominal cavity.* | ponction ascite |
| **paracentesis** *Insertion of a needle into the abdominal cavity to obtain fluid.* | paracentèse |
| **paracusia** *Any abnormality in the sense of hearing.* | paracousie |
| **paralysis agitans** *Synonym of Parkinson's disease.* | paralysie agitante |
| **paralytic** *1. Referring to paralysis. 2. A person who is paralyzed.* | paralytique |
| **paramedian** *Situated toward the middle of the body.* | paramédian |
| **paramedical** *Hospital support staff excluding physicians.* | paramédical |
| **parametritis** *Inflammation of the parametrium.* | paramétrite |
| **parametrium** *The connective tissue and smooth muscle between the broad ligament serous layers.* | paramètre |
| **paramnesia** *A condition exhibited by a person's belief they have memory for an event that never happened.* | paramnésie |
| **paranasal sinus** *Any of the sinuses (ethmoidal, frontal, maxillary or sphenoidal) that communicate with the nasal cavity.* | sinus de la face |
| **paranasal** *Situated next to the nose.* | paranasal |
| **paranoia** *A mental condition exhibited by delusions of persecution.* | paranoïa |
| **paranoid** *A person who has paranoia.* | paranoïde |
| **paraphimosis** *A condition in which the foreskin is retracted but cannot be replace because of a restricted foreskin.* | paraphimosis |
| **paraplegia** *Paralysis of the lower extremities.* | paraplégie |
| **parapraxis** *1. Unable to perform purposeful movements. 1. Irrational behavior.* | acte manqué |
| **pararectal** *Adjacent to the rectum.* | pararectal |
| **parasite** *An organism that lives on or within another organism without benefit to the latter.* | parasite |
| **parasympathetic** *Part of the autonomic nervous system that opposes sympathetic stimulation.* | parasympathique |
| **parathormone** *Synonym for parathyroid hormone.* | parathormone |
| **parathyroid** *Positioned adjacent to the thyroid.* | parathyroïde |
| **paravertebral** *Positioned adjacent to the vertebra.* | paravertébral |
| **parenchyma** *The functional elements of an organ.* | parenchyme |
| **parenteral** *Other than the alimentary canal.* | parentéral |
| **paresis** *Incomplete paralysis.* | parésie |
| **paresthesia** *An abnormal sensation usually described as pins and needles.* | paresthésie |
| **parietal** *Referring to the wall of a part or cavity.* | pariétal |
| **parietal cell** *Acid secreting cells of the stomach.* | cellule bordante |
| **Parkinson's disease** *A progressive neuromuscular disease exhibited by masklike facial expression, resting tremor, cogwheel rigidity and abnormal gait.* | Parkinson, maladie de |

| English | French |
|---|---|
| **paronychia** *Inflammation of the tissue bordering a fingernail* | paronychie |
| **parosmia** *An alteration in the sense of smell.* | parosmie |
| **parotid** *A gland near the ear.* | parotide |
| **parotiditis** *Inflammation of the parotid gland.* | parotidite |
| **paroxysmal** *Occurring in sudden attacks.* | paroxysmal |
| **parthenogenesis** *Reproduction that occurs without an egg being fertilized by sperm.* | parthénogenèse |
| **parting** | séparation |
| **parturition** *The process of giving birth.* | parturition |
| **passing medications** *Giving medications to each patient on a ward.* | délivrance de médicaments |
| **passive** *Not achieved through active effort.* | passif |
| **past history** *Prior medical problems experienced by a patient.* | antécédents |
| **paste** | pâte |
| **patch test** *A test used to determine which substances provoke an allergic response in a patient.* | test percutané |
| **patella** *The bone situated in the anterior portion of the knee.* | rotule |
| **patellectomy** *Surgical excision of the patella.* | patellectomie |
| **patent ductus arteriosus** *A condition exhibited by failure of the ductus arteriosus (communication between the aorta the the pulmonary artery normally noted in a fetus) to close.* | canal artériel systémique |
| **patent foramen ovale** *A congenital anomaly in which there is a defect in the wall between the right and left atria; this can be a benign condition or result in cryptogenic strokes.* | perméabilité du foramen ovale |
| **pathogenesis** *The course of a disease.* | pathogenèse |
| **pathogenic** *Referring to an organism that can cause disease.* | 1. pathogène 2. pathogénique |
| **pathognomonic** *Characteristic of something.* | pathognomonique |
| **pathological** *Referring to pathology.* | 1. pathologique 2. anatomopathologique |
| **pathology** *1. The branch of medicine dealing with the study of tissues and the forensic application. 2. Referring to a condition that is abnormal.* | 1. anatomopathologie 2. pathologie |
| **patient** | 1. malade 2. patient |
| **patient chart** | dossier de soin |
| **peak flow** *A measurement of lung function used in asthma.* | débit de pointe |
| **pectineal ligament** *A continuation of the lacunar ligament along the pectineal line in the pubis.* | ligament de Cooper |
| **pectoral** *Referring to the pectoral muscle.* | pectoral |
| **pediatrician** *Physician who is a specialist in pediatrics.* | pédiatre |
| **pediatrics** *Medical specialty concerned with the treatment and prevention of childhood disease.* | pédiatrie |
| **pedicle** *Part of a skin/tissue graft temporarily left connected to the original site.* | pédicule |

| English | French |
|---|---|
| **pediculated** *Referring to pedicle.* | pédiculé |
| **pediculosis** *Lice infestation.* | 1. pédiculose 2. phtiriase |
| **peduncle** *1. A stalk-like protrusion. 2. A bundle of nerve fibers connecting two parts of the brain.* | pédoncule |
| **pellagra** *A deficiency in nicotinic acid exhibited by diarrhea and dermatitis.* | pellagre |
| **pelvic** *Referring to the pelvis.* | pelvien |
| **pelvimetry** *Measurement of the dimensions of the pelvis to determine whether a patient is capable of natural childbirth.* | pelvimétrie |
| **pelvis** *The bony structure at the base of the spine.* | pelvis |
| **pemphigus** *A skin disorder with large bullous lesions.* | pemphigus |
| **penetration** | pénétration |
| **penicillin** *A synthetic antibiotic originally produced from blue mold.* | pénicilline |
| **penis** *Male genital organ used for the transfer of sperm and elimination of urine.* | 1. pénis 2. verge |
| **pentosuria** *The presence of pentose in the urine (a monosaccharide with five carbon atoms in the molecule).* | pentosurie |
| **pepsin** *A proteolytic gastric enzyme.* | pepsine |
| **peptic** *Referring to pepsin or concerning digestion.* | 1. pepsique 2. peptique |
| **peptide** *A compound with low molecular weight and containing two or more amino acids.* | peptide |
| **percussion** *A manual procedure involving tapping a body part to determine the size or density (liquid or air) of a part.* | percussion |
| **perforation** *Presence of a hole.* | perforation |
| **periaqueductal gray matter** *Refers to the brain gray matter adjacent to the periaqueductal.* | substance grise périaqueducale |
| **periarthritis** *Inflammation of the tissues around a joint.* | périarthrite |
| **pericardial** *Referring to around the heart.* | péricardique |
| **pericarditis** *Inflammation of the pericardium.* | péricardite |
| **pericardium** *The structure enclosing the heart which contains a fibrous outer layer and serous inner layer.* | péricarde |
| **perichondritis** *Inflammation of the perichondrium.* | périchondrite |
| **perichondrium** *The membrane that encloses a cartilage.* | périchondre |
| **pericolitis** *Inflammation of the membrane covering the colon.* | péricolite |
| **pericorneal ring** *Also known as Kayser-Fleischer rings exhibited by presence of brown or grey-green rings on the cornea. This is from the deposition of copper and seen in Wilson's disease.* | anneau de Kayser-Fleicher |
| **perilymph** *The fluid separating the membranous and osseous labyrinth.* | périlymphe |
| **perinatology** *The study of disease in the period just before and right after birth.* | médecine périnatale |
| **perineal** *Referring to the perineum.* | périnéal |
| **perineorrhaphy** *Surgical repair of the perineum.* | périnéorraphie |
| **perinephric** *Around the kidney.* | périnéphrétique |

| English | French |
|---|---|
| **perineum** *The area between the anus and scrotum or anus and vulva.* | périnée |
| **periodontal disease** *Present around to a tooth.* | parodontopathie |
| **periosteal** *Referring to the periosteum.* | périostal |
| **periosteal** *Referring to the periosteum.* | périostique |
| **periosteum** *A layer of connective tissue covering the bones.* | périoste |
| **periostitis** *Inflammation of the periosteum.* | périostite |
| **peripheral** *Referring to an outward part or surface.* | périphérique |
| **periproctitis** *Inflammation of the tissue encircling the anus and rectum.* | périproctite |
| **peristalsis** *The contraction of the longitudinal and circular muscle fibers of the alimentary canal so food is propelled.* | péristaltisme |
| **peritomy** *Surgically creating an opening of the periosteum.* | péritomie |
| **peritoneal** *Referring to the peritoneum.* | péritonéal |
| **peritoneum** *The serous membrane covering the abdominal organs and lining the abdominal walls.* | péritoine |
| **peritonitis** *Inflammation of the peritoneum.* | péritonite |
| **peritonsillar** *Surrounding the tonsils.* | périamygdalien |
| **periurethral** *Surrounding the urethra.* | périurétral |
| **permanent teeth** | dents permanentes |
| **pernicious** *1. Having a detrimental effect. 2. Pernicious anemia is a reduced red blood cell count due to Vitamin B12 deficiency.* | pernicieux |
| **pernio** *A localized area of erythema on the toes, fingers, and ears that is pruritic and tender.* | érythème pernio |
| **peroneal** *Referring to the fibula or the outer part of the leg.* | péronier |
| **peroneal atrophy** *Progressive muscle atrophy in the peroneal region.* | amyotrophie péronière de Charcot-Marie |
| **personality** | constitution |
| **perspiration** | perspiration |
| **pertussis** *Synonym for whooping cough.* | coqueluche |
| **pes cavus** *Excessive height of the longitudinal arch of the foot.* | pied creux |
| **pes valgus** *Abnormal longitudinal arch- it is flat.* | pied plat |
| **pessary** *A supportive device placed in the rectum or vagina.* | pessaire |
| **pet** | animal familier |
| **PET scan** *Positron emission tomography.* | tomographie par émission de positons |
| **petechia** *A small red or purple macule on the skin caused by bleeding.* | pétéchie |
| **petrissage** *Massage using a kneading action.* | pétrissage |
| **petrous bone** *Very hard bone, resembling a rock.* | rocher |
| **petrous** *Possessing a density of a stone.* | pétreux |
| **phagocyte** *A cell capable of surrounding and digesting microorganisms.* | phagocyte |
| **phagocytosis** *The action of a phagocyte.* | phagocytose |

| English | French |
|---|---|
| **pharmacist** *A professional who prepares and sells medicine through various systems, including governmental organizations like the Veterans Administration.* | pharmacien |
| **pharmacokinetics** *The study of the distribution, absorption and excretion of drugs within the body.* | pharmacocinétique |
| **pharmacology** *The study of all aspects of medicines.* | pharmacologie |
| **pharmacy** | pharmacie |
| **pharyngeal pouch** *A lateral diverticulum of the pharynx.* | poche pharyngée |
| **pharyngeal** *Referring to the pharynx.* | pharyngé |
| **pharyngectomy** *Surgical excision of part of the pharynx.* | pharyngectomie |
| **pharyngitis** *Inflammation of the pharynx.* | pharyngite |
| **pharyngolaryngectomy** *Surgical removal of part of the pharynx and larynx.* | pharyngolaryn-gectomie |
| **pharyngotympanic tube** *Synonym for eustachian tube.* | trompe d'Eustache |
| **pharynx** *The membranous cavity from the mouth to esophagus.* | pharynx |
| **phenotype** *The visual expression exhibited by a person from the association of the genotype with the environment.* | phénotype |
| **phenylketonuria** *A hereditary condition in which a person cannot excrete phenylalanine; untreated it causes brain and spinal cord dysfunction.* | phénylcétonurie |
| **phlebectomy** *Surgical excision of a vein.* | phlébectomie |
| **phlebitis** *Inflammation of a vein.* | phlébite |
| **phlebothrombosis** *Presence of a clot in a vein, without associated inflammation.* | phlébothrombose |
| **phlegmasia alba dolens** *Phlebitis of the femoral vein that can occur after pregnancy or typhoid fever.* | phlegmatia alba doens |
| **phlegmasia** *Inflammation or fever.* | phlegmatia |
| **phlyctenular** *Related to the formation of small vesicles on the cornea or conjunctiva.* | phlycténulaire |
| **phobia** *An profound fear of something.* | phobie |
| **phonation** *The vocalization of sounds.* | phonation |
| **phoniatrics** *The treatment of speech abnormalities.* | phoniatrie |
| **phosphaturia** *Presence of phosphates in the urine.* | phosphaturie |
| **phospholipid** *A substance, such as lecithin, that when hydrolyzed produces fatty acids, glycerin, and a nitrogen compound.* | phospholipide |
| **phosphonecrosis** *The breakdown of the mandible caused by excessive exposure to phosphorus.* | phosphonécrose |
| **photophobia** *Abnormal sensitivity to light.* | photophobie |
| **photosensitization** *The process of reacting to sunlight by developing edema and dermatitis.* | photosensibilisation |
| **phrenic** *Referring to the diaphragm.* | 1. diaphragmatique 2. phrénique |
| **phrenicectomy** *Surgical excision of the phrenic nerve.* | phrénicectomie |

| English | French |
|---|---|
| **phrenoplegia** *Paralysis of the diaphragm.* | 1. paralysie diaphragmatique 2. phrénoplégie |
| **physical exam** | examen physique |
| **physical therapy** *Treatment of disease by heat, massage and exercise as opposed to medications.* | kinésithérapie |
| **physician** | médecin |
| **physicist** *A person who is trained in the field of physics.* | physicien |
| **physiological saline** *0.9% normal saline.* | sérum physiologique |
| **physiology** *A subspecialty of biology that studies the normal functioning of the body.* | physiologie |
| **physiotherapy** *Physical therapy.* | physiothérapie |
| **pia mater** *The first layer of three covering the brain and spinal cord.* | pie-mère |
| **pica** *A desire for unusual substances as occurs in pregnancy and some psychological conditions.* | pica |
| **pigeon chest** *Abnormal protrusion of the sternum.* | thorax en carène |
| **pill** | pilule |
| **pillow** | oreiller |
| **pilonidal cyst** *A small cone-shaped cluster of tissue situated posterior to the third ventricle of the brain.* | sinus pilonidal |
| **pin; wire** | broche |
| **pineal gland** *A small body posterior to the third ventricle of the brain.* | épiphyse |
| **pinguecula** *The yellow tissue on the bulbar conjunctiva adjacent to the sclerocorneal junction.* | pinguécula |
| **pinning** | embrochage |
| **pinocytosis** *The absorption of fluid into a cell by the formation of vesicles on the cell membrane.* | pinocytose |
| **pinworm** *Common term for Enterobius vermincularis; a nematode worm that is a parasite.* | oxyure |
| **pipet** *A slender tube with a bulb used for transferring liquids.* | pipette |
| **pityriasis rosea** *A skin disease characterized by dry pink oval papulosquamous eruptions.* | pityriasis rosé de Gibert |
| **placebo controlled** *When a study is placebo controlled it means part of the group received an inactive treatment while the other group received active therapy.* | contre-placebo |
| **placenta** *The vascular tissue that nourishes a fetus through an umbilical cord.* | placenta |
| **placenta praevia** *A condition in which the placenta covers the cervical os.* | placenta praevia |
| **placental** *Referring to the placenta.* | placentaire |
| **placental barrier** *The semipermeable membrane of the placenta.* | barrière placentaire |
| **plagiocephaly** *A condition characterized by an asymmetric skull because the cranial sutures do not close normally.* | plagiocéphalie |
| **plantar** *Referring to the bottom of the foot.* | plantaire |

| English | French |
|---|---|
| **plantar fibromatosis** *Deep fascia nodules on the plantar aspect of the feet.* | aponévrosite plantaire |
| **plantar wart** *A viral epidermal growth on the bottom of the foot.* | verrue plantaire |
| **plasma cell** *A cell that produces only one type of antibody.* | plasmocyte |
| **plasmacytosis** *The existence of plasma cells in the blood.* | plasmocytose |
| **plasmapheresis** *A method of removing blood and reinfusing it after the elimination of antibodies.* | plasmaphérèse |
| **plaster** *Dehydrated gypsum that has water added to it in order to immobilize fractured extremities.* | 1. emplâtre 2. plâtre |
| **platelet** *An oval cell without a nucleus used in coagulation; also called a thrombocyte.* | 1. plaquette 2. thrombocyte |
| **platelet clumping** *Aggregation of platelets.* | agrégation plaquettaire |
| **platelet suppressive agent** *A substance that reduces the normal thrombotic effect of platelets.* | antiagrégant plaquettaire |
| **pledget** *A small plug of cotton or other synthetic material inserted into a wound.* | tampon d'ouate |
| **pleomorphism** *The ability of an organism or substance to attain distinct forms.* | pléomorphisme |
| **plethora** *An excess of something.* | pléthore |
| **plethysmograph** *A device used to measure the amount of blood flowing through a body part; impedance plethysmography is used to check for deep venous thrombosis.* | pléthysmographe |
| **pleura** *The serous membrane lining each lung.* | plèvre |
| **pleurisy** *Inflammation of the pleura.* | pleurésie |
| **plica** *A fold, as in a fold in the peritoneum.* | 1. plicature 2. repli |
| **pneumaturia** *Presence of air or gas in the urine.* | pneumaturie |
| **pneumoatocele** *1. A hernia-like protrusion of lung tissue. 2. A collection of gas in a sac such as the scrotum.* | pneumatocèle |
| **pneumococcus** *A bacterium causing pneumonia and meningitis. A common type is Streptococcus pneumoniae.* | pneumocoque |
| **pneumoconiosis** *Fibrosis of the lung due to dust inhalation.* | pneumoconiose |
| **pneumonectomy** *Surgical excision of all or part of a lung.* | pneumonectomie |
| **pneumonia** *Inflammation of the lung due to an infection caused by a virus or bacterium.* | pneumonie |
| **pneumoperitoneum** *Abnormal or induced presence of air or gas in the peritoneum.* | pneumopéritoine |
| **pneumothorax** *Abnormal presence of air between the lung and chest wall.* | pneumothorax |
| **poikilocytosis** *The presence of abnormally shaped erythrocytes.* | poïkilocytose |
| **poison** | poison |
| **polioencephalitis** *Polio infection of the brain.* | polioencéphalite |
| **poliomyelitis** *An infectious viral disease exhibited by constitutional symptoms that can lead to quadriplegia.* | poliomyélite |
| **polyarteritis nodosa** *A systemic necrotizing vasculitis that effects medium sized arteries.* | périartérite noueuse |

| English | French |
|---|---|
| **polychondritis** *Inflammation of the cartilage at more than one site.* | polychondrite |
| **polycystic** *Possessing more than one cyst.* | polykystique |
| **polycythemia** *Excess in the number of erythrocytes in the blood.* | 1. polycythémie 2. polyglobulie |
| **polycythemia vera** *Condition characterized by increase in erythrocytes, thrombocytes and leukocytes, as well as, splenomegaly.* | polyglobulie essentielle |
| **polydactyly** *Congenital anomaly exhibited by more than 5 digits on the hands and/or feet.* | polycactylie |
| **polydipsia** *Profound thirst.* | polydipsie |
| **polymenorrhea** *Increase in the frequency of menstruation.* | polyménorrhée |
| **polymyositis** *Inflammation of several muscle groups at once.* | polymyosite |
| **polyneuritis** *Inflammation of more than one nerve.* | polynévrite |
| **polyneuropathy** *A condition involving more than one nerve.* | polyneuropathie |
| **polyopia** *A condition in which one object is seen abnormally as two or more.* | polyopie |
| **polyposis** *The formation of multiple polyps.* | polypose |
| **polypus** *Synonym of polyp (a prominent growth from a mucous membrane).* | polype |
| **polysaccharide** *A carbohydrate that upon hydrolysis forms more than ten monosaccharides.* | polyoside |
| **polysialia** *Abnormal increase in saliva.* | 1. polysialie 2. ptyalisme |
| **polytrauma** *A condition exhibited by multiple injuries from blunt or penetrating trauma.* | polytraumatisme |
| **polyuria** *Abnormal increase in volume of urine excreted.* | polyurie |
| **pompholyx** *A condition exhibited by interdigital vesicles of the hands and feet.* | 1. dyshidrose 2. pompholyx |
| **pons** *The part of the brainstem that connects the medulla oblongata with the thalamus.* | protubérance annulaire |
| **pontine** *Referring to the pons.* | protubérantiel |
| **popliteal** *Referring to the posterior knee.* | poplité |
| **porphyria** *A hereditary condition currently classified based on the specific enzyme deficiency. The most common form is porphyria cutanea tarda that causes blistering lesions.* | porphyrie |
| **porphyrin** *A class of pigments that contain a flat ring of four heterocyclic groups.* | porphyrine |
| **portal** *Referring to an entrance such as porta hepatis.* | portail |
| **positive** | positif |
| **post-mortem changes** | phénomènes cadavériques |
| **post-term pregnancy** *A pregnancy that has gone beyond the expected length of time.* | grossesse prolongée |
| **post-voiding** *After urinating. A post-void residual is a measurement of the urine in the bladder after one urinates.* | post-mictionnel |
| **postabortal** *The period immediately after an abortion.* | post-abortum |

112

| English | French |
|---|---|
| posterior | postérieur |
| posterior chamber of the eye *An aqueous filled space between the cornea and the lens.* | chambre postérieure de l'œil |
| posterior columns *The dorsal portion of the gray matter of the spinal cord.* | voies cordonales postérieures |
| postmaturity *Generally referring to a pregnancy that goes beyond the due date.* | post-maturité |
| postpartum psychosis *A serious mental condition that occurs following pregnancy.* | psychose puerpérale |
| postpone | différer |
| postponement | ajournement |
| postural *Referring to position or posture.* | postural |
| potassium *A chemical of the alkali metal group.* | potassium |
| potency *Strength or power.* | puissance |
| pounding | martelage |
| powder | poudre |
| pox *A general term for fluid filled papules that upon rupturing leave pockmarks.* | vérole |
| preauricular *Anterior to the ear.* | préauriculaire |
| precancerous *Referring to an early stage in cancer development.* | précancéreux |
| precipitin *An antibody-antigen reaction producing a precipitate.* | précipitine |
| precordialgia *Pain in the precordium.* | précordialgie |
| precordium *The area occupying the epigastrum and lower sternum.* | 1. précordium 2. région précordiale |
| premature *Occurring earlier than expected.* | prématuré |
| premenstrual *Occurring prior to the onset of menstruation.* | prémenstruel |
| premolar *The teeth anterior to the molars.* | prémolaire |
| prenatal care *Medical care received while one is pregnant.* | hygiène de la grossesse |
| prenatal *Referring to the time prior to birth.* | prénatal |
| presbyacusia *An age related, progressive hearing loss.* | presbyacousie |
| presbyophrenia *Also called Wernicke's dementia, it is exhibited by confusion, amnesia and confabulation.* | presbyophrénie |
| presbyopia *Farsightedness associated with aging.* | presbytie |
| prescriber | prescripteur |
| prescription | 1. ordonnance 2. prescription |
| presenting symptom *The initial subjective complaint that initiated a visit.* | symptôme révélateur |
| pressure reducer *Anti-hypertensive agent.* | détendeur |
| pressure ulcer *Loss in skin integrity due to a portion of the body being in the same position for too long and possibly other factors.* | escarre de pression |
| presystole *The time just before systole.* | présystole |
| prevent, to | éviter |
| priapism *A painful and abnormally prolonged erection.* | priapisme |

113

| English | French |
|---|---|
| **prickly heat** *A rash with small vesicles that is pruritic and associated with a warm moist environment.* | bourbouille |
| **primipara** *A woman giving birth for the first time.* | primipare |
| **prior status** *Referring to a person's previous state of health.* | état antérieur |
| **probing** | sondage |
| **problem** | 1. difficulté 2. problème |
| **proctalgia** *A chronic high, dull rectal pain worse with sitting position.* | proctalgie |
| **proctectomy** *Surgical excision of the rectum.* | proctectomie |
| **proctitis** *Inflammation of the rectum.* | 1. proctite 2. rectite |
| **proctocele** *A hernia-type protrusion of the rectum into the vagina.* | proctocèle |
| **proctoscopy** *Inspection of the rectum with a scope.* | proctoscopie |
| **progeria** *A childhood disorder exhibited by signs of aging including gray hair, wrinkled skin and short height.* | progérie |
| **progesterone** *A steroid hormone that prepares the uterus for pregnancy.* | progestérone |
| **proglottis** *Any segment of a tapeworm.* | proglottis |
| **prognosis** | pronostic |
| **progressive** | 1. évolutif 2. progressif |
| **prolactin** *A pituitary hormone that facilitates milk production.* | prolactine |
| **prolapse** *The slipping downward of a body part, such as rectal prolapse.* | 1. procidence 2. prolapsus |
| **promonocyte** *An intermediate cell stage between monocyte and monoblast.* | 1. monoblaste 2. promonocyte |
| **promontory** *A protruding eminence.* | promontoire |
| **pronation** *Turning posteriorly. When the hand is pronated, it is turned medially until the palm is facing posteriorly (when the body was initially in the anatomic position).* | pronation |
| **prone** *Lying with the abdomen and face downward.* | procubitus |
| **prophylaxis** *That which is done to prevent disease.* | prophylaxie |
| **proprioceptor** *A receptor that responds to sensory input including position sense.* | propriocepteur |
| **proptosis oculi** *Synonym of exophthalmos; bulging of the eye.* | protrusion oculaire |
| **prostacyclin** *A prostaglandin that functions as an anticoagulant and vasodilator.* | prostacycline |
| **prostaglandin** *A compound first found in semen (thus "prosta" in the name from prostate) with many effects including uterine contraction.* | prostaglandine |
| **prostate** *A gland found in men that surrounds the neck of the urethra and bladder.* | prostate |
| **prostatectomy** *Surgical excision of the prostate.* | prostatectomie |
| **prosthesis** *An artificial body part.* | prothèse |
| **prostration** *Profound exhaustion.* | abattement |
| **protein** *A class of nitrogenous organic compound.* | protéine |
| **proteinuria** *The presence of protein in the urine.* | protéinurie |
| **proteolysis** *Enzyme action on proteins to form amino acids.* | protéolyse |

114

| English | French |
|---------|--------|
| **prothrombin** *A compound converted to thrombin during coagulation of blood.* | prothrombine |
| **protoplasm** *The cytoplasm, organelles and nucleus of a living cell.* | protoplasme |
| **protozoa** *A single celled microscopic organism including amoebas among others.* | protozoaire |
| **provoke, to** | provoquer |
| **proximal** *Situated closer to the center of the body (opposed to that which is farther away, as in distal).* | proximal |
| **pruritis** *A general term for conditions exhibited by itching.* | prurit |
| **pseudarthrosis** *Deossification of weight bearing long bones.* | pseudarthrose |
| **pseudobulbar palsy** *Sudden outbursts of laughter or tearfulness sometimes seen in amyotrophic lateral sclerosis.* | paralysie pseudobulbaire |
| **pseudomnesia** *Sensing the memory of an event that has never happened.* | déjà-vu |
| **psittacosis** *A chlamydial pneumonia that is transmitted by birds.* | psittacose |
| **psoitis** *Inflammation of the psoas muscle.* | psoïtis |
| **psoriasis** *A chronic papulosquamous dermatosis characterized by silver plaques.* | psoriasis |
| **psychasthenia** *Essentially any non-hysterical neuroses.* | psychasthénie |
| **psychiatry** *A branch of medicine specializing in the treatment of mental disorders.* | psychiatrie |
| **psychologist** *A professional specializing in psychology.* | psycholgue |
| **psychology** *The study of the human mind and emotions.* | psychologie |
| **psychoneurosis** *A mental disorder that could include depression or anxiety but does not include hallucinations.* | psychonévrose |
| **psychopathology** *Scientific examination of mental disease.* | psychopathologie |
| **psychosis** *A profound mental disorder that can include delusions and hallucinations.* | psychose |
| **psychosomatic** *Physical ailments arising from mental disease.* | psychosomatique |
| **psychotherapy** *Treatment of mental disease with cognitive-behavioral approaches.* | psychothérapie |
| **pterygium** *A membrane in the interpalpebral fissure present from the conjunctiva to the cornea.* | ptérigion |
| **ptosis** *Drooping of the upper eyelid usually due to paralysis of the third cranial nerve.* | ptose |
| **ptyalin** *An enzyme found in saliva.* | 1. amylase salivaire 2. ptyaline |
| **puberty** *The time when adolescents become capable of sexual reproduction.* | puberté |
| **pubis** *The anterior inferior part of the hip bone on each side that articulates at the pubic symphysis.* | pubis |
| **pudendal** *Referring to the female genitalia* | 1. honteux 2. vulvaire 3. pudendal |
| **pudendum muliebre vulva** *The mons, pubis, labia majora, labia minora and the vagina.* | vulve |
| **puerpera** *A woman who just gave birth.* | accouchée |

| English | French |
|---|---|
| **puerperium** *The six week period after childbirth.* | 1. puerpéralité 2. suite de couches 3. puerpérum |
| **puffed** | essoufflé |
| **puffiness** | bouffissure |
| **pull, to** | tirer |
| **pulmonary** *Referring to the lungs.* | pulmonaire |
| **pulmonary stenosis** *A stricture between the pulmonary artery and the right ventricle.* | rétrécissement pulmonaire |
| **pulp** *The tissue filling the root canals of a tooth.* | pulpe |
| **pulpitis** *Dental pulp inflammation.* | pulpite |
| **pulsation** | pulsation |
| **pulse** *The rhythmic throbbing of arteries felt at major vessels.* | pouls |
| **pulsus alternans** *A regular alternation of weak and strong beats of the pulse.* | pouls alternant |
| **pupil** *The opening at the center of the iris.* | pupille |
| **purpura** *The presence of patches of ecchymosis or petechiae.* | purpura |
| **purulent** *Referring to pus.* | 1. purulent 2. suppuré |
| **pus** | pus |
| **putrefaction** *The rotting or decaying of organic matter.* | putréfaction |
| **pyelitis** *Renal pelvis inflammation.* | pyélite |
| **pyelography** *Roentgenography of the renal pelvis and ureters after administration of contrast media.* | pyélographie |
| **pyelolithotomy** *Surgical excision of a calculus from the renal pelvis.* | pyélolithotomie |
| **pyemia** *Sepsis characterized by the presence of secondary abscesses.* | 1. pyémie 2. septicopyohémie |
| **pyknic** *Possessing a short, stocky physique.* | pycnique |
| **pyknosis** *The degeneration of a cell with the nucleus shrinking.* | pycnose |
| **pyloric** *Referring to the pylorus.* | pylorique |
| **pyloroplasty** *Surgical enlargement of a pylorus that previously was stenotic.* | pyloroplastie |
| **pylorus** *The opening at the distal stomach that opens into the duodenum.* | pylore |
| **pyoderma** *A purulent skin infection.* | pyodermite |
| **pyogenic** *Referring to the formation of pus.* | pyogène |
| **pyonephrosis** *Injury to the renal parenchyma due to pus.* | pyonéphrose |
| **pyorrhea** *Emission of pus.* | pyorrhée |
| **pyosalpinx** *Purulent material in the oviduct.* | pyosalpinx |
| **pyramidal** *A term that is used to describe various spinal tracts that originate in the cerebral cortex.* | pyramidal |
| **pyrexia** *Fever.* | pyrexie |
| **pyridoxine** *Synonym for vitamin B6.* | pyridoxine |
| **pyrogen** *A fever producing substance released by bacteria.* | pyrogène |
| **pyrosis** *Synonym for heartburn.* | pyrosis |

| English | French |
|---|---|
| **pytalism** *Synonym of polysialia.* | sialorrhée |
| **pyuria** *Presence of purulent material in the urine.* | pyurie |
| **Q fever** *A disease caused by rickettsiae from the ingestion of unpasteurized milk.* | fièvre Q |
| **quadriceps jerk (reflex)** | réflexe rotulien |
| **quadriceps** *The anterior thigh muscle composed of four muscles.* | quadriceps |
| **quadrigeminal bodies** *The cranial and caudal colliculi.* | tubercules quadrijumeaux |
| **quadriplegia** *Paralysis of all four extremities.* | 1. quadriplégie 2. tétraplégie |
| **qualify** | qualifier |
| **quarantine** *A place of isolation for infectious persons until it can be certain it is safe to let them mingle.* | quarantaine |
| **querulousness** *Whining or complaining.* | quérulence |
| **quiescent** *A time of inactivity.* | dormant |
| **quiet** | calme |
| **quinsy** *Peritonsillar inflammation or abscess.* | angine phlegmoneuse |
| **rabbeting** *The interlocking of two sections of a fractured bone.* | engrènement |
| **rabies** *An infectious viral disease transmitted through the bite of a mammal. Symptoms include hydrophobia, pharyngeal spasms and hyperactivity.* | rage |
| **racemose** *A gland having the form of a cluster.* | racémeux |
| **radial** *Referring to the radius.* | radial |
| **radiation** *1. The emission of energy in the form of electromagnetic waves. 2. Divergence from a common point.* | radiation |
| **radiculitis** *Inflammation of a spinal nerve root.* | radiculite |
| **radioactive** *Referring to the emission of ionizing particles or radiation.* | radioactif |
| **radioactive isotope** *An isotope with an unstable nucleus that is used in diagnostic imaging.* | isotope radioactif |
| **radiobiology** *The study of the effects of radiation on organisms.* | radiobiologie |
| **radioepithelitis** *The injury to epithelial cells due to effects of radiation.* | radiomucite |
| **radiography** *The department where images are produced on sensitive film by x-rays.* | radiographie |
| **radiologist** *A physician specializing in radiology.* | radiologiste |
| **radiology** *The branch of medicine concerned with roentgenography and other high-energy radiation.* | radiologie |
| **radionuclide** *A radioactive nuclide.* | 1. isotopique 2. radionucléide |
| **radiosensitivity** *The susceptibility of the skin to radiation.* | radiosensibilité |
| **radiotherapy** *Treatment of cancer with radiation.* | radiothérapie |
| **rage** | fureur |
| **raise** | élever |
| **rale** *An abnormal lung sound noted during auscultation.* | râle |

| English | French |
|---|---|
| **ramus** *A branch; a term used to describe a smaller vessel branching off from a larger one.* | rameau |
| **ramus** *Branch.* | branche |
| **ranula** *A retention cyst formed because of obstruction of a salivary gland in the floor of the mouth.* | 1. grenouillette 2. ranula |
| **rape** *Forced sexual relations.* | viol |
| **Rapid Eye Movement** *The movement of a person's eyes during this period of sleep.* | mouvement oculaire rapide |
| **rash** | rash |
| **rat bite fever** *As the name implies, it is a condition exhibited by fever, nausea and skin erythema after one is bitten by a rat.* | sodoku |
| **reactive** *Reagent.* | réactif |
| **rebound** *A term used to describe a type of tenderness found with peritonitis.* | rebond |
| **receptor** *A cell or organ that accepts stimuli and transmits data to a sensory nerve.* | récepteur |
| **recessive** *This refers to genetic controlled traits that are only inherited when code from both parents is the same.* | récessif |
| **recollection** *Memory.* | souvenir |
| **rectal tube placement** | sondage rectale |
| **rectal digital examination** *Use of a gloved finger to assess the rectal vault.* | toucher rectal |
| **rectal** *Referring to the rectum.* | rectal |
| **rectocele** *A herniation of the wall between the rectum and vagina.* | rectocèle |
| **rectoscopy** *Visualization of the rectum with a scope.* | rectoscopie |
| **rectosigmoidectomy** *Surgical resection of the rectum and sigmoid colon.* | rectosigmoïdectomie |
| **rectovesical septum** *The wall between the rectum and the urinary bladder.* | aponévrose de Denonvilliers |
| **rectus abdominis muscle** *The pair of long, flat muscles that connect the sternum with the pubis.* | 1. grand droit de l'abdomen 2. rectus abdominis muscle |
| **recumbent** *Lying down.* | couché |
| **red nucleus** *A collection of gray matter near the subthalamus that receives data from the superior cerebellar peduncle.* | noyau rouge |
| **reduction** *Return of a dislocated joint or fractured bone to its proper position.* | réduction |
| **referred pain** *Pain felt in an area distinct from the original source.* | douleur projetée |
| **regardless of** | quel que soit |
| **regurgitation** *1. Backflow of blood in the heart. 2. Movement of gastric contents into the mouth.* | régurgitation |
| **relapse** | rechute |
| **relapsing fever** *A recurrent bacterial infection, with fever, caused by Spirochetes.* | borréliose |
| **related to** | en rapport avec |

| English | French |
|---|---|
| **relation** *1. A person who has a blood or marriage connection. 2. Intercourse (if sexual, that is defined).* | relation |
| **relaxant** *Term generally used to refer to a muscle relaxant.* | décontracturant |
| **relaxin** *A hormone secreted by the placenta which dilates the cervix.* | relaxine |
| **releasing hormone** *Hormones that come from one gland such as the thalamus that cause release of hormones from another gland such as the pituitary.* | libération, hormone de |
| **reliability** | fiabilité |
| **relief** | soulagement |
| **relieve, to** | soulager |
| **REM (rapid eye movement) sleep** *This period of sleep is associated with irregular respirations and heart rate, involuntary movements and dreaming.* | sommeil à mouvements oculaires rapides (MOR) |
| **remission** *A decrease in severity or a temporary resolution.* | rémission |
| **removal** | 1. ablation 2. enlèvement |
| **renal** *Referring to the kidney.* | rénal |
| **renal colic** *Pain caused by passage of a calculus through the ureter.* | colique néphrétique |
| **renal failure** *Diminution of kidney function.* | insuffisance rénale |
| **renal pelvis** *The kidney collecting system.* | bassinet rénal |
| **renal threshold** *The level of glucose in the blood that the kidneys begin to excrete glucose in the urine.* | seuil rénal |
| **renin** *A renal enzyme that facilitates the production of angiotensin.* | rénine |
| **resection** *The removal of tissue.* | résection |
| **residual urine** *The amount of urine remaining in the bladder after a person voids.* | résidu vésical |
| **residual volume (RV)** *The amount of air left in the lung after a maximal exhalation.* | 1. air résiduel 2. volume résiduel |
| **resilient nystagmus** *A type of nystagmus in which there is slow movement in one direction and a quick movement in the other.* | nystagmus à ressort |
| **resin** *An organic substance that is insoluble in water. There are many types. Cholestyramine resin is used for hypercholesterolemia.* | résine |
| **resorbable suture (chromic)** | fil résorbable (chromic) |
| **respirator** *A device used to artificially ventilate a patient.* | respirateur |
| **respiratory** *Referring to respiration or the organs of respiration.* | respiratoire |
| **respiratory dead space** *The area between the mouth and the alveoli.* | espace mort respiratoire |
| **respiratory distress syndrome** *A disease in infants that is caused by a surfactant deficiency.* | détresse respiratoire, syndrome de |
| **respiratory rate** *The number of breaths per minute.* | fréquence respiratoire |
| **rest** | repos |
| **resting potential** *The electrical capability of a neuron compared to its surroundings.* | potentiel de repos |

119

| English | French |
|---|---|
| **restless legs** *Associated with a syndrome exhibited by continuous movement of the legs from uncertain etiology.* | impatiences |
| **resumption of menses** *A phrase used to describe the time when menstruation begins for the first time after childbirth.* | retour de couches |
| **retching** *Spasm of the stomach without presence of gastric material.* | haut-le-cœur |
| **reticular** *Referring to a matrix of membranous tubules inside the cytoplasm of a eukaryotic cells.* | réticulaire |
| **reticulo-endothelial** *Referring to the system of phagocytes involved in the immune system.* | réticulo-endothélial |
| **reticulocyte** *A red blood cell without a nucleus.* | 1. hématie granuleuse 2. réticulocyte |
| **reticulocytosis** *An abnormal increase in circulating reticulocytes.* | réticulocytose |
| **retina** *The innermost of three layers of the eyeball; it surrounds the vitreous body and is continuous with the optic nerve.* | rétine |
| **retinal detachment** *A tear or hole in the retina caused by vitreous traction.* | décollement de rétine |
| **retinitis** *Inflammation of the retina.* | rétinite |
| **retinoblastoma** *A tumor consisting of retinal germ cells.* | rétinoblastome |
| **retinopathy** *Any one of a number of retinal inflammatory conditions.* | rétinopathie |
| **retraction** *Being drawn back.* | rétraction |
| **retractor** *A device for pulling back tissue during surgery.* | 1. écarteur 2. rétracteur |
| **retrobulbar optic neuritis** *An inflammatory, demyelinating condition in the retrobulbar region.* | névrite optique rétrobulbaire |
| **retroflexed uterus** *Bending back of the uterus so that the top portion pushes against the rectum.* | utérus rétrofléchi |
| **retrograde** *Referring to backward movement.* | rétrograde |
| **retroperitoneal** *Situated or referring to the area posterior to the peritoneum.* | rétropéritonéal |
| **retropharyngeal** *Referring to the area posterior to the pharynx.* | rétropharyngé |
| **rhagade** *Fissures in the skin, particularly adjacent to body orifices.* | rhagade |
| **rheumatic** *Referring to rheumatism.* | rhumatismal |
| **rheumatic fever** *A febrile streptococcal disease causing pain and joint swelling.* | rhumatisme articulaire aigu |
| **rheumatic heart disease** *A manifestation of rheumatic fever, frequently causing valvular dysfunction.* | cardiopathie rhumatismale |
| **rheumatism** *Any condition exhibited by inflammation and pain in the joints and muscles.* | rhumatisme |
| **rheumatoid arthritis** *A symmetric peripheral polyarthritis.* | polyarthrite rhumatoïde |
| **rhinitis** *A viral infection or allergic reaction exhibited by nasal mucosal inflammation.* | rhinite |
| **rhinoplasty** *Plastic surgery performed on the nose.* | rhinoplastie |
| **rhinorrhea** *Abundant nasal mucosal drainage.* | rhinorrhée |
| **rhinoscopy** *Examination of the nasal passages.* | rhinoscopie |

| English | French |
|---|---|
| **rhizotomy** *Interruption of the spinal nerve roots within the spinal canal.* | 1. radicotomie 2. rhizotomie |
| **rhodopsin** *A reddish purple light sensitive pigment in the human retina.* | 1. pourpre rétinien 2. rhodopsine |
| **rhomboid** *A back muscle that elevates, retracts and adducts the scapula.* | rhomboïde |
| **rhonchus** *A coarse, dry sound heard on auscultation of the lungs.* | ronchus |
| **rhythm** | rythme |
| **rib** | côte |
| **rib cage** | cage thoracique |
| **riboflavin** *Also called vitamin B2, this essential vitamin is present in food such as eggs and is synthesized in the small bowel.* | 1. lactoflavine 2. riboflavine 3. vitamine B2 |
| **ribonucleic acid** *An acid present in all living cells, it is a messenger for DNA.* | ribonucléique acide |
| **ribosomal RNA** *Four chains designated by their appropriate coefficients.* | ARN ribosomal |
| **rickets** *A condition exhibited by softening and bowing of the long bones; caused by Vitamin D deficiency.* | rachitisme |
| **rickettsia** *A disease transmitted by ticks or fleas, caused by a bacterium from the genus Rickettsieae. Rocky Mountain Spotted fever is one of many diseases caused by this bacterium.* | rickettsie |
| **rigor mortis** *The normal stiffening of the muscles and joints that occurs a few hours after death.* | rigidité cadavérique |
| **ring** | anneau |
| **ringworm** *A fungal skin infection exhibited by pruritic well circumscribed patches on the scalp or feet.* | dermatophytose |
| **risus sardonicus** *A spasm of the facial muscles causing what appears to be a smile on one's face.* | rictus sardonique |
| **rocking** | balancement |
| **Rocky Mountain spotted fever** *A Rickettsial disease transmitted by ticks exhibited by fever, malaise and rash.* | fièvre pourprée des Montagnes Rocheuses |
| **rodent** | rongeur |
| **Roentgen** *One unit of ionizing radiation named after the German physicist Wilhelm Conrad Röntgen.* | Roentgen |
| **room; chamber** | chambre |
| **root** | racine |
| **rotation** | rotation |
| **rotator cuff** *The structure around the capsule of the shoulder joint formed by the infraspinatus, supraspinatus, teres minor and subscapularis muscles.* | coiffe des rotateurs |
| **round ligament** *The supporting structure of the uterus.* | ligament rond |
| **rubefacient** *A substance that reddens the skin.* | rubéfiant |
| **rude** | grossier |
| **rugine** *A surgical instrument that resembles a rasp.* | rugine |

| English | French |
|---|---|
| **ruling out** | excluant |
| **running suture** *A method of sewing a wound in which there is a knot at each end and continuous otherwise.* | surjet |
| **rupia** *A sign of tertiary syphilis in which there are bullae or vesicles formed on the skin that erupt and form crusts.* | rupia |
| **rupture** | rupture |
| **sacral** *Referring to the sacrum.* | sacré |
| **sacral canal** *The portion of the vertebral canal that progresses into the sacrum.* | canal sacré |
| **sacralization** *The fusion of the fifth lumbar vertebra to the sacrum.* | sacralisation |
| **sacrum** *The bone formed by five fused vertebrae that is situated between the two hip bones.* | sacrum |
| **saddle joint** *A joint that exhibits two saddle type surfaces at a 90 degree angle to each other, such as the carpometacarpal joint.* | articulation en selle |
| **sadness** | tristesse |
| **sagittal suture** *The line where the two parietal bones meet.* | suture sagittale |
| **Saint Vitus' dance** *A childhood chorea associated with rheumatic fever.* | Saint-Guy, danse de |
| **saline** *A solution of sodium chloride.* | 1. salin 2. solution salée |
| **saliva** | salive |
| **salivary gland** *The parotid, submandibular and sublingual glands that secrete saliva.* | gland salivaire |
| **salivation** *The process of secreting saliva.* | salivation |
| **salpingectomy** *Surgical resection of the fallopian tubes.* | salpingectomie |
| **salpingitis** *Inflammation of the fallopian tubes.* | salpingite |
| **salpingography** *Roentgenography of the fallopian tubes after administration of contrast media.* | salpingographie |
| **salpingostomy** *A surgical procedure involving cutting the fallopian tube.* | salpingostomie |
| **salt** | sel |
| **saluretic** *An agent that promotes excretion of sodium and chloride in the urine.* | salidiurétique |
| **sampling** | échantillonnage |
| **sandfly fever** *A febrile illness transmitted by a sandfly, from the genus Phlebotomus, and found in the Mediterranean.* | fièvre à phlébotome |
| **sanitary cordon** | cordon sanitaire |
| **saphena** *Referring to either of the two superficial saphenous veins.* | saphène |
| **saponify** *The creation of soap from oil using an alkali.* | saponification |
| **saprophyte** *Any organism living on dead organic material.* | saprophyte |
| **sarcoid** *Referring to sarcoidosis.* | sarcoïde |
| **sarcoidosis** *A chronic disease characterized by lymphadenopathy and widespread granulomas.* | 1. sarcoïdose 2. maladie de Besnier-Boeck-Schaumann |
| **sarcolemme** *The sheath that covers skeletal muscle fibers.* | sarcolemme |

| English | French |
|---|---|
| **sarcoma** *A non-epithelial malignant tumor.* | sarcome |
| **sartorius muscle** *The thigh muscle that runs from the pelvis to the proximal, medial aspect of the tibia.* | 1. couturier muscle 2. sartorius muscle |
| **saturation** *An amount, expressed in a percentage, that expresses the degree something is absorbed versus the maximal absorption possible.* | saturation |
| **saw** | scie |
| **scabies** *A skin condition exhibited by intense pruritis and a macular rash commonly in the perineal and interdigital spaces.* | 1. gale 2. scabies |
| **scabietic** *Referring to scabies.* | psorique |
| **scalding** *A burn injury from extremely hot water.* | bouillant |
| **scale** *A device to check a person's weight.* | balance |
| **scalp** | 1. cuir chevelu 2. scalp |
| **scalpel** *A knife used during surgery for incision of skin and tissue.* | scalpel |
| **scaphocephaly** *A condition exhibited by a long narrow skull because of early closure of the sagittal sutures.* | scaphocéphalie |
| **scaphoid bone** *The most lateral of the carpal bones; it articulates with the radius.* | scaphoïde carpien |
| **scapula** *Medical term for the shoulder blade.* | 1. omoplate 2. scapulaire |
| **scapulalgia** *Scapular pain.* | scapulalgie |
| **scarification** *Multiple small scratches of the skin, as is sometimes used for vaccine administration.* | scarification |
| **scarlet fever** *A condition caused by streptococci that is exhibited by fever and a bright red (scarlet) rash.* | scarlatine |
| **scatter** | dispersion |
| **scheme** | plan |
| **schistocyte** *Part of a red blood cell seen in hemolytic anemia.* | 1. schistocyte 2. schizocyte |
| **schistosomiasis** *A condition, sometimes known as bilharzia, which involves infestation with flukes of the genus Schistosoma.* | schistosomiase |
| **schizophrenia** *A chronic mental condition exhibited by delusions, hallucinations, and faulty perception.* | schizophrénie |
| **sciatica** *Pain radiating from the buttock down the back of the leg; it is caused by a compressed spinal nerve root.* | sciatalgie |
| **scimitar syndrome** *Part or all of the right lung venous outflow goes into the inferior vena cava.* | syndrome du cimeterre |
| **scirrhus** *A cancer that is hard to palpation.* | squirrhe |
| **scissors** | ciseaux |
| **sclera** *The white outer covering of the eyeball.* | sclérotique |
| **scleritis** *Inflammation of the eyeball.* | sclérite |
| **sclerodactylia** *Scleroderma of the digits.* | sclérodactylie |
| **scleroderma** *A systemic disease of the connective tissues.* | sclérodermie |
| **sclerotomy** *Surgical incision of the sclera.* | sclérotomie |
| **scolex** *The front end of a tapeworm.* | scolex |

| English | French |
|---|---|
| **scoliosis** *A lateral curvature of the spine.* | scoliose |
| **scopophilia** *Sexual please attained by viewing sexual organs.* | scopophilie |
| **scotoma** *A blind spot within an otherwise normal visual field.* | scotome |
| **scrape** | éraflure |
| **scratch** | égratignure |
| **screening** | dépistage |
| **scrotal** *Referring to the scrotum.* | scrotal |
| **scrotal hydrocele** *A benign collection of fluid in the scrotum.* | hydrocèle vaginale |
| **scrotum** *The sac which contains the testes.* | scrotum |
| **scurvy** *A disease of vitamin C deficiency exhibited by bleeding gums.* | scorbut |
| **scutulum** *A crust of tinea capitis.* | godet |
| **scybalum** *A hard, dry formation of stool in the bowel.* | scybales |
| **seals** | scellés |
| **sebaceous** *Referring to a sebaceous gland or what it secretes.* | sébacé |
| **sebaceous gland** *A gland in the skin that secretes sebum.* | gland sébacée |
| **seborrhea** *Abnormal amount of sebum production.* | séborrhée |
| **secretin** *A hormone that increases secretion from the pancreas and liver.* | sécrétine |
| **secretion** *The discharge of substances from cells or glands.* | sécrétion |
| **sedative** *A medication used to facilitate sleep or calm a person.* | 1. calmant 2. sédatif |
| **seeding** *A term used to describe planting of microbes into various parts of the body during an infection.* | ensemencement |
| **seizure** *An episode of tonic/clonic movement noted in epilepsy.* | ictus |
| **self-regulation** *An organ that functions without external input.* | autorégulation |
| **semen analysis** *Evaluation of semen used as part of a fertility workup.* | spermogramme |
| **semicircular canal** *The anterior, posterior and lateral canals in the inner ear that assist in balance control.* | canal semi-circulaire |
| **seminiferous tubules** *Used for transport of semen.* | tubes séminifères |
| **seminoma** *A malignant tumor of the testis.* | séminoma |
| **senescence** *The normal process of deterioration with age.* | sénescence |
| **senile** *Generally referring to mental deterioration associated with aging.* | sénile |
| **senility** *The process of being senile.* | sénilité |
| **sensation** *A perception when one is touched.* | sensation |
| **sensibility** *Ability to feel or perceive.* | sensibilité |
| **sensible** | sensé |
| **sensitization** *The change in an organ by a hormone so it will respond to another stimulus.* | sensibilisation |
| **sensitized** *Being abnormally sensitive to a substance.* | sensibilisé |
| **sensory nerve** *A nerve that receives input from various receptors.* | sensitif nerf |
| **sepsis** *A condition exhibited by overwhelming inflammation due to infection.* | 1. infection bactérienne 2. sepsie |
| **septic** *Referring to a state of sepsis.* | septique |

| English | French |
| --- | --- |
| **septicemia** *A systemic disease in which microorganisms or their toxins are in the blood stream.* | septicémie |
| **septum** *A wall separating two chambers, the nasal septum for example.* | 1. cloison 2. septum |
| **sequela** *A medical problem related to an initial injury or disease.* | séquelle |
| **sequestrum** *Necrotic bone present in an injured or diseased bone.* | séquestre |
| **serial** | sérié |
| **series** | série |
| **serotonin** *A neurotransmitter that constricts blood vessels.* | sérotonine |
| **serous** *Referring to serum or similar to serum.* | séreux |
| **serpiginous** *A skin lesion having wavy margin.* | serpigineux |
| **serum** *The fluid that isolates out when blood coagulates.* | sérum |
| **sessile** *Having a broad base with no stalk.* | sessile |
| **severe** | grave |
| **sex** | sexe |
| **sexual intercourse** | rapport sexuel |
| **sexually transmitted disease (STD)** *A condition one obtains from another during sexual relations.* | malade sexuellement transmissible (MST) |
| **shaking** | ébranlement |
| **sharp pain** | douleur exquise |
| **sheath** *A covering.* | gaine |
| **sheet** | drap |
| **shellfish** | coquillage |
| **shield** | écran |
| **shock** *A condition characterized by systemic hypoperfusion.* | choc |
| **shoe** | chaussure |
| **shortening** | raccourcissement |
| **shoulder** | épaule |
| **shunt** *An alternate path for blood or fluid.* | shunt |
| **sialadenitis** *Inflammation of a salivary gland.* | sialadénite |
| **sialogogue** *A substance that increase salivary flow.* | sialagogue |
| **sialolith** *A calculus in a salivary duct.* | sialolithe |
| **siblings** | fratrie |
| **sickle-cell anemia** *A hereditary type of anemia characterized by crescent shaped red blood cells.* | drépanocytose |
| **side** | côté |
| **side effect** | effet secondaire |
| **siderosis** *Excess iron in the blood or a pulmonary disease from iron inhalation called Pneumoconiosis.* | sidérose |
| **sigh, to** | soupir |
| **sigmoid** *Referring to the portion of the colon that leads into the rectum.* | sigmoïde |
| **sigmoidoscopy** *Visualization of the sigmoid colon with a scope.* | sigmoïdoscopie |
| **sigmoidostomy** *Formation of an opening in the sigmoid colon that communicates with the outside of the body.* | sigmoïdostomie |

| English | French |
|---|---|
| silent | silencieux |
| silicosis *Grinders's disease; fibrotic lung disease caused by inhalation of silica.* | silicose |
| silly | bête |
| silver | argent |
| silver nitrate stick *A medical device used to treat hypergranulation tissue.* | nitrate d'argent crayon |
| simultaneous | simultané |
| single | seul |
| single (not married) | célibataire |
| single use *A phrase used to indicate only one dose should be given.* | usage unique |
| sinistrocardia *Location of the heart toward the left (more than normally seen).* | 1. lévocardie 2. sinistrocardie |
| sinistrotorsion *Distorsion toward the left; in reference to the eye generally.* | lévorotation |
| sinoatrial   *Referring to the cardiac node of the same name.* | sino-auriculaire |
| sinoatrial node *A mass of cardiac tissue that acts as the pacemaker.* | Keith et Flack, nœud de |
| sinus arrhythmia *Cardiac dysrhythmias related to sinoatrial nodal dysfunction.* | arythmie sinusale |
| sinusitis *Inflammation of the sinuses.* | sinusite |
| sinusoid *An irregular vessel having almost no adventitia that is found in the liver, heart, parathyroid, spleen and pancreas.* | sinusoïdal |
| sip, to | siroter |
| site | lieu |
| sitting | assis |
| size | grandeur |
| skeleton | squelette |
| skin | peau |
| skin fold | pli cutané |
| skin lesion | lésion cutanée |
| skin rash | éruption cutanée |
| sleep | sommeil |
| sleep apnea *Episodic apnea during sleep that is exhibited by daytime symptoms of fatigue, difficulty concentrating and sleepiness.* | apnée de sommeil |
| sleeping sickness *Also called Trypanosomiasis, this disease is caused by a parasitic protozoa and transmitted by the tsetse fly.* | sommeil, maladie du |
| slice | tranche |
| slide *A thin, rectangular piece of glass used for viewing specimen under a microscope.* | lame |
| slight | 1. frêle 2. léger |
| sling | écharpe 2. fronde |
| slow | lent |
| sludge *A viscous fluid.* | fango |

| English | French |
|---|---|
| **slurring** | empâtement |
| **smallpox** *Variola.* | variole |
| **smear** *Used to refer to a specimen smeared on a slide.* | frottis |
| **smegma** *A thick curdled secretion found around the clitoris and the prepuce.* | smegma |
| **smoking** | tabagisme |
| **snapping finger** *Also called trigger finger and stenosing flexor tenosynovitis; one complains of a snapping sensation when the affected digit is flexed.* | doigt à ressort |
| **sneeze** | éternuement |
| **sniffing** | reniflement |
| **snore, to** | ronfler |
| **soap** | savon |
| **sob** | sanglot |
| **sock** | chaussette |
| **socket** *An anatomical hollow that is part of an articulation or where the eyeball rests.* | 1. cavité articulaire 2. douille 3. fourreau |
| **sodium chloride** | chlorure de sodium |
| **soft** | mou |
| **solar plexus** *A cluster of ganglia and nerves, located at the base of the sternum, that surround the celiac trunk.* | plexus solaire |
| **sole** | plante du pied |
| **soleus muscle** *Assists with ankle plantar flexion.* | soléaire muscle |
| **solvent** *Able to dissolve with other chemicals.* | solvant |
| **somatic** *Referring to the body.* | somatique |
| **somnambulism** *Sleepwalking.* | somnambulisme |
| **somnolence** *Drowsiness.* | somnolence |
| **soporific** *Promoting drowsiness or sleep.* | soporifique |
| **sore throat** | angine |
| **sorrow** | peine |
| **soul** | âme |
| **sour** | aigre |
| **span** | empan |
| **sparing** | économe |
| **spasmolytic** *A substance that diminishes spasms.* | spasmolytique |
| **spastic** *Stiff, awkward movement of the muscles.* | spastique |
| **spasticity** *Refers to continuous spastic movement.* | spasticité |
| **specific** | spécifique |
| **specimen** | 1. échantillon 2. spécimen |
| **spectrometry** *The use of a device to measure spectra.* | spectrométrie |
| **spectroscope** *A device for producing and recording spectra.* | spectroscope |
| **speculum** *A device used to open a canal, like the vagina, for inspection.* | spéculum |

| English | French |
|---|---|
| speech | discours |
| speech therapist | orthophoniste |
| sperm | sperme |
| spermatic cord *The structure containing the ductus deferens, testicular artery, and nerves that goes from the inguinal ring to the testis.* | cordon spermatique |
| spermatocele *A cyst in the epididymis containing spermatozoa.* | spermatocèle |
| spermatogenesis *The production of spermatozoa.* | spermatogenèse |
| spermatozoon *A mature male germ cell that is capable of fertilizing an ovum.* | spermatozoïde |
| spermicide *A substance capable of killing sperm.* | spermicide |
| sphenoidal sinus *Part of the sphenoid bone; it communicates with the most superior aspect of the nasal meatus.* | sinus sphénoïdal |
| spherocyte *An erythrocyte without the usual central pallor; it is noted in spherocytosis and some hemolytic anemias.* | sphérocyte |
| spherocytosis *The presence of spherocytes in the blood.* | sphérocytose |
| sphincterotomy *Surgical incision of the anal sphincter.* | sphinctérotomie |
| sphygmomanometer *Device for measuring blood pressure.* | sphygmomanomètre |
| spica *A figure of eight bandage.* | spica |
| spicule *A sharp, slender part.* | spicule |
| spider nevus *A papule with telangiectases radiating from the center.* | 1. angiome stellaire 2. araignée |
| spinal *Referring to the spine.* | spinal |
| spinal cord *The bundle of nerves that with the brain comprise the central nervous system.* | moelle épinière |
| spinal ganglion *The ganglion located on the dorsal root of each spinal nerve.* | ganglion rachidien |
| spinal nerve *The term for each of the thirty pairs of nerves that originate in the spine and traverse between the vertebrae. There are eight cervical, twelve thoracic, five lumbar, five sacral and one coccygeal nerve pairs.* | rachidien nerf |
| spinal reflex *A reflex that has an arc passing through the spine.* | réflexe médullaire |
| spinal shock *Hypotension related to injury or intervention of the spine.* | 1. choc spinal 2. sidération médullaire |
| spine *The spinal column or a thorny protrusion.* | 1. épine 2. rachis |
| spine of vertebra | apophyse épineuse |
| spirograph *A device used to record respiratory movements.* | spirographe |
| spirometer *A device used to measure pulmonary capacity.* | spiromètre |
| spit | cracher |
| splanchnic nerves *The nerves supplying the abdominal viscera and blood vessels.* | splanchniques nerfs |
| spleen *The visceral organ that is involved with production and removal of blood cells.* | spleen |
| splenectomy *Surgical excision of the spleen.* | splénectomie |
| splenic flexure of the colon | angle gauche du côlon |

| English | French |
|---|---|
| **splenic** *Referring to the spleen.* | splénique |
| **splenomegaly** *An abnormally enlarged spleen.* | splénomégalie |
| **splint** *A rigid support used to immobilize and extremity.* | gouttière |
| **splinter** *A small, thin object; usually refers to the object being imbedded in the body.* | esquille |
| **spoiled** | avarié |
| **spondylitis** *Inflammation of the vertebrae.* | spondylite |
| **spondylolisthesis** *The overlapping of one vertebra over another.* | spondylolisthésis |
| **spondylolysis** *Dissolution of the vertebra.* | spndylolyse |
| **sponge** | éponge |
| **spongiosis** *Edema of the spongy layer of the skin.* | spongiose |
| **spontaneous** | spontané |
| **spoonful** | cuillérée |
| **sporotrichosis** *A Sporotrichum schenckii infection manifested by formation of lymphatic and subcutaneous nodules.* | sporotrichose |
| **sprain** | 1. entorse 2. foulure |
| **spray** | pulvérisation |
| **sputum** *A mixture of respiratory tract secretions and saliva.* | crachat |
| **squama** *A scale or platelike body.* | 1. écaille 2. squame |
| **squamous** *Scaly.* | squameux |
| **square root** | racine carrée |
| **squeeze, to** | comprimer |
| **squirt, to** | gicler |
| **stab wound** | plaie par arme blanche |
| **stabbing pain** | douleur enn coup de poignard |
| **staggering** | titubant |
| **staging** *Refers to a stratification of cancer for example.* | stadification |
| **stamina** *Ability to maintain physical or mental exertion for a long period.* | vigueur |
| **stammering** *The impulse to repeat the first letter of words and involuntary pauses while speaking.* | balbutiement |
| **standing** | debout |
| **stapedectomy** *Surgical excision of the stapes.* | stapédectomie |
| **stapedius muscle** *Located in the tympanic interior, it reduces stapedial movement.* | 1. étrier, muscle de l' 2. stapedius muscle |
| **stapes** *This auditory ossicle is the innermost of three ossicles and is shaped like a stirrup.* | stapes |
| **staphyloma** *Protrusion of the cornea due to inflammation.* | staphylome |
| **staphylorrhaphy** *Surgical repair of a defect between the soft palate and uvula.* | staphylorraphie |
| **starvation** | famine |
| **starved** | affamé |

129

| English | French |
|---|---|
| **stasis** *Lack of movement.* | stase |
| **state** | état |
| **statement** | affirmation |
| **static** *Not changing.* | statique |
| **status** | status |
| **status of illness** | état de mal |
| **steady state** *In equilibrium.* | état d'équilibre |
| **steatoma** *A sebaceous cyst or lipoma.* | stéatome |
| **steatorrhea** *Excrement with an abnormally high fat content.* | stéatorrhée |
| **steatosis** *Fatty degeneration; when referring to the liver it involves invasion of fat into hepatocytes.* | stéatose |
| **stellate ganglion** *Formed by the seventh cervical, eighth cervical and first thoracic ganglia.* | stellaire ganglion |
| **stenosis** *Narrowing of an orifice.* | sténose |
| **stercobilin** *A substance created by the reduction of bilirubin and gives excrement the brown hue.* | stercobiline |
| **stereognosis** *The ability to identify an object by touch.* | stéréognosie |
| **sterile** *1. Infertile 2. Refers to equipment that is free of contamination.* | stérile |
| **sterilization** *A procedure done to prevent production of offspring.* | stérilisation |
| **sternal** *Referring to the sternum.* | sternal |
| **sternocleidomastoid** *The pair of muscles that connect the sternum, clavicle and mastoid process.* | sternocleidomastoïdien |
| **sterocolith** *A fecal calculus.* | sterocolithe |
| **sterol** *Unsaturated steroid alcohols such as cholesterol.* | stérol |
| **stethoscope** *Device used to auscultate the heart, lungs and over arteries to assess for abnormalities.* | stéthoscope |
| **stiff** | engourdi |
| **stiff-neck** | raideur de la nuque |
| **stillborn** *Refers to a newborn that died in utero.* | mort-né |
| **sting** | dard |
| **stirrup** *An attachment to an exam table where a woman puts her legs to assist examination of the genitalia.* | étrier |
| **stomach** | estomac |
| **stomach pain** | brûlure gastrique |
| **story** | histoire |
| **strabismus** *An anomaly of ocular movement.* | strabisme |
| **strabismus** *Also called esotropia or commonly "cross-eyed".* | strabisme convergent |
| **straight leg raising test** *One leg is raised while the patient is supine, presence of radicular pain indicates a possible lumbar disc disorder.* | Lassègue, manœuvre |
| **strait-jacket** *A device used to temporarily restrain the arms of patients who are psychotic and violent.* | camisole de force |
| **strange** | étrange |
| **strength** | force |

| English | French |
|---|---|
| stress | contrainte |
| stress fracture *A long bone fracture caused by repetitive mechanical stress.* | fracture de fatigue |
| stretcher *A device used to carry a patient in the supine position.* | 1. brancard 2. civière |
| stria *A narrow bandlike body.* | vergeture |
| stricture | stricture |
| stride | enjambée |
| string | ficelle |
| stroke volume *The amount of blood ejected from the ventricle with each contraction.* | volume d'éjection |
| stroma *A term used to describe the framework of an organ.* | stroma |
| strong | fort |
| stump *Term used to designate what remains of an amputated extremity.* | moignon |
| stupor | stupeur |
| stuttering *Involuntary repetition of the first consonant.* | 1. bégaiement 2. palisyllabie |
| stylet *A thin wire within a catheter that is removed after the catheter is in place.* | stylet |
| subacute *A stage between acute and chronic.* | subaigue |
| subarachnoid *The layer of the brain covering between the arachnoid and pia mater.* | sous-arachnoïdien |
| subclavian *Refers to the area under the clavicle; the subclavian vein runs below the clavicle.* | sous-clavier |
| subclavian steal syndrome *Retrograde vertebral artery flow due to ipsilateral subclavian artery stenosis.* | syndrome du vol de la sous-clavière |
| subdural *The area between the dura mater and the arachnoid membrane.* | sous-dural |
| subdural hematoma *Formation of a blood clot between the dura mater and the arachnoid membrane.* | hémorragie sous-durale |
| suberosis *A type of hypersensitivity pneumonitis related to inhalation of moldy cork dust.* | subérose |
| sublingual *Situated under the tongue.* | sublingual |
| submaxillary *Situated below the maxilla.* | sous-maxillaire |
| subphrenic *Referring to below the diaphragm.* | sous-diaphragmatique |
| success | réussite |
| succussion *The presence of a splashing sound when a body cavity is moved indicating presence of both air and fluid.* | succussion |
| sucking | succion |
| sudamina *White vesicles noted because of retained sweat in the layers of the epidermis.* | sudamina |
| sudden infant death syndrome *A leading cause of death of infants from one month to one year; the etiology is unknown.* | mort subite dunourrisson |
| suffer, to | souffrir |
| sugar | sucre |

| English | French |
|---|---|
| **sugar-coated tablet** | dragée |
| **suicide** | suicide |
| **sulcus** *A groove, like in the brain.* | 1. sillon 2. sulcus |
| **sulfonamide** *A class of drugs derived from sulfanilamide that are antibacterial.* | sulfamide |
| **sulfur** | soufre |
| **superciliary arch** *The area superior to the upper border of each orbit.* | arcade sourcilière |
| **superfecundation** *The fertilization of two different ova by spermatozoa of two different males.* | superfécondation |
| **superficial inguinal ring** *The opening of the aponeurosis of the external oblique muscle for the round ligament or spermatic cord.* | anneau inguinal superficiel |
| **superior** | supérieur |
| **supination** *Turning the sole of the foot or the palm of the hand upward..* | supination |
| **supine** | couché sur le dos |
| **supplies** | 1. fournitures 2. provisions |
| **suppository** | suppositoire |
| **suppuration** *Formation of purulent material.* | suppuration |
| **supraorbital** *Situated above the orbit.* | sus-orbitaire |
| **suprapubic** *Situated above the pubis.* | sus-pubien |
| **sural** *Referring to the calf of the leg.* | sural |
| **surfactant** *A substance that reduces surface tension in the lungs.* | surfactant |
| **surgeon** | chirurgien |
| **surgery** | chirurgie |
| **surgical** *Referring to surgery.* | chirurgical |
| **surgical suite** *The group of rooms reserved for surgical procedures.* | bloc opératoire |
| **surname** | nom de famille |
| **sustained** | soutenu |
| **sustained release** *Describes a medicine that is slowly dispersed so it has a lasting effect.* | libération, prolongée |
| **suture** | suture |
| **swab** | écouvillon |
| **swallow** | gorgée |
| **swallowing** | avalement |
| **sweat** | sueur |
| **swollen** | gonflé |
| **sycosis** *A bacterial infection affecting the hair follicles on a person's face.* | impétigo sycosiforme |
| **symbiosis** *The living together of two organisms.* | symbiose |
| **symmetry** *Being equally bilaterally.* | symétrie |
| **sympathectomy** *The surgical resection of a sympathetic nerve to reduce undesired effects.* | sympathectomie |

| English | French |
|---|---|
| **sympathetic nervous system** *The nerves responsible for the flight or fight response.* | système sympathique |
| **symptom** | symptôme |
| **synapse** *The intersection of two nerve cells.* | synapse |
| **synarthrosis** *Adjacent bones connected by a joint but the joint is fixed.* | synarthrose |
| **synchondrosis** *A joint with little motion that uses cartilage such as the vertebral bodies.* | synchondrose |
| **syncope** *Sudden loss of consciousness.* | syncope |
| **synechia** *The adhesion of two body parts, such as synechia vulvae in which the labia minora are congenitally adherent.* | synéchie |
| **synovectomy** *Surgical resection of a synovial membrane.* | synovectomie |
| **synovial fluid** *The fluid that surrounds, for example, the knee within a capsule.* | liquide synovial |
| **synovitis** *Inflammation of the synovium.* | synovite |
| **syphilis** *A infectious disease caused by Treponema pallidum that causes a painless penile ulcer in the primary stage but can lead to irreversible brain damage in the untreated tertiary stage.* | syphilis |
| **syringe** | seringue |
| **syringomelia** *A condition exhibited by fluid-filled cavities in the spinal cord.* | syringomyélie |
| **syrup** | sirop |
| **systole** *The phase of the cardiac cycle in which the ventricles contract.* | systole |
| **systolic** *Referring to systole or that which occurs during systole.* | systolique |
| **tablespoon** | cuillère à soupe |
| **tablet** | 1. comprimé 2. tablette |
| **tachycardia** *Heart rate higher than physiologic normal.* | tachycardie |
| **tactile** *Able to be felt.* | tactile |
| **talipes calcaneus** *A foot deformity exhibited by abnormal dorsiflexion.* | pied bot talus |
| **talipes equinus** *A foot deformity exhibited by abnormal plantar flexion.* | pied varus équin |
| **talipes** *Medical term for what is commonly known as club foot.* | pied bot |
| **talon** *The ball of the ankle joint.* | astragale os |
| **talus** *The most superior tarsal bone that articulates with the tibia.* | talus |
| **tamponade** *1. Stopping bleeding during surgery with a cotton pledget. 2. When referring to cardiac tamponade, it is the limitation of cardiac contraction because of blood or fluid accumulation in the pericardial sac.* | tamponnade |
| **tap** | robinet |
| **tape measure** | toise |
| **tapeworm** *A parasitic, intestinal flatworm.* | tænia |
| **target** | cible |
| **target cell** *An abnormal cell that is present in liver disease and certain hemoglobinopathies.* | cellule-cible |
| **tarsal** *Referring to any bone in the tarsus.* | 1. tarsal 2. tarsien |
| **tarsalgia** *Pain in any of the tarsal bones.* | tarsalgie |

| English | French |
|---|---|
| **tarsectomy** *Surgical excision of all or part of the tarsus.* | tarsectomie |
| **tarsoplasty** *Plastic surgery involving the eyelid.* | tarsoplastie |
| **tarsorrhaphy** *Suturing the eyelids in order to tighten the palpebral fissure.* | tarsorraphie |
| **tarsus** *The group of seven bones of the ankle or foot (three cuneiform bones, talus, calcaneus, navicular, cuboid bones).* | tarse |
| **task** | tâche |
| **taste** | 1. goût 2. saveur |
| **taste bud** | bourgeon du goût |
| **taurocholic acid** *A bile acid composed of cholic acid and taurine.* | taurocholique acide |
| **tear** | larme |
| **tear** *Referring to a vaginal tear after childbirth.* | déchirure |
| **teaspoon** | cuillère à café |
| **tectum** *A roof-like body.* | toit |
| **tectum mesencephali** *The posterior portion of the mesencephalon including the sup. and inf. colliculi and tectal lamina.* | lame quadrijumelle |
| **telangiectasis** *A condition exhibited by red, dilated capillaries on the skin.* | télangiectasie |
| **telemetry** *Use of radio signals to transmit patient data. The most common form is for electrocardiography in a patient who is ambulatory.* | télémétrie |
| **temperature** | température |
| **temporomandibular joint** *The hinged joint of the temporal bone and mandible.* | articulation temporo-mandibulaire |
| **tendinitis** *Inflammation of a tendon.* | tendinite |
| **tendon** | tendon |
| **tendon reflex** *A deep reflex elicited by gently tapping the tendon.* | réflexe tendineux |
| **tenesmus** *The attempt to defecate but attempts elicit pain and are ineffective.* | ténesme |
| **tennis elbow** *Inflammation at the lateral aspect of the epicondyle where the muscle and tendon join; lateral epicondylitis.* | coude du joueur de tennis |
| **tenoplasty** *Surgical repair of a tendon.* | ténoplastie |
| **tenorrhaphy** *The surgical repair with suture of a separated tendon.* | ténorraphie |
| **tenosynovitis** *Inflammation and swelling of an articulation.* | ténosynovite |
| **tenotomy** *Incision of a tendon as is done for strabismus.* | ténotomie |
| **tepid** | tiède |
| **teratogen** *A substance that induces fetal anomalies.* | tératogène |
| **teratoma** *A tumor made up of tissue not usually at the location (a mass of hair, teeth and gingival tissue in a leg tumor for instance).* | tèratome |
| **terebrant** *Having a piercing quality.* | térébrant |
| **terminally ill patient** | patient en fin de vie |
| **tertian fever** *A febrile syndrome caused by Plasmodium vivax which produces a fever spike every 48 hours.* | fièvre tierce |
| **tertiary** | tertiaire |

| English | French |
|---|---|
| **test strip (ie. glucose)** *A material used for various lab tests, mostly commonly glucose.* | bandelette diagnostique |
| **test tube** | éprouvette |
| **testicle** *One of a pair of organs in the male scrotum that produces sperm.* | testicule |
| **testosterone** *This steroid hormone produces secondary male sexual characteristics.* | testostérone |
| **tetanus** *A condition caused by Clostridium tetani which produces spasm and rigidity of voluntary muscles.* | tétanos |
| **tetany** *A condition caused by the hypocalcemic effect of hypoparathyroidism, exhibited by periodic muscle spasms, convulsions, and peri-oral numbness.* | tétanie |
| **tetracycline** *An antibiotic used for gram positive and gram negative infections.* | tétracycline |
| **tetradactylous** *Referring to a condition of having only four digits on a hand or foot.* | tétradactyle |
| **thalamus** | thalamus |
| **thalassemia** *A hereditary hemolytic anemia first observed in people from the Mediterranean area.* | thalassémie |
| **thalidomide** *A drug used originally as a sedative, after it was found to cause congenital anomalies, its use was restricted. Now it is used for a few conditions such as multiple myeloma.* | thalidomide |
| **theca** *A tendon or ovarian follicle sheath.* | thèque |
| **thecoma** *A tumor composed of theca cells.* | thécome |
| **thenar eminence** *Formed by the bellies of the abductor pollicis brevis, flexor pollicis brevis and opponens pollicis.* | éminence thénar |
| **therapeutic range** | fourchette thérapeutique |
| **thermometer** | thermomètre |
| **thiamine** *Also called vitamin B1; a deficiency causes beriberi.* | thiamine |
| **thigh** | cuisse |
| **thin** | maigre |
| **thirst** | soif |
| **thoracentesis** *Insertion of a needle into the pleural space to drain and or obtain a specimen for analysis.* | ponction pleurale |
| **thoracentesis** *Insertion of a needle into the pleural space to drain and or obtain a specimen for analysis.* | thoracentèse |
| **thoracic** *Referring to the thorax.* | thoracique |
| **thoracoplasty** *Surgical removal of ribs.* | thoracoplastie |
| **thoracoscopy** *Visualization of the thoracic cavity with a scope.* | thoracoscopie |
| **thoracotomy** *Surgical incision of the thorax.* | thoracotomie |
| **thorax** *The part of the body between the neck and abdomen.* | thorax |
| **three way foley** *A urinary tube used for irrigation of the bladder.* | sonde Foley 3 voies |
| **threonine** *An amino acid needed for the growth in infants.* | thréonine |
| **throat** | gorge |

| English | French |
|---|---|
| **throbbing** | pulsatile |
| **thrombectomy** *Excision of a thrombus from a vein or artery.* | thrombectomie |
| **thrombin** *An enzyme that is a catalyst for the conversion of fibrinogen to fibrin in the formation of a clot.* | thrombine |
| **thromboangiitis** *Inflammation and thrombosis in a blood vessel.* | thrombangéite |
| **thromboarteritis** *Thrombosis of an inflammed artery.* | thromboartérite |
| **thrombocytopenia** *Abnormal decrease in the number of blood platelets.* | thrombocytopénie |
| **thrombophlebitis** *Inflammation of a venous wall associated with a thrombus.* | thrombophlébite |
| **thrombosis** *Formation of a clot in a vein or artery.* | thrombose |
| **throughout** | partout |
| **thumb** | pouce |
| **thymectomy** *Surgical excision of the thymus.* | thymectomie |
| **thymine** *A chemical with a pyrimidine base found in DNA.* | thymine |
| **thymocyte** *A lymphocyte located in the thymus.* | thymocyte |
| **thymoma** *A tumor composed of thymic tissue and is sometimes associated with myasthenia gravis.* | thymome |
| **thymus** *A body organ located in the neck and it produces T cells to improve immune function.* | thymus |
| **thyroglossal cyst** *A common congenital growth in the thyroglossal duct.* | kyste thyréoglosse |
| **thyroid** *A gland in the neck that secretes hormones regulating metabolism.* | thyroïde |
| **thyroid stimulating hormone (TSH)** *A thyroid secreted by the pituitary that regulates the thyroid.* | thyréotrope hormone |
| **thyroidectomy** *Surgical resection of all or part of the thyroid.* | thyroïdectomie |
| **thyrotoxicosis** *Abnormal increase in thyroid activity exhibited by thinning hair, hypertension, tachycardia and at times atrial fibrillation.* | thyréotoxicose |
| **thyroxine** *An iodine containing hormone, referred to T4.* | thyroxine |
| **tibia** *The larger of two long bones in the lower leg.* | tibia |
| **tick bite** | morsure de tique |
| **tick-borne fever** *A relapsing fever caused by a spirochete of the genus Borrelia.* | fièvre à tiques |
| **tickle** | chatouillement |
| **tidal volume** *The amount of air inspired with each breath. One can set a ventilator to deliver a preset number of milliliters of oxygenated air with each breath.* | volume courant |
| **tight junction** *An intercellular junction with an impermeable membrane.* | nexus |
| **tincture** *1. A very small amount of something. 2. A medicine dissolved in alcohol.* | teinture |
| **tinea** *Medical term for ringworm.* | teigne |
| **tingling** | 1. fourmillement 2. picotement |

| English | French |
|---------|--------|
| **tinnitus** *Medical term for ringing in the ears. It is associated with Meniere's syndrome among other conditions.* | 1. acouphène 2. bourdonnement d'oreille 3. tinnitus |
| **tired** | fatigué |
| **tocopherol** *Vitamin E.* | tocophérol |
| **tongs** *A medical device used for holding or grasping.* | pinces |
| **tongue** | langue |
| **tongue depressor; tongue blade** *As the name implies, the stick pushes the tongue down so the posterior aspect of the mouth can be viewed more readily.* | abaisse-langue |
| **tonometer** *A device used to measure ocular pressure in glaucoma.* | tonomètre |
| **tonsil** *A rounded mass of lymphoid tissue, most commonly referring to the pharyngeal tonsil.* | amygdale |
| **tonsillectomy** *Excision of the tonsils.* | 1. adéno-amygdalectomie 2. amygdalectomie 3. tonsillectomie |
| **tonsillitis** *Inflammation of the tonsils.* | 1. amygdalite 2. tonsillite |
| **tooth** | dent |
| **toothless** | édenté |
| **torn** | déchiré |
| **torpor** *Unresponsiveness to normal stimuli.* | torpeur |
| **torsade de pointe** *Ventricular cardiac rhythm disturbance.* | torsade de pointe |
| **torsion** *Refers to twisting. Testicular torsion is the twisting of the spermatic cord that can lead to ischemia and gangrene of the testicle.* | torsion |
| **torsion spasm** *Also called dystonia musculorum deformans, a genetic condition exhibited by twisting contortions sideways and forward while walking.* | spasme de torsion |
| **torso** *The trunk of the body.* | torse |
| **torticollis** *A condition exhibited by the head being turned to one side continuously.* | torticolis |
| **touch** | attouchement |
| **tourniquet** *A device tied tightly around an extremity to diminish blood flow or blood loss.* | 1. garrot 2. tourniquet |
| **toxemia** *The release of toxic substances into the blood stream from a local infection. Toxemia of pregnancy is a synonym for preeclampsia.* | toxémie |
| **toxic** | toxique |
| **toxicology** *The study of the nature, effects and detection of poisons.* | toxicologie |
| **toxin** *A poison of plant or animal origin.* | toxine |
| **toxoid** *A chemically modified toxin that can be used as a vaccine.* | anatoxine |
| **toxoplasmosis** *A disease caused by the* | toxoplasmose |
| **trabecule** *A connective tissue strand that goes from a capsule to the enclosed organ.* | trabécule |
| **trabeculotomy** *A surgery for open angle glaucoma.* | trabéculotomie |

| English | French |
|---|---|
| **trachea** *The ringed canal between the pharynx and bronchi.* | trachée |
| **tracheitis** *Inflammation of the trachea.* | trachéite |
| **trachelorrhaphy** *Surgical repair of a lacerated cervix.* | trachélorraphie |
| **tracheobronchitis** *Inflammation of the trachea and bronchi.* | trachéobronchite |
| **tracheostomy** *Creation of a surgical opening in the trachea so a tube could be placed in the trachea.* | trachéostomie |
| **tracheotomy** *Surgical incision of the trachea.* | trachéotomie |
| **trachoma** *An infection of the cornea and conjunctiva caused by Chlamydia.* | trachome |
| **tragus** *The fleshy prominence anterior to the opening of the ear.* | tragus |
| **tranquilizer** *A medication used to diminish anxiety.* | tranquillisant |
| **transabdominal** *Through the abdominal wall.* | transabdominal |
| **transaminase** *An enzyme that facilitates the transfer of an amino group to an amino acid.* | transaminase |
| **transdermal** *Through the skin.* | 1. percutané 2. transdermique |
| **transfusion** *Administration of blood products intravenously.* | transfusion |
| **transient ischemic attack** *Cerebral ischemic changes resulting from transitory hypoperfusion.* | accident ischémique transitoire |
| **transpire, to** *To happen or occur.* | avérer, s' |
| **transplant** *To move a body part from one location to another.* | transplant |
| **transplantation** *The grafting of tissues.* | transplantation |
| **transudation** *The movement of body tissue through a membrane that is usually the result of inflammation.* | transsudation |
| **trapezium** *The lateral bone in the distal row of carpal bones.* | trapèze |
| **trapezius muscle** *The muscle with an origin of occipital bone and seventh cervical vertebra, insertion of clavicle and scapula, and it draws the scapula backward.* | muscle trapèze |
| **trapezoid** *The bone between the trapezium and capitate bones.* | trapézoïde |
| **trauma** | trauma |
| **treadmill** | tapis roulant |
| **treatment** | traitement |
| **treatment failure** *A phrase indicating the prior interventions have been unsuccessful.* | échec thérapeutique |
| **treatment regimen** | protocole thérapeutique |
| **treatment withdrawal** *The cessation of active management; this is done for instance, when the patient is terminal.* | arrêt du traitement |
| **trematoda** *A parasitic fluke such as Schistosoma.* | trématode |
| **tremor** | tremblement |
| **trephining** *Cutting away a circular disc of bone or the cornea.* | trépanation |
| **triceps** *Referring to something having three heads like the triceps muscle.* | triceps |

| English | French |
|---|---|
| **triceps reflex** *A tendon reflex causing extension of the arm when the triceps tendon is gently tapped.* | réflexe tricipital |
| **trichiasis** *Inversion of the eyelashes.* | trichiasis |
| **trichinosis** *A disease caused by meat infected by Trichinella spiralis causing fever and gastrointestinal effects.* | trichinose |
| **trichophytosis** *A skin or nail fungal infection caused by Trichophyton.* | trichophytie |
| **tricuspid valve** *The cardiac valve located between the right atrium and right ventricle.* | valvule tricuspide |
| **trigeminal** *Generally refers to the fifth cranial nerve.* | trigéminal |
| **trigeminal nerve** *The fifth cranial nerve which supplies the motor function of mastication and has three sensory branches, the ophthalmic, maxillary and mandibular.* | trijumeau nerf |
| **trigeminal neuralgia** *Pain in the region of one or more branches of the fifth cranial nerve sensory branches.* | névralgie faciale |
| **trigger** | gâchette |
| **trigone** *Usually refers to the area at the base of the bladder between the openings of the ureters and the urethra.* | 1. triangle 2. trigone |
| **triplegia** *Paralysis of three extremities.* | triplégie |
| **triplets** | triplés |
| **triploid** *Referring to a cell with three homologous sets of chromosomes.* | triploïde |
| **trismus** *Commonly called lockjaw, it is a spasm of the muscles supplied by the trigeminal nerve and is an early symptom of tetanus.* | trismus |
| **trisomy 21** *A congenital anomaly in which chromosome 21 is effected and results in Down's syndrome.* | trisomie 21 |
| **trisomy** *A general category of congenital anomalies in which there is an extra set of chromosomes in the cell nucleus.* | trisomie |
| **trivial** | banal |
| **trocar** *A device enclosed in a catheter that is used to withdraw fluid from a body cavity.* | trocart |
| **trochanter** *Refers to the greater or lesser trochanter; the prominences on the femoral neck.* | trochanter |
| **trochlea** *A pulley-shaped structure such as the groove at the distal humerus.* | trochlée |
| **trochlear** *Referring to a trochlea.* | trochléaire |
| **trochlear nerve** *The fourth cranial nerve that supplies the superior oblique muscle of the eyeball.* | pathétique nerf |
| **trophoblast** *A layer of endodermal tissue that helps attach an ovum to the uterine wall.* | trophoblaste |
| **truncal** *Referring to the trunk of a body or a nerve.* | tronculaire |
| **truss** *A synthetic device for containing a hernia within the abdomen.* | bandage herniaire |
| **truth** | vérité |
| **trypanosomiasis** *A disease caused by a protozoa of the genus Trypanosoma that can cause sleeping sickness and Chagas' disease.* | trypanosomiase |
| **trypsin** *An enzyme whose precursor is secreted by the pancreas that breaks down proteins in the intestine.* | trypsine |

| English | French |
|---|---|
| **trypsinogen** *The precursor to trypsin that is secreted by the pancreas.* | trypsinogène |
| **tryptophan** *An amino acid that is a precursor of serotonin. If present in the body in appropriate levels it can prevent pellegra even if niacin levels are low.* | tryptophane |
| **tsetse fly** *An insect that transmits the protozoa trypanosoma and can cause sleeping sickness.* | mouche tsé-tsé |
| **tubal** *Referring to a tube, as in fallopian tube.* | tubaire |
| **tubercle** *1. A granulomatous nodule produced by Mycobacterium tuberculosis. 2. A small prominence on a bone.* | tubercule |
| **tuberculin** *A solution containing M. tuberculosis or M. bovis that is used to test for tuberculosis by injecting the solution intradermally and looking for a reaction.* | tuberculine |
| **tuberculoma** *1. A tuberculous growth in the brain. 2. A mass that is produced from enlargement of a caseous tubercle.* | tuberculome |
| **tuberculosis** *Any infectious disease caused by Mycobacterium.* | tuberculose |
| **tuberculous** *Referring to tuberculosis.* | tuberculeux |
| **tuberosity** *A protuberance. For instance the iliac tuberosity is a prominence on the surface of the ilium.* | tubérosité |
| **tuberous sclerosis** *An inherited neurocutaneous disorder exhibited by benign hamartomas of the brain, lung, kidney, skin and other organs.* | Bourneville |
| **tubo-ovarian** *Referring to the fallopian tube or ovary.* | tubo-ovarien |
| **tubular** *Referring to a hollow, round-shaped organ.* | tubulaire |
| **tularemia** *An infectious disease caused by Francisella tularensis. The symptoms range from mild constitutional complaints to septic shock.* | tularémie |
| **tumefaction** *An area of swelling.* | tuméfaction |
| **tumor** *A benign or malignant overgrowth of tissue.* | tumeur |
| **tunica** *Generally a covering of a body part or organ. The tunica mucosa nasi is the mucous membrane lining the nasal cavity.* | tunique |
| **tuning fork** *A device used to distinguish between perceptive and conductive hearing loss.* | diapason |
| **turbinate bones** *The three curved shelves in the nasal cavity.* | cornets des fosses nasales |
| **turbinectomy** *Surgical excision of a turbinate bone.* | turbinectomie |
| **turgid** *Congested and swollen.* | 1. enflé 2. turgescent |
| **turgor** *Referring to the elasticity of skin. If one pinches skin and it remains in place the patient is dehydrated.* | turgescence |
| **twins** | jumeaux |
| **twitch** | secousse musculaire |
| **two times** | deux fois |
| **tympanic** *Referring to the tympanic membrane or having a resonant quality to percussion.* | tympanique |
| **tympanic membrane** *The membrane between the external and middle ear.* | 1. tympan 2. membrane du tympan |
| **tympanoplasty** *Restoration of the tympanic membrane's continuity.* | tympanoplastie |

| English | French |
|---|---|
| **typhoid fever** *A condition caused by ingestion of food or water containing salmonella typhi that is exhibited by fever and abdominal signs and symptoms.* | typhoïde fièvre |
| **typhus fever** *A rickettsiae infection exhibited by rash, fever, headache and myalgia.* | typhus |
| **tyrosine** *An amino acid important in the synthesis of hormones.* | tyrosine |
| **ulcer** *A concave wound caused by a break in the integrity of skin or mucous membrane.* | ulcère |
| **ulcerative** *Referring to ulceration.* | ulcératif |
| **ulcerative colitis** *Recurrent episode of inflammation of the membranous layer of the colon.* | rectocolite ulcéro-hémorragique |
| **ultrasonography** *Visualization of body structures with the echoes of ultrasound pulses.* | ultrasonographie |
| **ultrasound** *A sound or vibration of ultrasonic frequency.* | ultrason |
| **ultraviolet rays** *Electromagnetic radiation with wavelength longer than x rays.* | rayons ultraviolets |
| **umbilicated** *Referring to depressed areas that resemble the umbilicus.* | ombiliqué |
| **umbilicus** *The scar that denotes the end of the umbilical cord.* | 1. nombril 2. ombilic |
| **unciform** *Another term for hamate bone in the wrist.* | 1. crochu 2. unciforme |
| **uncinariasis** *Hookworm infestation of genus Uncinaria.* | uncinariose |
| **uncinate bone** *Hamate bone.* | hamatum |
| **unconsciousness** *Unable to respond to sensory stimuli.* | inconscience |
| **under; infra** *Sometimes used when indicating a patient is "under treatment" for a condition (active treatment).* | sous |
| **underlying** | sous-jacent |
| **undulant** *Wave-like appearance.* | ondulant |
| **unexpected** | inattendu |
| **unicellular** *A term describing organisms like protozoans that only have cell.* | unicellulaire |
| **unilateral** *One side only.* | unilatéral |
| **uniovolar** *Referring to one fertilized ovum.* | uniovulaire |
| **uniparous** *Refers to a single birth.* | unipare |
| **unknown** | inconnu |
| **unstable knee** *A condition with giving way of the knee due to ligamentous or cartilaginous dysfunction.* | genou instable |
| **unsteady** | instable |
| **upper limb** | membre supérieur |
| **upper respiratory tract** *Generally considered the part of the respiratory tract superior to the vocal cords.* | voies respiratoires supérieures |
| **upright** | position debout |
| **urachus** *A connection between the bladder and the allantois in the fetus.* | ouraque |
| **urate** *The salt of uric acid.* | urate |
| **urea** *A nitrogenous product of protein metabolism; excreted in urine.* | 1. urée 2. uréique |
| **uremia** *An excess of urea and creatinine in the blood.* | urémie |

| English | French |
|---|---|
| **ureter** *The conduit between each kidney and the urinary bladder.* | uretère |
| **ureteral** *Referring to one of two tubes from the kidneys to the bladder that carry urine.* | 1. urétéral 2. urétérique |
| **ureterectomy** *Surgical resection of one or both ureters.* | urétérectomie |
| **ureteritis** *Inflammation of the ureter.* | urétérite |
| **ureterocele** *Protrusion of the distal portion of the ureter into the bladder.* | urétérocèle |
| **ureterolith** *Presence of a stone in the ureter.* | urétérolithe |
| **ureterolithotomy** *Removal of a ureteral stone.* | urétérolithotomie |
| **ureterovaginal** *Referring to the ureter and vagina.* | urétérovaginal |
| **ureterovesical** *Referring to the ureter and urinary bladder.* | urétérovésical |
| **urethra** *The canal connecting the urinary bladder with the outside of the body.* | urètre |
| **urethral** *Referring to the urethra.* | urétral |
| **urethritis** *Inflammation of the urethra.* | urétrite |
| **urethrocele** *A prolapse of the urethra through the meatus.* | urétrocèle |
| **urethrography** *Imaging of the urethra after instillation of contrast media.* | urétrography |
| **urethroplasty** *Surgical repair of the urethra.* | urétroplastie |
| **urethroscope** *A scope used to visualize the inside of the urethra.* | urétroscope |
| **urethrotomy** *A surgical opening of the urethra.* | urétrotomie |
| **urgency** | besoin impérieux |
| **uric** *Uric acid is a purine-derived product of nitrogen metabolism that can increase the risk of gout and calculi.* | urique |
| **urinalysis** *Chemical and microscopic examination of the urine.* | analyse urinaire |
| **urinary** *Referring to the urine.* | urinaire |
| **urinary bladder** *The organ collecting urine from the ureters prior to discharge via the urethra.* | vésicule urine |
| **urinary bladder** *The organ collecting urine from the ureters prior to discharge via the urethra.* | vessie |
| **urinary casts** *A protein precipitated from renal tubules and excreted in the urine.* | cylindres urinaires |
| **urinary drainage bag** *The bag that is attached via tube to an indwelling or condom catheter to collect urine.* | sac à urine |
| **urinary sediments** *The debris that settles in a urine sample when left undisturbed.* | culot urinaire |
| **urinary tract** *The organs and canals associated with urine secretion including the kidneys, ureters, bladder and urethra.* | voie urinaires |
| **urine** | urine |
| **urinometer** *A device for measuring urine specific gravity.* | urinomètre |
| **urobilin** *A brownish pigment that is an oxidized form of urobilinogen.* | urobiline |
| **urobilinogen** *A colorless substance produced in the intestines when bilirubin is reduced.* | urobilinogène |
| **urochrome** *A yellow pigment in the urine that gives urine its color.* | urochrome |

142

| English | French |
|---|---|
| **urogenital** *Referring to the urinary and genital systems.* | 1. génito-urinaire 2. urogénital |
| **urography** *Roentgenography of the urinary tract after administration of contrast media.* | urographie |
| **urolith** *Urinary calculi.* | 1. calcul urinaire 2. urolithe |
| **urology** *Surgical specialty involving medical and surgical treatment of the urogenital system.* | urologie |
| **urticaria** *A diffuse pruritic macular rash, caused by an allergy.* | urticaire |
| **usual** | habituel |
| **uterine** *Referring to the uterus.* | utérin |
| **uterine bleeding** | hémorragie utérine |
| **uterine fibroid** *A benign tumor made up of muscular and fibrous tissue in the uterus.* | fibrome utérin |
| **uterovesical** *Referring to the uterus and urinary bladder.* | utérovésical |
| **uterus** *The hollow organ in the female pelvis where a fertilized ovum embeds and grows.* | utérus |
| **utricle** *A small sac. It can refer to a division of the membranous labyrinth.* | utricule |
| **uveal tract** *A vascular structure of the eye that includes the choroid, ciliary body and iris.* | 1. tractus uvéal 2. uvée |
| **uveitis** *Inflammation of the uvea.* | uvéite |
| **uvula** *A fleshy pendent at the back of the soft palate.* | 1. luette 2. uvula |
| **uvulectomy** *Excision of the uvula.* | uvulectomie |
| **uvulitis** *Inflammation of the uvula.* | 1. ourantie 2. uvulite |
| **vaccination** *The act of receiving a vaccine.* | vaccination |
| **vaccine** *A solution of attenuated microorganisms given to prevent or treat a disease.* | vaccin |
| **vaccine status** | statut vaccinal |
| **vacuole** *A cavity that develops in a cell.* | vacuole |
| **vagal** *Referring to the vagus nerve.* | vagal |
| **vagina** *The canal in a female that extends from the vulva to the cervix.* | vagin |
| **vaginal** *Referring to the vagina.* | vaginal |
| **vaginismus** *Involuntary contraction of the vagina muscles that causes a painful spasm.* | vaginisme |
| **vagitus** *An infant cry that can be further defined as vagitus vaginalis in which the infant cries while its head is in the vaginal canal.* | vagissement |
| **vagotomy** *Incision of the vagus nerve.* | vagotomie |
| **vagus nerve** *The tenth cranial nerve that supplies the heart, lungs visceral organs; its function is tested by assessment of elevation of the uvula.* | pneumogastrique nerf; vague nerf |
| **valgus** *Refers to a joint being abnormally angulated away from the midline of the body.* | valgus |
| **valine** *An essential amino acid that assists with nitrogen equilibrium.* | valine |

| English | French |
|---|---|
| **Valsalva's maneuver** *A technique in which one attempts to exhale with the mouth and nose closed; this equalizes pressure in the ears.* | manœuvre de Valsalva |
| **valvulotomy** *Surgical incision of a valve.* | valvulotomie |
| **varicella** *A virus that causes chickenpox and shingles. Also called herpes zoster.* | varicelle |
| **varicocele** *A cluster of varicose veins in the scrotum.* | varicocèle |
| **varicose** *Referring to an abnormally distended, irregular vein.* | variqueux |
| **varix** *A twisted, distended vein, artery or lymph vessel.* | varice |
| **varus** *Refers to a joint being abnormally angulated toward the midline of the body.* | varus |
| **vascular** *Referring to a blood vessel.* | vasculaire |
| **vasculitis** *Inflammation of a blood vessel.* | vascularite |
| **vasectomy** *The surgical separation of each vas deferens with the intent of producing a sterile person.* | vasectomie |
| **vasoconstriction** *The process of making the blood vessels smaller which increases blood pressure.* | vasoconstriction |
| **vasodilatation** *The process of making the blood vessels larger which decreases blood pressure.* | vasodilatation |
| **vasomotor** *Referring to the constriction or dilation of vessels.* | vasomoteur |
| **vasopressin** *A hormone secreted by the pituitary that facilitates the retention of sodium and water and also increases blood pressure.* | vasopressine |
| **vasospasm** *The abrupt constriction of a blood vessel.* | vasospasme |
| **vasovagal** *Referring to overstimulation of the vagus nerve, exhibited by hypotension, pallor, nausea and diaphoresis.* | vasovagal |
| **vector** *An organism that transmits disease.* | vecteur |
| **vegetation** *Abnormal growth, such as cardiac valve vegetations as found in endocarditis.* | végétation |
| **velum** *A veil-like part.* | voile |
| **vena cava** *The large vein that carries deoxygenated blood to the right atrium.* | veine cave |
| **venereal disease** *A condition transmitted via sexual intercourse.* | malade vénérienne |
| **venography** *Roentgenography of a vein after administration of contrast media.* | 1. phlébographie 2. veinographie |
| **venom** | venin |
| **venous** *Referring to the veins.* | veineux |
| **ventilation** *The movement of air into the lungs; generally meant to suggest by an artificial process.* | ventilation |
| **ventral** *Referring to the underside but in humans, a ventral hernia, for example, refers to an abdominal hernia.* | ventral |
| **ventricle** *1. One of two chambers of the heart. 2. The four inter-connected cavities in the center of the brain.* | ventricule |
| **ventricular septal defect** *An abnormal communication between the right and left ventricles via a hole in the septum.* | communication interventriculaire |
| **ventriculography** *Roentgenography of the ventricles after administration of contrast media.* | ventriculographie |

| English | French |
|---|---|
| **venula** *The vessels that connect the capillary plexuses to veins.* | veinule |
| **verminous** *Referring to presence of worms.* | vermineux |
| **verruca** *A hyperplastic epidermal lesion, sometimes referred to as plantar wart.* | verrue |
| **vertebra** *A term for each bone surrounding the spine.* | vertèbre |
| **vertebral column** | colonne vertébrale |
| **vertebrobasilar insufficiency** *Diminished flow to the vertebral and basilar arteries causing posterior fossa symptoms.* | insuffisance vertébrobasilaire |
| **vertex** *The crown of the head.* | vertex |
| **vertigo** *A sensation of imbalance with many possible causes.* | vertige |
| **vesical** *Referring to the urinary bladder.* | vésical |
| **vesicovaginal** *Referring to the urinary bladder and vagina.* | vésicovaginal |
| **vesiculitis** *Inflammation of the urinary bladder.* | vésiculite |
| **vestibular** *Referring to a vestibule.* | vestibulaire |
| **vestigial** *Rudimentary.* | vestigial |
| **viable** *Referring to a fetus that can survive childbirth.* | viable |
| **vial** | flacon |
| **vibration** | vibration |
| **villous** *Covered with many villi.* | villeux |
| **villus** *A small vascular prominence from a membrane surface.* | villosité |
| **virilization** *The result of androgen; a process of development of masculine characteristics.* | masculinisation |
| **virology** *The study of viruses.* | virologie |
| **virulence** *The potential severity of a disease or poison.* | virulence |
| **viscera** *Referring to the organs in the abdominal or thoracic cavity.* | viscère |
| **viscometer** *A device used to measure viscosity.* | viscomètre |
| **viscous** *Having a thick, sticky consistency.* | visqueux |
| **vision** | vision |
| **visual field** *The complete area a person can see with their eyes in a fixed position.* | champ visuel |
| **vital capacity (VC)** *The maximal amount of air exhaled after a maximal inhalation.* | capacité vitale |
| **vital signs** *The designation for blood pressure, pulse, respirations and temperature.* | signes vitaux |
| **vitelline** *Referring to the yolk of an egg or ovum.* | vitellin |
| **vitreous** *Glass appearance; used to describe the vitreous body of the eye.* | 1. corps vitré 2. vitré |
| **vivisection** *Animal surgery done for purposes of research.* | vivisection |
| **vocal** | vocal |
| **voice** | voix |
| **voiding cystography** *Roentgenography of the bladder and urethra after administration of contrast media.* | cystographie mictionnelle |
| **volunteer** | bénévole |

| English | French |
|---|---|
| **volvulus** *Twisting of the bowel leading to obstruction and sometimes perforation.* | volvulus |
| **vomit, to** | vomir |
| **vulval cleft** *The area between the labia majora where the vagina and urethra rest.* | fente vulvaire |
| **vulvectomy** *Surgical resection of the vulva.* | vulvectomie |
| **vulvitis** *Inflammation of the vulva.* | vulvite |
| **vulvovaginitis** *Inflammation of the vulva and vagina.* | vulvovaginite |
| **waddling gait** *Walking in short steps in a swaying fashion.* | démarche dandinante |
| **walker** | déambulateur |
| **walking cast** *A cast used for simple fractures of the lower leg.* | botte de marche |
| **ward** | salle d'hôpital |
| **wasp** | guêpe |
| **water** | eau |
| **wax** | cire |
| **weak** | 1. faible 2. chétif |
| **weakness** | faiblesse |
| **weekly** | toutes les semaines |
| **weepy** | larmoyant |
| **well fed** | bien nourri |
| **wet** | mouillé |
| **wheelchair** | fauteuil roulant |
| **wheeze** | sifflement respiratoire |
| **whiplash** | coup du lapin |
| **whipworm** *A parasitic, intestinal nematode worm of the genus Trichuris.* | trichocéphale |
| **whisper** | bruit respiratoire |
| **whisper, to** | chuchoter |
| **whistle** | sifflement |
| **white** | blanc |
| **white matter** *The brain tissue consisting of myelin sheaths and nerve fibers.* | substance blanche |
| **whitlow** *An abscess occurring on the palmar surface of the fingertips.* | panaris |
| **wick; drain** | mèche |
| **widening** | élargissement |
| **width** | largeur |
| **wisdom tooth** | dent de sagesse |
| **wise** | sage |
| **withdrawal** | sevrage |
| **withhold** | abstenir |
| **wooden belly** *A rigid abdomen.* | ventre de bois |
| **World Health Organization (WHO)** | Organisation mondiale de la santé (OMS) |

| English | French |
|---------|--------|
| worm | ver |
| worry | souci |
| worsen | aggraver, s' |
| wound | plaie |
| wound care | parage |
| wrist | poignet |
| **xanthine** *A purine derivative that is found in the blood and urine after the metabolism of nucleic acids to uric acid.* | xanthine |
| **xanthochromia** *A yellow tone to the skin or spinal fluid.* | xanthochromie |
| **xanthoma** *A lipid deposition on the skin exhibited by an irregular yellow patch.* | xanthome |
| **xerodermia** *A mild form of ichthyosis.* | xérodermie |
| **xerophthalmia** *A manifestation of Vitamin A deficiency exhibited by dryness of the cornea and conjunctiva.* | xérophtalmie |
| **xeroradiography** *A form of radiography using photoelectric cells.* | xéroradiographie |
| **xerostomia** *A dry mouth from salivary gland hypofunction.* | xérostomie |
| **xiphoid process** *The inferior segment of the sternum.* | appendice xiphoïde |
| **yawn, to** | bâiller |
| **year** | année |
| **yearly** | annuel |
| **yeast** | levure |
| **yell, to** | hurler |
| **yellow** | jaune |
| **yellow fever** *A viral, hemorrhagic fever transmitted by mosquitos.* | 1. fièvre jaune 2. amarillose |
| **young** | jeune |
| **youth** | jeunesse |
| **zeiosis** *Resembling a bubbling activity.* | zéiose |
| **zero** | zéro |
| **Ziehl-Neelsen carbolfuchsin stain** *A stain used to detect acid-fast bacilli that appear red on the methylene blue background.* | colorant de Ziehl-Neelsen |
| **zinc** | zinc |
| **zonula** *A small zone or junction.* | zonule |
| **zoology** *The study of animals.* | zoologie |
| **zoonosis** *An animal-born disease that can be transmitted to humans, such as rabies.* | zoonose |
| **zoopsia** *A hallucination exhibited by the apparent visualization of animals.* | zoopsie |
| **zygomatic bone** *The triangular cheek bone.* | malaire os |
| **zygote** *A fertilized ovum.* | zygote |
| **zymogen** *An inactive compound that is metabolized to an active state.* | 1. proenzyme 2. zymogène |

| French | English |
| --- | --- |
| abaisse-langue | tongue depressor; tongue blade |
| abaissement | lowering |
| abattement | prostration |
| abcès | abscess |
| abcès alvéolaire | gumboil |
| abcès gingival | gumboil |
| abdomen | abdomen |
| abducens nerf | abducens nerve |
| abducteur | abducent |
| aberrant | aberrant |
| ablation | removal |
| abondant | bulky |
| abord | access |
| aboutissement | end point |
| absence | absence |
| absence d'utérus | ametria |
| absolu | absolute |
| abstenir | withhold |
| abus | abuse |
| abus sexuel | sexual abuse |
| acalculie | acalculia |
| acanthome | acanthoma |
| acanthose | acanthosis |
| acapnie | acapnia |
| acariase | acariasis |
| acaricide | acaricide |
| acarien | acarus |
| acariose | acariasis |
| acatalasie | acatalasia |
| acathisie | acathisia |
| accepter | comply |
| accès | attack; fit |
| accès maniaque aigu | acute manic attack |
| accessoire | accessory |
| accident | accident |
| accident ischémique transitoire | transient ischemic attack (TIA) |
| accident vasculaire cérébral | cerebrovascular accident (stroke) |
| accidenté | casualty |
| acclimatization | acclimatation |
| accommodation | accommodation |

| French | English |
|---|---|
| accompagnement | coaching |
| accompli | achieved |
| accord | agreement |
| accouchée | puerpera |
| accouchement | childbirth |
| accoucheur | obstetrician |
| accrétion | accretion |
| accroissement | increment |
| acéphale | acephalous |
| acétabulaire | acetabular |
| acétonémie | acetonemia |
| acétonurie | acetonuria |
| acétylcholine | acetylcholine |
| acétylsalicylique (acide) | acetylsalicylic acid |
| achalasie | achalasia |
| achlorhydrie | achlorhydria |
| acholie | acholia |
| achondroplasie | achondroplasia |
| achromatopsie | achromatopsia |
| achylie | achylia |
| acide | acid |
| acide gras | fatty acid |
| acide nicotinique | nicotinic acid |
| acidémie | acidemia |
| acidité | acidity |
| acidophilie | eosinophilia |
| acinite | acinitis |
| acné | acne |
| acné rosacée | acne rosacea |
| acorée | acorea |
| acouphène | tinnitus |
| acoustique | acoustic |
| acrocéphalie | acrocephaly |
| acrocyanose | acrocyanosis |
| acrodermatite | acrodermatitis |
| acrodynie | acrodynia |
| acromégalie | acaromegaly |
| acromio-claviculaire | acromioclavicular |
| acropathie ulcéromutilante | acrodystrophic neuropathy |
| acrotique | acrotic |
| acte manqué | parapraxis |
| actine | actin |

| French | English |
|---|---|
| acinodermatose | actinic dermatosis |
| action immédiate | immediate-acting |
| action prolongée | long acting |
| activité | activity |
| actomyosine | actomyosin |
| actuel | current |
| actuellement | currently |
| acuité | acuity |
| acupuncture | acupuncture |
| adactylie | adactylia |
| adaptation à la lumière | light adaptation |
| adaptation à l'obscurité | dark adaptation |
| adapté | convenient |
| addiction | addiction |
| Addison, maladie d' | Addison's disease |
| adducteur | adductor |
| adduction | adduction |
| adénectomie | adenectomy |
| adénite | adenitis |
| adéno-amygdalectomie | tonsillectomy |
| adénocarcinome | adenocarcinoma |
| adénofibrome | adenofibroma |
| adénoïde | adenoid |
| adénoïdectomie | adenoidectomy |
| adénoïdite | adenoiditis |
| adénolymphome | adenolymphoma |
| adénomyome | adenomyoma |
| adénomyose | adenomyosis |
| adénopathie | adenopathy |
| adénopathie, localisée | localized adenopathy |
| adénopathie, généralisée | generalized adenopathy |
| adénosine diphosphate (ADP) | adenosine diphosphate |
| adénosine monophosphate (AMP) | adenosine monophosphate |
| adénosine triphosphate (ATP) | adenosine triphosphate |
| adénovirus | adenovirus |
| adéquat | adequate |
| adhérence | adherence |
| adhésion | adhesion |
| adipeux | adipose |
| adiposité | fatness |
| aditus | aditus |
| adjuvant | adjuvant |

| French | English |
|---|---|
| ADN | DNA |
| adolescence | adolescence |
| adoucissant | demulcent |
| adrénalectomie | adrenalectomy |
| adrénaline | adrenaline (epinephrine) |
| adrénergique | adrenergic |
| adrénocorticotrope hormone | adrenocorticotrophic hormone (ACTH) |
| adventice | adventitia |
| aérobie | aerobe |
| aérodontalgie | aerodontalgia |
| aéroembolisme | air embolism |
| aérophagie | aerophagy |
| afébrile | afebrile |
| affamé | starved |
| affect | affect |
| affection démyélinisante | demyelinating disease |
| afférent | afferent |
| affinité | affinity |
| affirmation | statement |
| aflatoxine | aflatoxin |
| agacer | needle |
| agar | agar |
| âge | age |
| âge gestationnel | gestational age |
| agénésie | agenesis |
| agenouillé | kneeling |
| agglutination | agglutination |
| aggraver, s' | worsen |
| agitation | agitation |
| agnathie | agnathia |
| agnosie | agnosia |
| agonie | agony |
| agoniste | agonist |
| agoraphobie | agoraphobia |
| agrafe | clasp |
| agrandissement | enlargement |
| agranulocytose | agranulocytosis |
| agraphie | agraphia |
| agrégation plaquettaire | platelet clumping |
| agrément | approval |
| agression | aggression |
| agrippement | grasping |

| French | English |
| --- | --- |
| aidant | caregiver |
| aide | assistance |
| aigre | sour |
| aigu (masculine) aiguë (féminine) | acute |
| aiguille | needle |
| aiguille hypodermique | hypodermic needle |
| aiguille à ponction lombaire | needle for lumbar puncture |
| aile blanche interne | hypoglossal triangle |
| aimant | magnet |
| aine | groin |
| air complémentaire | inspiratory reserve volume |
| air de réserve | expiratory reserve volume |
| air résiduel | residual volume (RV) |
| aisselle | axilla |
| ajournement | postponement |
| ajouter | add |
| ajustement | adjustment |
| akathisie | akathisia |
| akinésie | acinesia |
| albinisme | albinism |
| albinos | albino |
| albumine | albumin |
| albuminurie | albuminuria |
| alcali | alkali |
| alcalin | alkaline |
| alcalinurie | alkalinuria |
| alcaloïde | alkaloid |
| alcalose | alkalosis |
| alcaptonurie | alkaptonuria |
| alcool | alcohol |
| alcool éthylique | ethanol |
| alcoolémie | blood alcohol level |
| alcoolique | alcoholic |
| alcoolisme | alcoholism |
| alcootest | breath test (for alcohol) |
| aldéhyde | aldehyde |
| aldostérone | aldosterone |
| aldostéronisme | aldosteronism |
| alèse | drawsheet |
| alexie | alexia |
| algide | algid |
| algie vasculaire de la face | cluster headache |

| French | English |
|---|---|
| algogène | algogenic |
| algue | alga |
| aliénation mentale | insanity |
| aliéné | insane |
| alignement dentaire défectueux | malalignment (dental) |
| aliment | food |
| alimentaire | alimentary |
| alimentation parentérale | enteral feeding |
| alitement | bed rest |
| allaitement maternel | breast feeding |
| allantoïde | allantois |
| allèle | allele |
| allergène | allergen |
| allergie | allergy |
| allogreffe | allograft |
| allongement | lengthening |
| allopathie | allopathy |
| allure | pace |
| alopécie | alopecia |
| alpha-fœtoprotéine (AFP) | alpha-fetoprotein |
| altération | impairment |
| altéré | impaired |
| alvéolaire | alveolar |
| alvéole pulmonaire | alveolus |
| Alzheimer, maladie d' | Alzheimer's disease |
| amalgame | amalgam |
| amarillose | yellow fever |
| amastie | amastia |
| amaurose | amaurosis |
| ambidextre | ambidextrous |
| amblyopie | amblyopia |
| ambulation | ambulation |
| ambulatoire | ambulatory |
| âme | soul |
| amélie | amelia |
| amélioration | amelioration |
| aménorrhée | amenorrhea |
| amer | bitter |
| amétrie | ametria |
| amétropie | ametropia |
| amiante | asbestos |
| amibe | ameba |

| French | English |
|---|---|
| amibiase | amebiasis |
| aminé acide | amino acid |
| ammoniac | ammonia |
| amnésie | amnesia |
| amnésie antérograde | amnesia, antegrade |
| amniocentèse | amniocentesis |
| amniographie | amniography |
| amnios | amnion |
| amoebicide | amebicide |
| amoebome | ameboma |
| amorphe | amorphous |
| ampliation | expansion |
| ampoule | ampulla; blister |
| amputation orthopédique | kineplasty |
| amygdale | tonsil |
| amygdalectomie | tonsillectomy |
| amygdalite | tonsillitis |
| amylase | amylase |
| amylase salivaire | ptyalin |
| amyloïdose | amyloidosis |
| amyotonie | amyotonia |
| amyotrophie | amyotrophy; muscular atrophy |
| amyotrophie péronière de Charcot-Marie | peroneal atrophy |
| anabolisme | anabolism |
| anacrote | anacrotic |
| anaérobie | anaerobe |
| analeptique | analeptic |
| analgésie | analgesia |
| analgésique | analgesic |
| analogue | analogous |
| analyse urinaire | urinalysis |
| anaphase | anaphase |
| anaphorèse | anaphoresis |
| anaphylaxie | anaphylaxis |
| anaplasie | anaplasia |
| anasarque fœtoplacentaire | hydrops fetalis |
| anastomose | anastomosis |
| anatomie | anatomy |
| anatomique | anatomical |
| anatomopathologie | pathology |
| anatomopathologique | pathological |
| anatoxine | toxoid |

| French | English |
|---|---|
| ancien | former |
| androgène | androgen |
| androstérone | androsterone |
| anémie | anemia |
| anémie aplasique | aplastic anemia |
| anémie ferriprive | iron-deficiency anemia |
| anémie hémolytique | hemolytic anemia |
| anencéphalie | anencephaly |
| anéroïde | aneroid |
| anesthésie | anesthesia |
| anesthésie en gant | glove anesthesia |
| anesthésie par bloc nerveux | nerve-block anesthesia |
| anesthésie péridurale | epidural analgesia |
| anesthésique | anesthetic |
| anesthésiste | anesthetist |
| anévrisme | aneurysm |
| anévrisme atrério-veineux | arteriovenous aneurysm |
| anévrisme disséquant | dissecting aneurysm |
| angéite | angiitis |
| angiectasie | angiectasie |
| angine | sore throat |
| angine de poitrine | angina pectoris |
| angine de Vincent | Vincent's angina |
| angine herpétiforme | herpangina |
| angine phlegmoneuse | quinsy |
| angiocardiographie | coronary angiography |
| angiocholite | cholangitis |
| angiogramme | angiogram |
| angiographie | angiography |
| angiome | angioma |
| angiome caverneux | cavernous hemangioma |
| angiome plan | capillary nevus |
| angiome stellaire | spider nevus |
| angioneurotique | angioneurotic |
| angioplastie | angioplasty |
| angiosarcome | angiosarcoma |
| angiospasme | angiospasm |
| angiotensine | angiotensin |
| angle | flexure |
| angoisse | anguish |
| angor d'effort | exercised induce angina |
| anhidrose | anhidrosis |

| French | English |
| --- | --- |
| anhidrotique | anhidrotic |
| anhydre | anhydrous |
| anhydride carbonique | carbon dioxide gas |
| animal familier | pet |
| animé | brisk |
| aniséiconie | aniseikonia |
| anisochromatopsie | anisochromatopsia |
| anisocorie | anisocoria |
| anisocytose | anisocytosis |
| anisomélie | anisomelia |
| anisométropie | anisometropia |
| ankyloglossie | ankyloglossia |
| ankylose | ankylosis |
| ankylostome | hookworm |
| ankylostomiase | ancylostomiasis |
| anneau | ring |
| anneau de Kayser-Fleicher | pericorneal ring |
| année | year |
| annexes | adnexa |
| annuel | yearly |
| annulaire | annular (ring finger) |
| annuler | cancel |
| anodin | harmless |
| anomalie congénitale | birth defect |
| anomie | anomia |
| anonychie | anonychia |
| anopérinéal | anoperineal |
| anorchide | anorchous |
| anorectal | anorectal |
| anorexie | anorexia |
| anorexie mentale | anorexia nervosa |
| anorganique | inorganic |
| anormal | abnormal |
| anosmie | anosmia |
| anovulation | anovulation |
| anoxémie | anoxemia |
| anoxie | anoxia |
| anse afférente, syndrome de l' | afferent loop syndrome |
| antagoniste | antagonist |
| antebrachium | forearm |
| antécédents | past history |
| antécédents familiaux | family history |

| French | English |
|---|---|
| antéhypophyse | adenohypophysis |
| anténatal | antenatal |
| antérieur | anterior |
| antérograde | anterograde |
| antéro-inférieur | anteroinferior |
| antérolatéral | anterolateral |
| antéromédian | anteromedian |
| antéropostérieur | anteroposterior |
| antérosupérieur | anterosuperior |
| antéversion | anteversion |
| anthelminthique | anthelmintic |
| anthracose | anthracosis |
| anthrax | anthrax |
| antiacide | antacid |
| antiagrégant plaquettaire | platelet suppressive agent |
| antibiotique | antibiotic |
| anticholinergique | anticholinergic |
| anticholinestérase | anticholinesterase |
| anticoagulant | anticoagulant |
| anticodon | anticodon |
| anticonceptionnel | contraceptive |
| anticonvulsivant | anticonvulsant |
| anticorps | antibody |
| anticorps tréponémiques fluorescents (test FTA) | FTA test |
| antidépresseur | antidepressant |
| anti-diabétiques oraux | oral anti-diabetic |
| antidiurétique hormone | antidiuretic hormone (vasopressin) |
| antidote | antidote |
| antifongique | antimycotic |
| antigène | antigen |
| antihistaminique | antihistamine |
| antihypertenseur | antihypertensive |
| anti-inflammatoire | anti-inflammatory |
| antilymphocytaire | antilymphocyte |
| antimétabolite | antimetabolite |
| antimigraineux | antimigraine |
| antimitotique | antimitotic |
| antimycosique | antimycotic |
| antinion | glabella |
| antipaludique | antimalarial |
| antipéristaltique | antiperistaltic |
| antiprurigineux | antipruritic |

| French | English |
|---|---|
| antipyrétique | antipyretic |
| antiseptique | antiseptic |
| antisérum | antiserum |
| antispasmodique | antispasmodic |
| antithrombine | antithrombin |
| antithyroïdien | antithyroid |
| antitoxine | antitoxin |
| antitussif | antitussive |
| antivenin | antivenin |
| antre | antrum |
| antrotomie | antrotomy |
| anurie | anuria |
| anus | anus |
| anxiété | anxiety |
| anxieux | anxious |
| aorte | aorta |
| aortique | aortic |
| aoûtat | chigger |
| apathie | apathy |
| aperception | apperception |
| apéristaltisme | aperistalsis |
| Apgar, indice d' | Apgar score |
| aphagie | aphagia |
| aphakie | aphakia |
| aphasie | aphasia |
| aphonie | aphonia |
| aphte buccal | aphthous stomatitis |
| apicectomie | apicetomy |
| aplasie médullaire | bone marrow aplasia |
| aplatir | flatten |
| apnée | apnea |
| apnée de sommeil | sleep apnea |
| aponévrose | aponeurosis |
| aponévrose de Denonvilliers | rectovesical septum |
| aponévrosite plantaire | plantar fibromatosis |
| apophyse | apophysis |
| apophyse épineuse | spine of vertebra |
| apophyse mastoïde | mastoid process |
| apoplexie | apoplexy |
| appareil autopiqueur | fingerstick device |
| appareil juxtaglomérulaire | juxtaglomerular apparatus |
| appareil orthopédique | brace |

| French | English |
| --- | --- |
| appariement | matching |
| apparition | emergence |
| appendice | appendix |
| appendice xiphoïde | xiphoid process |
| appendicectomie | appendectomy |
| appendicite | appendicitis |
| applicateur | applicator |
| application | application |
| apport alimentaire | food intake |
| apport hydrique | fluid intake |
| apporter | bring |
| appréhension | apprehension |
| apprentissage | learning |
| approximatif | approximate |
| approximativement | approximately |
| apraxie | apraxia |
| apte | apt |
| aptitude | aptitude |
| aptylisme | aptyalism |
| aprétique | afebrile |
| aqueux | aqueous |
| arachnodactylie | arachnodactyly |
| arachnoïde | arachnoid |
| araignée | spider nevus |
| arbovirus | arbovirus |
| arc | arcus |
| arcade sourcilière | superciliary arch |
| arceau | cradle |
| aréole | areola |
| argent | silver |
| argininosuccinurie | argininosuccinicaciduria |
| argumenter | argue |
| argyrie | argyria |
| ARN ribosomal | ribosomal RNA |
| arrêt cardiaque | cardiac arrest |
| arrêt du traitement | treatment withdrawal |
| arrhénoblastome | arrhenoblastoma |
| arriération profonde | amentia |
| arriéré | feeble minded |
| arrière-faix | after-birth |
| arrière-goût | after-taste |
| artefact | artifact |

| French | English |
|---|---|
| artère | artery |
| artériectomie | arteriectomy |
| artériel | arterial |
| artériographie | arteriography |
| artérioplastie | arterioplasty |
| artériosclérose | arteriosclerosis |
| artériotomie | arteriotomy |
| artérite | arteritis |
| arthralgie | arthralgia |
| arthrite | arthritis |
| arthrodèse | arthrodesis |
| arthrodynie | arthrodynia |
| arthrographie | arthrography |
| arthropathie des hémophiles | hemophilic arthropathy |
| arthroplastie | arthroplasty |
| arthroscopie | arthroscopy |
| arthrose | osteoarthritis |
| arthrotomie | arthrotomy |
| articulaire | articular |
| articulation cox-fémorale | hip joint |
| articulation en selle | saddle joint |
| articulation temporo-mandibulaire | temporomandibular joint |
| articulation tibio-astragalienne | ankle joint |
| artificiel | artificial |
| aryténoïde | arytenoid |
| arythmie | arrhythmia |
| arythmie sinusale | sinus arrhythmia |
| asbeste | asbestos |
| asbestose | asbestosis |
| ascaricide | ascaricide |
| ascaris | ascaris (round worm) |
| ascite | ascites; ascitic fluid |
| ascorbique acide | ascorbic acid |
| asepsie | asepsis |
| aseptique | aseptic |
| asexué | asexual |
| aspect | appearance |
| aspermie | aspermia |
| asphyxie | asphyxia |
| aspirateur | aspirator |
| aspiration | aspiration |
| aspirine | aspirin |

| French | English |
|---|---|
| assis | sitting |
| assistance cardiorespiratoire | cardiorespiratory assistance |
| assoupissement | drowsiness |
| assurer de, s' | ensure |
| astéatose | asteatosis |
| astéréognosie | astereognosis |
| asthénie | asthenia |
| asthénopie | asthenopia |
| asthme | asthma |
| asthme hyperéosinophilique | hypereosinophilic asthma |
| astragale os | talon |
| astringent | astringent |
| astrocytome | astrocytoma |
| astroglie | astroglia |
| asymétrie | asymmetry |
| asymptomatique | asymptomatic |
| asynclitisme | asynclitism |
| atavisme | atavism |
| ataxie | ataxia |
| atélectasie | atelectasis |
| athérogène | atherogenic |
| athérome | atheroma |
| athétose | athetosis |
| athlète, pied d' | athlete's foot |
| atlas | atlas |
| atomiseur | atomizer |
| atonie | atony |
| atrésie | atresia |
| atrial | atrial |
| atrioventriculaire | atrioventricular |
| atrium | atrium |
| atrophie | atrophy |
| atrophie sclérosante de la vulve | kraurosis vulvae |
| atrophique | atrophic |
| atropine | atropine |
| attaque | attack, seizure |
| atteint | affected |
| atteinte | disorder; impairment |
| attelle | brace; splint |
| attelle pour dorsiflexion du poignet | cock-up splint |
| attendre | expect |
| attente en | on hold |

| French | English |
|---|---|
| attentif | alert |
| atténuer | alleviate |
| attouchement | touch |
| atypique | atypical |
| au-delà | beyond |
| au-dessus de la normale | above normal |
| audiogramme | audiogram |
| audiologiste | audiologist |
| audiomètre | audiometer |
| auditif | auditory |
| audition | hearing |
| augmentation de volume | enlargement |
| aural | aural |
| auriculaire | auricular |
| auricule | auricle |
| auriculotemporal | auriculotemporal |
| auriculoventriculaire | atrioventricular |
| auscultation | auscultation |
| autisme | autism |
| autiste | autistic |
| auto-anticorps | autoantibody |
| auto-antigen | autoantigen |
| autochtone | indigenous |
| autoclave | autoclave |
| autogène | autogenous |
| autogreffe | autograft |
| autohypnose | autohypnosis |
| auto-immunisation | autoimmunization |
| autolyse | autolysis |
| autopsie | autopsy |
| autorégulation | self-regulation |
| autosomique | autosomal |
| autotransfusion | autotransfusion |
| autour | around |
| avalement | swallowing |
| avancé | advanced |
| avant en | forwards |
| avant la mort | antemortem |
| avant-bras | forearm |
| avarié | spoiled |
| avasculaire | avascular |
| avérer, s' | transpire |

| French | English |
|---|---|
| aveugle | blind |
| aviaire | avian |
| avitaminose | avitaminosis |
| avortement | abortion |
| avortement provoqué | induced abortion |
| axe | axis |
| axillaire | axillary |
| axone | axon |
| azoospermie | azoospermia |
| azote | nitrogen |
| azotémie | azotemia |
| azoturie | azoturia |
| bacillaire | bacillary |
| bacille | bacillus |
| bactéricide | bactericidal |
| bactériémie | bacteremia |
| bactérien | bacterial |
| bactéries | bacteria |
| bactériostatique | bacteriostatic |
| bactérurie | bacteriuria |
| bagassose | bagassois |
| bâiller | yawn |
| baisse | decline |
| balance | scale (like to check weight) |
| balancement | rocking |
| balanite | balanitis |
| balbutiement | stammering |
| ballonnement | bloating |
| ballottement | ballottement |
| balnéologie | balneology |
| banal | trivial |
| bandage | bandage |
| bandage herniaire | truss |
| bande élastique | elastic bandage |
| bande plâtrée | casting gauze |
| bandelette diagnostique | test strip (ie. glucose) |
| bandelette longitudinale du côlon | longitudinal band of colon |
| banque de sang | blood bank |
| barrière hématoméningée | blood brain barrier |
| barrière placentaire | placental barrier |
| bas poids moléculaire | low-molecular weight |
| basal | basal |

| French | English |
|---|---|
| base de données | access |
| Basedow-Graves, maladie de | Graves' disease |
| basilaire | basilar |
| basophile | basophil |
| bassin androïde | android pelvis |
| bassin de lit | bedpan |
| bassinet rénal | renal pelvis |
| battement | beat |
| battement cardiaque | heart beat |
| baume | balm |
| baver | dribble |
| béance du col utérin | incompetent cervix |
| béant | gaping |
| beaucoup de | lots of |
| bébé | baby |
| bec-de-lièvre | cleft lip |
| bec-de-perroquet | beaked osteophyte |
| bégaiement | stuttering |
| Behçet, maladie de | Behçet's syndrome |
| bénévole | volunteer |
| bénin | benign |
| béquilles | crutches |
| berceau | cradle |
| bérylliose | berylliosis |
| Besnier-Boeck-Schaumann, maladie de | sarcoidosis |
| besoin | need |
| besoin impérieux | urgency (as in urinary urgency) |
| bêta-bloquant | betablocker |
| bête | silly |
| bézoard | bezoar |
| biaisé | biased |
| biauriculaire | binaural |
| biberon | bottle |
| bibliothèque | library |
| biceps | biceps |
| bicuspide | bicuspid |
| bien nourri | well fed |
| bien portant | healthy |
| bifide | bifid |
| bifurqué | bifurcate |
| bilan | assessment |
| bilatéral | bilateral |

| French | English |
|---|---|
| bile | bile |
| Bilharzia | Bilharzi (Schistosomiasis) |
| biliaire | biliary |
| bilieux | bilious |
| bilirubine | bilirubin |
| biliurie | biliuria |
| biliverdine | biliverdin |
| bimanuel | bimanual |
| binoculaire | binocular |
| biochimie | biochemistry |
| biodisponibilité | bioavailability |
| biologie | biology |
| biopsie | biopsy |
| biopsie à l'aiguille | needle biopsy |
| biopsie-exérèse | excisional biopsy |
| biotine | biotin |
| biovulé | binovular |
| bistouri | bistoury; scalpel |
| blanc | white |
| blastomycose | blastomycosis |
| blastomycose chéloïdienne | Lobo's disease |
| blennorrhée | blennorrhea |
| blénorragie | gonorrhea |
| blépharite | blepharitis |
| blépharospasme | blepharospasm |
| blessé | injured person |
| blesser | injure |
| blessure | injury |
| bleu | blue |
| bloc auriculo-ventriculaire | atrio-ventricular block |
| bloc cardiaque | heart block |
| bloc de branche | bundle branch block |
| bloc opératoire | surgical suite |
| blouse | gown |
| boire | drink |
| bol | bolus |
| bombé | bulging |
| bord | border; margin |
| borréliose | relapsing fever |
| bosse | lump |
| bosse sérosanguine | caput succedaneum |
| botte de marche | walking cast |

| French | English |
| --- | --- |
| bouche | mouth |
| bouche-à-bouche | mouth to mouth |
| bouchée | mouthful |
| boucle débit-volume | flow-volume loop |
| bouffée de chaleur | hot flash |
| bouffissure | puffiness |
| bougie | candle |
| bougirage | bougienage |
| bouillant | scalding |
| bouillon de culture | culture broth |
| boulimie | bulimia |
| bourbouille | prickly heat |
| bourdonnement d'oreille | tinnitus |
| bourgeon charnu | granulation tissue |
| bourgeon du goût | taste bud |
| Bourneville | tuberous sclerosis |
| bourrelet | labrum |
| bourse | bursa; scrotum |
| bout du doigt | fingertip |
| bouteille | bottle |
| bouton | button; pimple |
| bouton d'Alep | oriental sore |
| bouton de fièvre | cold sore |
| brachial | brachial |
| brachiale artère | brachial artery |
| brachycéphalie | brachycephaly |
| bradycardie | bradycardia |
| bradykinine | bradykinin |
| brancard | stretcher |
| branche | ramus; branch |
| branchial | branchial |
| bras | arm |
| bregma | bregma |
| brillant | bright |
| broche | pin; wire |
| bromhidrose | bromidrosis |
| bromisme | bromism |
| bronche | bronchus |
| bronchectasie | bronchiectasis |
| bronchiole | bronchiole |
| bronchiolite | bronchiolitis |
| bronchique | bronchial |

| French | English |
|---|---|
| bronchite | bronchitis |
| bronchite aiguë | acute bronchitis |
| bronchite chronitis | chronic bronchitis |
| bronchogénique | bronchogenic |
| bronchographie | bronchography |
| bronchopneumonie | bronchopneumonia |
| bronchoscope | bronchoscope |
| bronchoscopie | bronchoscopy |
| bronchospasme | bronchospasm |
| brosse | brush |
| broyé | ground |
| brucellose | brucellosis |
| bruit | bruit; sound |
| bruit respiratoire | whisper |
| brûlure | burn |
| brûlure gastrique | stomach pain |
| brûlures gastriques | heart burn |
| brûlures mictionnelles | burning on urination |
| brun | brown |
| brut | gross |
| bubon | bubo |
| buccal | buccal |
| buccinateur | buccinator |
| Budd-Chiari, syndrome de | Budd-Chiari syndrome |
| buisson | bush |
| bulbe rachidien | medulla oblongata |
| bulle | bulla |
| bursite | bursitis |
| byssinose | byssinosis |
| c.à.d. (c'est-à-dire) | i.e. (id est) |
| caca | excrement (slang) |
| cachexie | cachexia |
| cadavre | cadaver |
| caducée | caduceus |
| caduque | decidua |
| cæcum | cecum |
| cage thoracique | rib cage |
| caillot | clot |
| caillot sanguin | blood clot |
| caisson hyperbare | hyperbaric chamber |
| caissons, maladie des | caisson disease (decompression sickness) |
| cal | callus |

| French | English |
|---|---|
| cal vicieux | malunion |
| calcaire | calcareous |
| calcanéum | calcaneus |
| calcémie | calcemia |
| calciférol | calciferol |
| calcification | calcification |
| calcitonine | calcitonin |
| calcium | calcium |
| calcul | calculus (stone) |
| calcul biliaire | gallstone |
| calcul urinaire | urolith |
| calcul vésical | cystolithiasis |
| calibre | gauge |
| calibrer | calibrate |
| calice | calyx |
| callosité | callosity; callus |
| calmant | sedative |
| calme | quiet |
| calorie | calorie |
| calotte crânienne | calvaria |
| calvitie | alopecia |
| camisole de force | strait-jacket |
| canal artériel | ductus arteriosus |
| canal artériel systémique | patent ductus arteriosus |
| canal biliaire | bile duct |
| canal carpien, syndrome du | carpal tunnel syndrome |
| canal cystique | cystic duct |
| canal galactophore | lactiferous duct |
| canal ionique | ion channel |
| canal sacré | sacral canal |
| canal semi-circulaire | semicircular canal |
| canalicule | canaliculus |
| cancer | cancer; carcinoma |
| cancer bronchique | bronchial carcinoma |
| cancer du sein | breast cancer |
| cancroïde | cancroid |
| candidose, œsophagienne | esophageal candidosis |
| canine | canine teeth |
| cannabis | cannabis |
| canne anglaise | forearm crutch |
| canule | cannula |
| capacité respiratoire | lung capacity |

| French | English |
|---|---|
| capacité vitale | vital capacity (VC) |
| capillaire | capillary |
| capsulite | capsulitis |
| capsulotomie | capsulotomy |
| capuchon muqueux | pericoronal flap |
| carboxyhémoglobine | carboxyhemoglobin |
| carcinogène | carcinogenic |
| carcinoïde | carcinoid |
| carcinomatose | carcinomatosis |
| carcinome | carcinoma |
| cardia | cardia |
| cardiaque | cardiac |
| cardiologie | cardiology |
| cardiomyopathie | cardiomyopathy |
| cardiopathie congénitale | congenital heart disease |
| cardiopathie ischémique | ischemic heart disease |
| cardiopathie rhumatismale | rheumatic heart disease |
| cardiovasculaire | cardiovascular |
| cardite | carditis |
| carence affective | affective deprivation |
| carène | carina |
| carie | caries |
| carie dentaire | dental caries |
| carné | carneous |
| caroncule | caruncle |
| carotène | carotene |
| carotide | carotid |
| carpe | carpus |
| carpe, grand os du | capitate bone |
| carpométacarpien | carpometacarpal |
| cartographie | mapping |
| caryocinèse | karyokinesis |
| caryotype | karyotype |
| caséine | casein |
| Casoni, épreuve de | Casoni's test |
| cassé | broken |
| cassure | break |
| castration | castration |
| catabolisme | catabolism |
| catalepsie | catalepsy |
| cataphorèse | cataphoresis |
| cataplexie | cataplexy |

| French | English |
|---|---|
| cataracte | cataract |
| catarrhe | catarrh |
| catatonie | catatonie |
| catharsis | catharsis |
| cathartique | cathartic |
| cathéter | catheter |
| cauchemar | nightmare |
| caudal | caudal |
| caudé | caudate |
| causal | causative |
| caustique | caustic |
| cautère | cautery |
| caverne | cavity |
| cavité articulaire | socket |
| cécité | blindness |
| ceinture | belt; waist |
| ceinture pelvienne | hip girdle |
| célibataire | single (not married) |
| cellule | cell |
| cellule bordante | parietal cell |
| cellule ciliée | hair cell |
| cellule-cible | target cell |
| cellules caliciformes | goblet cells |
| cellulite | cellulitis |
| cellulose | cellulose |
| centigrade | centigrade |
| centimètre | centimeter |
| centre | center |
| centrifugeuse | centrifuge |
| centripète | centripetal |
| céphalée | headache |
| céphalée de tension | tension headache |
| céphalique | cephalic |
| cercaire | cercaria |
| cerclage | banding |
| cérébral | cerebral |
| cérébration | cerebration |
| cérumen | cerumen |
| cervicalgie | cervical (neck) pain |
| cerveau | brain; cerebrum |
| cerveau antérieur | forebrain |
| cerveau postérieur | hindbrain |

| French | English |
|---|---|
| cervelet | cerebellum |
| cervical | cervical |
| cervicectomie | cervicectomy |
| cervicite | cervicitis |
| cervico-vaginite | cervico-vaginitis |
| césarienne | caesarian section |
| cestode | tapeworm; cestode |
| cétone | ketone |
| cétonémie | ketonemia |
| cétonurie | ketonuria |
| cétose | ketosis |
| chagrin | grief |
| chair | flesh |
| chair de poule | goose bumps |
| chalazion | meibomian cyst |
| chaleur | heat |
| chambre | room; chamber |
| chambre postérieure de l'œil | posterior chamber of the eye |
| champ opératoire | drape |
| champ visuel | visual field |
| champignon | fungus |
| chancre | chancre |
| chancrelle | chancroid |
| changement | alteration |
| chaque | every |
| chat dans la gorge, avoir un | frog in the throat, to have |
| chatouillement | tickle |
| chaud | hot |
| chaussette | sock |
| chaussure | shoe |
| chef d'un muscle | caput |
| chéilite | chelilitis |
| chélateur | chelating agent |
| chéloïde | keloid |
| chémorécepteur | chemoreceptor |
| chémosis | chemosis |
| chétif | weak |
| cheveu | hair |
| cheville | ankle |
| chiasma | chiasma |
| chimère | chimera |
| chimiotactisme | chemotaxis |

| French | English |
|---|---|
| chimiothérapie | chemotherapy |
| chiropracteur | chiropractor |
| chiropraxie | chiropractic |
| chirurgical | surgical |
| chirurgie | surgery |
| chirurgien | surgeon |
| chlamydiase | chlamydiosis |
| chloasma | chloasma |
| chlorhydrate | hydrochloride |
| chlorhydrique acide | hydrochloric acid |
| chloroforme | chloroform |
| chlorome | chloroma |
| chlorure de sodium | sodium chloride |
| choanes | choanae |
| choc | shock |
| choc anaphylactique | anaphylactic shock |
| choc spinal | spinal shock |
| choc toxique | toxic shock |
| choix | choice |
| cholagogue | cholagogue |
| cholangogramme | cholangiogram |
| cholangite | cholangitis |
| cholécystectomie | cholecystectomy |
| cholécystenstérostomie | cholecystenterostomy |
| cholécystite | cholecystitis |
| cholécystolithiase | cholecystolithiasis |
| cholédocholithotomie | choledocholithotomy |
| cholélithiase | cholelithiasis |
| cholémie | cholemia |
| choléra | cholera |
| cholestéatome | cholesteatoma |
| cholestérol | cholesterol |
| cholinergique | cholinergic |
| cholinestérase | cholinesterase |
| cholurie | choluria |
| chondralgie | chondralgia |
| chondrite | chondritis |
| chondrodynie | chondralgia |
| chondromalacie | chondromalacia |
| chondrome | chondroma |
| chondrosarcome | chondrosarcoma |
| chordée | chordee |

172

| French | English |
|---|---|
| chordite | chorditis |
| chorée | chorea |
| choroïde | choroid |
| choroïdite | choroiditis |
| choroïdocyclite | choroidocyclitis |
| chromatine | chromatin |
| chromasome | chromosome |
| chronique | chronic |
| chuchoter | whisper |
| chuintement | hissing |
| chyle | chyle |
| chyleux | chylous |
| chylomicron | chylomicron |
| chyme | chyme |
| cible | target |
| cicatrice | cicatrix (scar) |
| cicatriciel | cicatricial |
| cicatrisation | healing |
| cil | eyelash |
| cils | cilia |
| cinéplastie | kineplasty |
| cinésie | kinesis |
| circadien | circadian |
| circoncision | circumcision |
| circonférence | circumference |
| circonflexe nerf | circumflex nerve |
| circonscrit | circumscribed |
| circulation sanguine | blood stream |
| cire | wax |
| cirrhose | cirrhosis |
| cirsoïde | cirsoid |
| ciseaux | scissors |
| citer | mention |
| citerne de Pecquet | ampulla chyli |
| civière | stretcher |
| clair | clear |
| clamp | forceps |
| claquement | click; snap |
| classement | grading |
| claudication | claudication; limp |
| claustrophobie | claustrophobia |
| clavicule | clavicle |

| French | English |
|---|---|
| clearance | clearance |
| cléidotomie | cleidotomy |
| clic | click |
| cliché thoracique | chest x-ray |
| clignement | blinking |
| clinique | clinic |
| clitoris | clitoris |
| cloison | septum |
| clonique | clonic |
| clonus du pied | ankle clonus |
| cloque | blister |
| clou | boil; clavus |
| coagulation | coagulation |
| coarctation | coarctation |
| cobalt | cobalt |
| cocaïne | cocaine |
| cocaïnomanie | cocaine addiction |
| coccus | coccus |
| coccygodynie | coccydynia |
| coccyx | coccyx |
| cochlée | cochlea |
| codéine | codeine |
| codon | codon |
| cœliaque | celiac |
| cœlioscope | laparoscope |
| cœlioscopie | laparoscopy |
| cœur | heart |
| cœur pulmonaire | cor pulmonale |
| cœur-poumon artificiel | heart lung machine |
| cognition | cognition |
| coiffe des rotateurs | rotator cuff |
| coït | coitus |
| col | neck |
| col de l'utérus | cervix uteri |
| colectomie | colectomy |
| colique | colic |
| colique néphrétique | renal colic |
| colite | colitis |
| colite pseudo-membraneuse | pseudomembranous colitis |
| collabé | collapsed |
| collagène | collagen |
| collapsus | collapse |

| French | English |
|---|---|
| colle | glue |
| collobome | colloboma |
| collodion | collodion |
| colloïde | colloid |
| collyre | eye drops |
| colobome | coloboma |
| côlon | colon |
| côlon ascendant | ascending colon |
| côlon irritable | irritable bowel syndrome |
| colonne vertébrale | vertebral column |
| coloration conjonctive | color of conjunctiva |
| colostomie | colostomy |
| colostrum | colostrum |
| colpite | colpitis |
| colpocèle | colpocele |
| colporraphie | colporrhaphy |
| colposcope | colposcope |
| colposcopie | colposcopy |
| columelle | modiolus |
| coma | coma |
| coma dépassé | brain death |
| comateux | comatose |
| comédons | comedones |
| commensal | commensal |
| commentaire | comment |
| commotion | concussion |
| commun | common |
| communication interauriculaire | atrial septal defect |
| communication interventriculaire | ventricular septal defect |
| compatibilité | compatibility |
| compatibilité sanguine, épreuve de | cross-matching (blood) |
| compliance | compliance |
| comportement alimentaire | feeding behavior |
| composé | compound |
| compréhension | comprehension |
| compresse | pad |
| compression | compression |
| compression médullaire | cord compression |
| comprimé | tablet |
| comprimer | squeeze |
| comptage | counting |
| compte | count |

175

| French | English |
|---|---|
| compte-gouttes | dropper |
| concavité | concavity |
| concentration | concentration |
| concentrique | concentric |
| conception | conception |
| concrétion | concretion |
| condom | condom |
| conduction osseuse | osteophony |
| conduit lactifère | lactiferous duct |
| condyle | condyle |
| condylome | condyloma |
| condylomes acuminés | condylomata acuminata |
| cône | cone |
| confabulation | confabulation |
| confiance | confidence |
| conflit | conflict |
| confusion | confusion |
| confusion mentale | delirium |
| congélation | freezing |
| congénital | congenital |
| congestif | congestive |
| conjonctif | conjunctiva |
| conjonctivite | conjunctivitis |
| connaissance | cognition |
| connu | known |
| conque | concha |
| consanguinité | consanguinity |
| conscient | conscious |
| conseil conjugal | marital counseling |
| conseiller | advise |
| conservateur | conservative |
| consolidation | consolidation |
| consommation d'oxygène | oxygen consumption |
| constant | consistent |
| constipation | constipation |
| constitution | personality |
| constriction | constriction |
| contage | contact |
| contagieux | contagious |
| contagion secondaire | cross-infection |
| contaminé | contaminated |
| contention | bracing |

| French | English |
|---|---|
| contenu | content |
| contondant | blunt |
| contraceptif | contraceptive |
| contraceptif oral | oral contraceptive |
| contracture ischémique | ischemia contracture |
| contradictoire | contradictory |
| contraignant | demanding |
| contrainte | stress |
| contre-indication | contraindication |
| contre-placebo | placebo controlled |
| contusion | contusion |
| convenable | adequate |
| conversion | conversion |
| convexe | convex |
| convulsion | convulsion |
| copulation | copulation |
| coque | coccus |
| coqueluche | pertussis; whooping cough |
| coquillage | shellfish |
| cor | clavus |
| coracoïde | coracoid |
| corde | cord; chorda |
| cordite | chorditis |
| cordon sanitaire | sanitary cordon |
| cordon spermatique | spermatic cord |
| cordons de la moelle spinale | funiculi of the spinal cord |
| corne | horn |
| corné | keratic |
| cornée | cornea |
| cornéen | corneal |
| cornets des fosses nasales | turbinate bones |
| coroner | coroner |
| coronoïde | coronoid |
| corps calleux | corpus callosum |
| corps cellulaire | cell body |
| corps ciliaire | ciliary body |
| corps étranger | foreign body |
| corps genouillé | geniculate body |
| corps jaune | corpus luteum |
| corps strié | striate body |
| corps vitré | vitreous |
| corpulence | corpulence |

| French | English |
|---|---|
| corpuscule | corpuscle |
| cortex | cortex |
| cortical | cortical |
| corticostéroïde | corticosteroid |
| corticosurrénale | adrenal cortex |
| corticotrope | corticotrophic |
| cortisol | cortisol |
| cortisone | cortisone |
| coryza | coryza |
| coryza spasmodique | hay fever |
| costochondrite | costochondritis |
| côte | rib |
| côté | side |
| cou | neck |
| couché | recumbent |
| couche de bébé | diaper |
| couché sur le dos | supine |
| coude | cubitus (elbow) |
| coude du joueur de tennis | tennis elbow |
| cou-de-pied | instep |
| coup de chaleur | heat stroke |
| coup de pied | kick |
| coup d'œil | glance |
| coup du lapin | whiplash |
| coupe transversale | cross-section |
| couper | cut |
| couperose | acne rosacea |
| courbure | flexure |
| couronne dentaire | corona dentis |
| cours en | on going |
| coussinet | cushion |
| coût | cost |
| couturier muscle | sartorius muscle |
| couveuse | incubator |
| coxalgie | coxalgia |
| coxarthrose | arthritis of the hip |
| crachat | sputum |
| cracher | spit |
| crainte | fear |
| crampe | cramp |
| crâne | cranium |
| crânien | cranial |

| French | English |
|---|---|
| cranioclaste | cranioclast |
| craniopharyngiome | craniopharyngioma |
| craniosynostose | craniosynostosis |
| craniotabès | craniotabes |
| craniotomie | craniotomy |
| créatine | creatine |
| créatinine | creatinine |
| crénothérapie | crenotherapy |
| crépitation | crepitus |
| crête ampullaire | acoustic crest |
| crête iliaque | iliac crest |
| crétinisme | cretinism |
| creux | hollow |
| crevasse | crevice |
| cri du chat, maladie du | cat cry syndrome |
| cribriforme | cribriform |
| cricoïde | cricoid |
| crise | crisis; seizure |
| cristallin | lens |
| cristallinien | lenticular |
| cristalloïde | crystalloid |
| cristallurie | crystalluria |
| crochu | unciform |
| crochu du carpe | hamate bone; uncinate bone |
| croissance | growth |
| croup | croup |
| croûte | crust |
| cruciforme | cruciform |
| crural | crural; femoral |
| crural nerf | femoral nerve |
| cryesthésie | cryesthesia |
| cryochirurgie | cryosurgery |
| cryothérapie | cryotherapy |
| cryptorchidie | cryptorchism |
| cryptococcose | cryptococcus |
| cubitus | ulna; cubitus |
| cuillère à café | teaspoon |
| cuillère à soupe | tablespoon |
| cuillérée | spoonful |
| cuir chevelu | scalp |
| cuisse | thigh |
| cuivre | copper |

| French | English |
|---|---|
| cul-de-sac de Douglas | Douglas' pouch |
| culdoscopie | culdoscopy |
| culot urinaire | urinary sediments |
| culture | culture |
| cunéiforme | cuneiform |
| curare | curare |
| curatif | curative |
| curetage | curettage |
| curette | curette |
| cutané | cutaneous |
| cuticule | cuticle |
| cuvette | basin |
| cyanocobalamine | cyanocobalamin |
| cyanose | cyanosis |
| cycle anovulatoire | anovulatory cycle |
| cycle de Krebs | Krebs' cycle |
| cyclite | cyclitis |
| cyclodialyse | cyclodialysis |
| cycloplégie | cycloplegia |
| cyclothymie | cyclothymia |
| cyclotomie | cyclotomy |
| cylindraxe | axon |
| cylindre épithélial | epithelial cast |
| cylindres urinaires | urinary casts |
| cyphoscoliose | kyphoscoliosis |
| cyphose | kyphosis |
| cystadénome | cystadenoma |
| cystectomie | cystectomy |
| cysticercose | cysticercosis |
| cystinose | cystinosis |
| cystinurie | cystinuria |
| cystique | cystic |
| cystite | cystitis |
| cystocèle | cystocele |
| cystographie | cystography |
| cystographie mictionnelle | voiding cystography |
| cystolithiase | cystolithiasis |
| cystocope | cystocope |
| cystoscopie | cystoscopy |
| cytologie | cytology |
| cytoplasme | cytoplasm |
| cytotoxine | cytotoxin |

| French | English |
|---|---|
| cytotoxique | cytotoxic |
| dacryoadénite | dacryoadenitis |
| dacryocysitite | dacryocystitis |
| dacryocystorhinostomie | dacryocystorhinostomy |
| dacryolithe | dacryolith |
| daltonisme | color blindness |
| dard | sting |
| date de péremption | expiration date |
| date limite | deadline |
| de première intention | first line |
| déambulateur | walker |
| débilité | debility |
| débit cardiaque | cardiac output |
| débit de pointe | peak flow |
| débit expiratoire | expiratory flow rate |
| déboîtement | dislocation |
| debout | standing |
| début | onset |
| décapitation | decapitation |
| décennie | decade |
| décérébré | decerebrate |
| décès | death |
| déchiré | torn |
| déchirure | laceration |
| décibel | decibel |
| decidua | decidua |
| déclin | decline |
| décollement de rétine | retinal detachment |
| décompensation | decompensation |
| décompression | decompression |
| déconnexion interhémisphérique, syndrome de | commissural syndrome |
| décontracturant | relaxant |
| décubitus | recumbent decubitus |
| décussation | decussation |
| dédoublement | duplication |
| défaut | defect |
| défécation | defecation |
| défense musculaire | guarding |
| défibrillateur | defibrillator |
| déficit | deficiency |
| déficit immunitaire | immunodeficiency |
| déficit musculaire | muscle weakness |

| French | English |
|---|---|
| déformation | deformity |
| dégénérescence maculaire | macular degeneration |
| déglutition | deglutition |
| degré | grade |
| déjà-vu | pseudomnesia |
| délai supplémentaire | extension |
| délirant | delusional |
| délire | delusion |
| delirium tremens | delirium tremens |
| délivrance | expulsion of placenta |
| délivrance de médicaments | passing medications |
| délivre | after-birth |
| deltoïde | deltoid |
| démangeaison | itch |
| démarcation | demarcation |
| démarche | gait |
| démarche dandinante | waddling gait |
| démarche festinante | festinating gait |
| démence | dementia |
| demi | half |
| demi-vie | half life |
| démographie | demography |
| dendrite | dendrite |
| dénégation | negation |
| dénervé | denervated |
| dengue | dengue |
| densité | density |
| dent | tooth |
| dents de lait | deciduous teeth |
| dent de sagesse | wisdom tooth |
| dent incluse | impacted tooth |
| dents permanentes | permanent teeth |
| dentaire | dental |
| dentier | denture |
| dentiforme | odontoid |
| dentiste | dentist |
| dentition | dentition |
| dépilatoire | depilatory |
| dépistage | screening |
| déplacement | displacement |
| dépliant | leaflet |
| dépourvu de | free of |

| French | English |
| --- | --- |
| dépression | depression |
| déprimé | depressed |
| dermaphyte | dermatophyte |
| dermatite | dermatitis |
| dermatite atopique | atopic dermatitis |
| dermatite medicamenteuse | drug eruption |
| dermatite séborrhéique | seborrheic dermatitis |
| dermatographie | dermatography |
| dermatologie | dermatology |
| dermatologiste | dermatologist |
| dermatome | dermatome |
| dermatoycose | dermatomycosis |
| dermatomyosite | dermatomyositis |
| dermatophyte | dermatophyte |
| dermatophytose | ringworm |
| dermatose | dermatosis |
| derme | dermis |
| dermographie | dermographia |
| dernier | last |
| désarticulation | disarticulation |
| descendant | descending |
| désensibilisation | desensitization |
| déséquilibre | disequilibrium |
| déshabiller | disrobe |
| déshydratation | dehydration |
| désinfectant | disinfectant |
| désintoxication | detoxication |
| désir obsédant | craving |
| desmoïde | desmoid |
| désorientation | disorientation |
| désoxyribonucléique acide | deoxyribonucleic acid (DNA) |
| desquamation | desquamation |
| dessiccation | desiccation |
| dessin | drawing |
| dessous | below |
| désuet | obsolete |
| détendeur | pressure reducer |
| détérioration | deterioration |
| détermination | assay |
| déterminer | ascertain |
| détresse respiratoire, syndrome de | respiratory distress syndrome |
| détritus | detritus |

| French | English |
| --- | --- |
| détroit inférieur du bassin | inferior pelvis strait |
| détrusor | detrusor urinae |
| deuil | mourning |
| deutéranomalie | deuteranomaly |
| deux fois | two times |
| déviation | deviation |
| dextran | dextran |
| dextrocardie | dextrocardia |
| diabète insipide | diabetes insipidus |
| diabète sucré | diabetes mellitus |
| diabétique | diabetic |
| diagnostic differentiel | differential diagnosis |
| diagnostique | diagnostic |
| diamètre promonto-rétropubien | conjugate diameter |
| diapason | tuning fork |
| diapédèse | diapedesis |
| diaphorétique | diaphoretic |
| diaphragmatique | phrenic |
| diaphragme | diaphragm |
| diaphyse | diaphysis |
| diarrhée | diarrhea |
| diarrhée des voyageurs | traveler's diarrhea |
| diarthrose | diarthrosis |
| diastase | diastase |
| diastole | diastole |
| diathermie | diathermy |
| diasthèse | diasthesis |
| diète | diet |
| diététicien | dietitian |
| différentiel | differential |
| différer | postpone |
| difficulté | problem |
| digestion | digestion |
| digitale | disaccharide |
| dilatateur | dilator |
| dilatation | dilatation |
| dilution | dilution |
| dimercaprol (BAL) | dimercaprol |
| dimidié | homolateral |
| diminution | decrease |
| d'involution | involutional |
| dioptrie | dipotre |

| French | English |
|---|---|
| dioxyde | dioxide |
| diphtérie | diphtheria |
| diplégie | diplegia |
| diplocoque | diplococcus |
| diploïde | diploid |
| diplopie | diplopia |
| dipsomanie | dipsomania |
| disaccharide | disaccharide |
| discours | speech |
| discret | discrete |
| discuter | argue |
| dislocation | dislocation |
| disparition | disappearance |
| dispersion | scatter |
| disponibilité | availability |
| disponible | available |
| disposé en réseau | cancellous |
| dispositif intra-utérin | intrauterine contraceptive device |
| disque optique | optic disk |
| dissection | dissection |
| dissémination | dissemination |
| dissolution | dissolution |
| distal | distal |
| distendu | distended |
| distichiase | distichiasis |
| distribution | distribution |
| diurèse | diuresis |
| diurétique | diuretic |
| diurne | diurnal |
| diverticule | diverticulum |
| diverticulite | diverticulitis |
| diverticulose | diverticulosis |
| doigt | digit; finger |
| doigt à ressort | snapping finger |
| doigt en marteau | mallet finger |
| dôme pleural | cervical pleura |
| donner naissance | bear, to |
| donneur | donor |
| dopamine | dopamine |
| dopa-réaction | dopa reaction |
| dorloter | pamper |
| dormant | quiescent |

| French | English |
|---|---|
| dorsal | dorsal |
| dorsalgie | back pain |
| dorsiflexion | dorsiflexion |
| dos | dorsum; back |
| dosage | dosage |
| dosage biologique | bioassay |
| dose | dose |
| dose létale médiane (DL 50) | median lethal dose (LD 50) |
| dose mortelle | lethal dose |
| dossier | file; backrest |
| dossier clinique | clinical record |
| dossier de soin | patient chart |
| dossier médical | medical record |
| doter | endow |
| d'où | hence |
| double | double |
| douille | socket |
| douleur | pain |
| douleur enn coup de poignard | stabbing pain |
| douleur exquise | sharp pain |
| douleur projetée | referred pain |
| douloureux | painful |
| douve | fluke |
| doux | mild |
| Down, syndrome de | Down's syndrome |
| dracunculose | dracunculosis |
| dragée | sugar-coated tablet |
| drain | drainage tube |
| drap | sheet |
| drépanocytose | sickle-cell anemia |
| drogue | drug |
| droit | dexter; right; straight; erect |
| duodénal | duodenal |
| dur | hard |
| durée | duration |
| durée de vie | lifetime |
| dure-mère | dura mater |
| durillon | callus |
| dysarthrie | dysarthria |
| dyschésie | dyschezia |
| dyschondroplasie | dyschondroplasia |
| dyscorie | dyscoria |

| French | English |
|---|---|
| dysdiadococinésie | dysdiadocokinesia |
| dysenterie | dysentery |
| dysesthésie | dysesthesia |
| dysfonction | dysfunction |
| dysgénésie gonadique | gonadal dysgenesis |
| dyshidrose | pompholyx |
| dyskinésie | dyskinesia |
| dyslalie | dyslalia |
| dyslexie | dyslexia |
| dysménorrhée | dysmenorrhea |
| dysostose cléido-crânienne | cleidocranial dysostosis |
| dypareunie | dyspareunia |
| dyspepsie | dyspepsia |
| dysphagie | dysphagia |
| dysplasie | dysplasia |
| dyspnée | dyspnea |
| dyspnée d'effort | exercise-induced dyspnea |
| dystocie | dystocia |
| dystrophie musculaire progressive | muscular dystrophy |
| dysurie | dysuria |
| eau | water |
| eau de javel | bleach |
| eau potable | drinking water |
| éblouissement | glare |
| ébranlement | shaking |
| ébriété | drunkenness |
| écaille | squama |
| écart | interval |
| écarteur | retractor |
| ecchondrome | ecchondroma |
| ecchymose | ecchymosis |
| échancrure | incisura |
| échantillon | specimen |
| échantillonnage | sampling |
| écharpe | sling |
| échec thérapeutique | treatment failure |
| échelle colorimétrique | color chart |
| échinocoque | Echinococcus |
| échocardiographic | echocardiographic |
| échocardiographie | echocardiography |
| échocardiographie transœsophagienne | transesophageal echocardiography |
| écholalie | echolalia |

| French | English |
|---|---|
| éclampsie | eclampsia |
| éclater | burst |
| éclosion | outbreak |
| ecmnésie | ecmnesia |
| économe | sparing |
| écoulement | flow |
| écoulement gazeux | air flow |
| écouvillon | swab |
| écran | shield |
| écran fluorescent | fluorescent screen |
| ectasie | ectasia |
| ectoderme | ectoderm |
| ectopique | ectopic |
| ectrodactylie | ectrodactylia |
| écumeux | frothy |
| eczéma | eczema |
| édenté | toothless |
| effecteur | effector |
| effet cumulatif | cumulative effect |
| effet indésriable | adverse effect |
| effet secondaire | side effect |
| efficace | efficacious |
| effleurage | effleurage |
| effort | effort |
| efforts expulsifs | bearing down |
| effusion | effusion |
| égal | equal |
| égocentrique | egocentric |
| égratignure | scratch |
| éjaculation | ejaculation |
| élargissement | widening |
| élastine | elastin |
| électif | elective |
| électrocardiogramme | electrocardiogram |
| électrochoc | electroconvulsive therapy |
| électrode | electrode |
| électroencéphalogramme | electroencephalogram |
| électrolyte | electrolyte |
| électromyographie | electromyography |
| électrophorèse | electrophoresis |
| électuaire | lincture |
| éléphantiasis | elephantiasis |

| French | English |
|---|---|
| éléphantiasis familial | Milroy's disease |
| élevé | high |
| élever | raise |
| élixir | elixir |
| éloigné de | away from |
| émaciation | emaciation |
| embole | embolus |
| embolectomie | embolectomy |
| embolie graisseuse | fat embolism |
| embolie pulmonaire septique | septic pulmonary embolism |
| embout auriculaire | ear mold |
| embout buccal | mouth piece |
| embrochage | pinning |
| embryologie | embryology |
| embryon | embryo |
| émétique | emetic |
| éminence hypothénar | hypothenar eminence |
| éminence thénar | thenar eminence |
| emmétropie | emmetropia |
| émollient | emollient |
| émotion | emotion |
| émoussé | blunt |
| empan | span |
| empâtement | slurring |
| empathie | empathy |
| emphysème | emphysema |
| emplâtre | plaster |
| empyème | empyema |
| émulsion | emulsion |
| en apparence | ostensibly |
| en conformité avec | in conformity with |
| en effet | indeed |
| en raison de | owing to |
| en rapport avec | related to |
| énarthrose | enarthrosis |
| enceinte | gravid; pregnant |
| encéphale | brain |
| encéphaline | enkephalin |
| encéphalique | encephalic |
| encéphalite | encephalitis |
| encéphalocèle | encephalocele |
| encéphalographie | encephalography |

| French | English |
|---|---|
| encéphalomacie | encephalomacia |
| encéphalomyélite | encephalomyelitis |
| encéphalopathie | encephalopathy |
| enchondrome | enchondroma |
| enclouage | nailing |
| enclume | incus |
| encoprésie | encopresis |
| enartérite | endarteritis |
| endémique | endemic |
| endocardite | endocarditis |
| endocervicite | endocervicitis |
| endocrine | endocrine |
| endocrinologie | endocrinology |
| endoderme | endoderm |
| endogène | endogenous |
| endolymphe | endolymph |
| endomètre | endometrium |
| endométriome | endometrioma |
| endométriose | endometriosis |
| endométrite | endometritis |
| endonèvre | endoneurium |
| endormi | asleep |
| endorphine | endorphin |
| endoscope | endoscope |
| endothéliome | endothelioma |
| endotrachéal | endotracheal |
| enfance | childhood |
| enfant | child |
| enflé | turgid |
| engourdi | stiff |
| engourdissement | numbness |
| engrènement | rabbeting |
| enjambée | stride |
| enlèvement | removal |
| énophtalmie | enophthalmos |
| énorme | enormous |
| énostose | enostosis |
| enrhumer, s' | catch a cold |
| enroué | hoarse |
| enseignement | education |
| ensemencement | seeding |
| entaille | nick |

| French | English |
|---|---|
| entérectomie | enterectomy |
| entérique | enteric |
| entérite | enteritis |
| entérocoque | enterococcus |
| entérolithe | enterolith |
| entéroptose | enteroptosis |
| entérotomie | enterotomy |
| entorse | sprain |
| entraînement électrosystolique | cardiac pacing |
| entraîneur | pacemaker |
| entrée | admission |
| entretien | maintenance |
| énucléation | enucleation |
| énurésie | enuresis |
| envie de l'ongle | hangnail |
| enzyme | enzyme |
| éosinophile | eosinophile |
| éosinophilie | eosinophilia |
| épaissi | inspissated |
| épanchement | extravasation |
| épaule | shoulder |
| épendyme | ependyma |
| épendymome | ependymoma |
| éphédrine | ephedrine |
| éphélide | macula solaris |
| épiblépharon | epiblepharon |
| épicarde | epicardium |
| épicondyle | epicondyle |
| épicondylite | epicondylitis |
| épicrâne | epicranium |
| épidémie | epidemic |
| épidémiologie | epidemiology |
| épiderme | epidermis |
| épidermophytose | epidermophytosis |
| épididymite | epididymitis |
| épididymo-orchite | epididymo-orchitis |
| épidural | epidural |
| épigastre | epigastrium |
| épiglotte | epiglottis |
| épilation | epilation |
| épilepsie | epilepsy |
| épileptiforme | epileptiform |

| French | English |
|---|---|
| épileptique crise | epileptic seizure |
| épileptogène | epileptogenic |
| épine | spine |
| épine calcanéenne | calcaneal spur |
| épinéphrine | epinephrine |
| épiphyse | pineal gland |
| épiphysite | epiphysitis |
| épiplocèle | omentocele |
| épiploon | omentum |
| épiploopexie | omentopexy |
| épisclérite | episcleritis |
| épisiotomie | episiotomy |
| épistaxis | epistaxis |
| épithélial | epithelial |
| épithéliome | epithelioma |
| épithélium | epithelium |
| épitrochlée | epitrochlea |
| éponge | sponge |
| éprouvette | test tube |
| épuisement par la chaleur | heat exhaustion |
| équilibre | equilibrium |
| équilibre acido-basique | acid-base balance |
| éraflure | scrape |
| ergomètre | ergometer |
| ergonomie | ergonomics |
| ergostérol | ergosterol |
| erthothérapie | occupational therapy |
| érosion | erosion |
| erreur | error |
| éructation | eructation |
| éruption cutanée | skin rash |
| érysipèlas | erysipelas |
| érythème fessier du nourrisson | diaper rash |
| érythème noueux | erythema nodosum |
| érythème pernio | pernio |
| érythème polymorphe | erythema mutliforme |
| érthyroblaste | erythroblast |
| érthyroblastose fœtale | erythroblastosis fetalis |
| érthyrocyanose | erythrocyanosis |
| érthyrocyte | erythrocyte |
| érthyrocytopénie | erythrocytopenia |
| érthyrocytose | erythrocytosis |

| French | English |
|--------|---------|
| érthyropoïèse | erythropoiesis |
| escarre | eschar |
| escarre de décubitus | decubitus ulcer |
| escarre de pression | pressure ulcer |
| ésérine | eserine |
| ésotropie | esotropia |
| espace mort | dead space |
| espace mort respiratoire | respiratory dead space |
| espérance de vie | life expectancy |
| esquille | splinter |
| essentiel | essential |
| essoufflé | puffed |
| estomac | stomach |
| estrogène | estrogen |
| étalonnage | calibration |
| étanche | impervious |
| étape terminale | end stage |
| état | state |
| état antérieur | prior status |
| état de mal | status of illness |
| état de stress post-traumatique | post-traumatic stress (the state of) |
| état d'équilibre | steady state |
| état nauséeux gravidique | morning sickness |
| éternuement | sneeze |
| ethmoïde | ethmoid |
| éthylique | alcoholic |
| étiologie | etiology |
| étouffer | choke |
| étourdissement | dizziness |
| étrange | strange |
| étranglement | constriction |
| étrier | stirrup |
| étrier, muscle de l' | stapedius muscle |
| étuve | incubator |
| eunuque | eunuch |
| euthanasie | euthanasia |
| évacuation | evacuation |
| évaluation | evaluation |
| évanouissement | faint |
| éveil | arousal |
| éventration | eventration |
| éversion | eversion |

| French | English |
| --- | --- |
| évident | evident; obvious |
| éviscération | evisceration |
| évitable | avoidable |
| éviter | prevent |
| évolué | advanced |
| évolutif | progressive |
| évolution de la maladie | disease outcome |
| évulsion | evulsion |
| exacerbation | exacerbation |
| examen | examination |
| examen physique | physical exam |
| exanthème | exanthema |
| excès | excess |
| excipient | excipient |
| excluant | ruling out |
| excoriation | excoriation |
| excrément | excrement |
| excreta | excreta |
| exentération | exenteration |
| exfoliation | exfoliation |
| exhumation | exhumation |
| exogène | exogenous |
| exomphale | exomphalos |
| exonération | defecation |
| exostose | exostosis |
| exotoxine | exotoxin |
| expectorant | expectorant |
| expectoration | expectoration |
| expiratoire | expiratory |
| expulsion | expulsion |
| exsanguino-transfusion | exchange transfusion |
| exsudat | exudate |
| extenseur | extensor |
| externe | external |
| exirper | extirpate |
| extracapsulaire | extracapsular |
| extracellulaire | extracellular |
| extrait | extract |
| extrasystole | extrasystole |
| extravasation | extravasation |
| extrémité | extremity |
| extrinsèque | extrinsic |

| French | English |
| --- | --- |
| face | face |
| facette | facet |
| facial nerf | facial nerve |
| faciès | facies |
| facteur antihémophilique | antihemophilic factor |
| facteur antinucléaire | antinuclear factor |
| facteur antirachitique | antirachitic factor |
| facteur de croissance | growth factor |
| facteur natriurétique auriculaire | atrial natriuretic factor |
| facture | bill |
| faible | weak |
| faiblesse | weakness |
| faim | hunger |
| faire craquer ses doigts | crack one's knuckles |
| faire face | cope |
| faisceau atrio-ventriculaire | atrioventricular bundle |
| faisceau de His | bundle of His |
| falciforme | falciform |
| familial | familial |
| famille | family |
| famine | starvation |
| fango | sludge |
| faradisation | faradism |
| fascia | fascia |
| fasciculation | fasciculation |
| fascicule | fascicle |
| fasciite | fascitis |
| fatal | fatal |
| fatigué | tired |
| fausse-couche | miscarriage |
| faute d'orthographe | misspelling |
| fauteuil roulant | wheelchair |
| faux du cerveau | falx cerebri |
| favus | favus |
| fébrile | febrile |
| fécalome | fecal impaction |
| fèces | feces |
| fécondité | fecundity |
| fêlure | crack |
| femelle | female |
| femme | female |
| fémoral nerf | femoral nerve |

| French | English |
|---|---|
| fémur | femur |
| fenêtre | fenestra; window |
| fente palatine | cleft palate |
| fente vulvaire | vulval cleft |
| fer | iron |
| fermé | closed |
| fertilisation | fertilization |
| fertilité | fertility |
| fesses | buttock |
| fessier muscle | gluteal muscle |
| fétichisme | fetichism |
| feuillet | layer |
| fiabilité | reliability |
| fibre grimpante | climbing fiber |
| fibre moussue | mossy fiber |
| fibre musculaire | smooth muscle fiber |
| fibre musculaire striée | striated muscle fiber |
| fibre nerveuse myélinisée | medullated nerve fiber |
| fibres afférentes musculaires rapides | fast muscle fibers |
| fibreux | fibroid |
| fibrillation | fibrillation |
| fibrillation auriculaire | atrial fibrillation |
| fibrine | fibrin |
| fibroadénome | fibroadenoma |
| fibroblaste | fibroblast |
| fibrochondrite | fibrochondritis |
| fibro-élastose | fibroelastosis |
| fibrome utérin | uterine fibroid |
| fibromyome | fibromyoma |
| fibrosarcome | fibrosarcoma |
| fibrose | fibrosis |
| fibrose pulmonaire | pulmonary fibrosis |
| fibrose rétropéritonéale | retroperitoneal fibrosis |
| fibrosite | fibrositis |
| fibula | fibula |
| ficelle | string |
| fièvre | fever |
| fièvre à phlébotome | sandfly fever |
| fièvre à tiques | tick-borne fever |
| fièvre aphteuse | foot and mouth disease |
| fièvre bileuse hémoglobinurique | blackwater fever |
| fièvre intermittente | ague |

| French | English |
|---|---|
| fièvre jaune | yellow fever |
| fièvre pourprée des Montagnes Rocheuses | Rocky Mountain spotted fever |
| fièvre prolongée inexpliquée | fever of unknown origin |
| fièvre Q | Q fever |
| fièvre tierce | tertian fever |
| fièvre typhoïde | typhoid fever |
| figure | face |
| filaire | filaria |
| filaire de Médine | guinea worm |
| filariose lymphatique | lymphatic filariasis |
| filiforme | filiform |
| fille | daughter |
| filum terminale | filum terminale |
| fimbria | fimbria |
| fiole | flask |
| fissure | fissure |
| fistule | fistula |
| fixation | fixation |
| flacon | vial |
| flagellation | flagellation |
| flagelle | flagellum |
| flambée | outbreak |
| flasque | flaccid |
| flatulence | flatulence |
| fléchisseur | flexor |
| flottant | floating |
| flou | hazy |
| fluidifiant | mucolytic |
| fluor | fluorine |
| fluoration | fluoridation |
| fluorescéine | fluoresceine |
| fluoroscopie | fluoroscopy |
| flutter | flutter |
| fœtal | fetal |
| foie | liver |
| folie | madness |
| folique acide | folic acid |
| folliculaire | follicular |
| follicule pileux | hair follicle |
| folliculostimulante hormone | follicle stimulating hormone (FSH) |
| fonction | function |
| fonction ventriculaire | ventricular function |

| French | English |
| --- | --- |
| fond d'œil | eyeground |
| fongicide | fungicide |
| fontanelle | fontanelle |
| foramen | foramen |
| force | strength |
| force de préhension | grip strength |
| forceps | forceps |
| foret | drill |
| formulaire | formulary |
| formule leucocytaire | differential leucocyte count |
| fornix | fornix |
| fort | strong |
| fosse | fossa |
| fou | insane |
| foudroyant | fulminating |
| foulure | sprain |
| fourchette thérapeutique | therapeutic range |
| fourmillement | tingling |
| fournitures | supplies |
| fourreau | socket |
| fovea | fovea |
| fracture | fracture |
| fracture de fatigue | stress fracture |
| fracture en bois vert | greenstick fracture |
| fracture ouverte | compound fracture |
| fragilité osseuse | fragilitas ossium |
| frais | cool |
| fraise | burr |
| frange | fimbria |
| frapper | hit |
| fratrie | siblings |
| frein | frenulum |
| frêle | slight |
| frémissement | fremitus |
| fréquence | frequency |
| fréquence cardiaque | heart rate |
| fréquence respiratoire | respiratory rate |
| friction | friction |
| frisson | chill |
| froid | cold |
| fronde | sling |
| front | forehead; front |

| French | English |
|---|---|
| frontal | frontal |
| frottement | friction rub |
| frottis | smear |
| fuite | leakage |
| fundus | fundus |
| funiculite | funiculitis |
| fureur | rage |
| furoncle | furuncle |
| furonculose | furunculosis |
| fuseau achromatique | achromatic spindle |
| fusiforme | fusiform |
| gâchette | trigger |
| gaïac | guaiac |
| gaine | sheath |
| galactocéle | galactocele |
| galactorrhée | galactorrhea |
| galactose | galactose |
| galactosémie | galactosemie |
| gale | scabies |
| gale des blanchisseurs | dhobie itch |
| galop (bruit ou rythme de) | gallop |
| galvanisme | galvanism |
| galvanomètre | galvanometer |
| gamète | gamete |
| gammaglobuline | gammaglobulin |
| gangliectomie | ganglionectomie |
| ganglion | node |
| ganglion gèniculè | geniculate ganglion |
| ganglion lymphatique | lymph node |
| ganglion rachidien | spinal ganglion |
| gangrène | gangrene |
| gangrène gazeuse | gas gangrene |
| gant | glove |
| gant chirurgical stériles | sterile surgical gloves |
| gant d'examen | exam (non-sterile) gloves |
| garde ne nuit | night shift |
| gargarisme | gargle |
| gargouillement | gurgling |
| gargoylisme | gargoylism |
| garrot | tourniquet |
| gastrectomie | gastrectomy |
| gastrine | gastrin |

| French | English |
|---|---|
| gastrique | gastric |
| gastrite | gastritis |
| gastrocèle | gastrocele |
| gastrocnemius muscle | gastrocnemius |
| gastro-entérite | gastroenteritis |
| gastro-entérostomie | gastroenterostomy |
| gastrojéjunostomie | gastrojejunostomy |
| gastropexie | gastropexy |
| gastroscope | gastroscope |
| gastrostomie | gastrostomy |
| gauche | left |
| gaucher | left handed |
| gavage | gavage |
| gaz carbonique | carbon dioxide gas |
| gaze | gauze |
| gazométrie artérielle | arterial blood gas |
| géant | giant |
| gel | gel |
| gel de contact échographie | echocardiography contact gel |
| gelé | frozen |
| gélose | agar |
| gélule | capsule |
| gelures | frostbite |
| gémir | groan |
| gencive | gum |
| gène | gene |
| gêne | discomfort |
| général | general |
| génétique | genetic |
| géniculé | geniculate |
| génitaux organes | genitalia |
| génito-urinaire | urogenital |
| génome | genome |
| genou | knee |
| genou instable | unstable knee |
| genoux cagneux | knock knees |
| genu valgum | outward bending of the knee |
| genu varum | inward bending of the knee |
| gériatrie | geriatrics |
| germe | germ |
| gérontologie | gerontology |
| gestation | gestation |

| French | English |
|---|---|
| giardiase | giardiasis |
| gibbosité | hunchback |
| gicler | squirt |
| gigantisme | gigantism |
| gingival | gingival |
| gingivite | gingivitis |
| ginglyme | ginglymus |
| glabelle | glabella |
| gland | glans |
| gland apocrine | apocrine gland |
| gland endocrine | endocrine gland |
| gland mammaire | mammary gland |
| gland pinéale | epiphysis cerebri |
| gland salivaire | salivary gland |
| gland sébacée | sebaceous gland |
| glaucome | glaucoma |
| glénoïde | glenoid |
| gliome | glioma |
| gliomyome | gliomyoma |
| globule rouge | erythrocyte |
| globule sanguin | blood cell |
| globuline antilymphocytaire | antilymphocyte globulin |
| glomangiome | glomus tumor |
| glomérule | glomerulus |
| glomérulonéphrite | glomerulonephritis |
| glomique tumeur | glomus tumor |
| glomus carotidien | carotid body |
| glossectomie | glossectomy |
| glossite | glossitis |
| glossocynie | glossodynia |
| glossopharyngien | glossopharyngeal |
| glotte | glottis |
| glucagon | glucagon |
| glucide | carbohydrate |
| glutéal | gluteal |
| gluteus muscle | gluteus muscle |
| glycémie | glycemia |
| glycérine | glycerin |
| glycogène | glycogen |
| glycogenèse | glycogenesis |
| glycolyse | glycolysis |
| glycoprotéine | glycoprotein |

| French | English |
|---|---|
| glycosurie | glycosuria |
| gnathique | gnathic |
| godet | scutulum |
| goitre | goiter |
| gomme | gumma |
| gonade | gonad |
| gonadotrophine | gonadotrophin |
| gonarthrose | arthritis of the knee |
| gonflé | swollen |
| gonocoque | gonococcus |
| gorge | throat |
| gorgée | swallow |
| gouge | gouge |
| goût | taste |
| goutte | drop |
| goutte-à-goutte | drop by drop |
| goutte épaisse | malaria screening test |
| gouttes par minute | drops per minute |
| gouttière | splint |
| grabataire | bedridden |
| graisse | fat |
| gramme | gram |
| grand droit de l'abdomen | rectus abdominis muscle |
| grandeur | size |
| granulocyte | granulocyte |
| granulome | granuloma |
| gras | fatty |
| grave | severe |
| gravide | gravid |
| greffe osseuse | bone graft |
| grenouille | frog |
| grenouillette | ranula |
| griffes du chat,maladie des | cat scratch fever |
| grippe | influenza |
| grippe aviaire | avian flu |
| grognement | grunting |
| grossesse | gestation; pregnancy |
| grossesse extra-utérine | ectopic pregnancy |
| grossesse prolongée | post-term pregnancy |
| grosseur | lump |
| grossier | rude |
| groupage sanguin | blood grouping |

| French | English |
|---|---|
| groupe sanguin | blood type |
| guêpe | wasp |
| guérison | cure |
| gustatif | gustatory |
| gynécologie | gynecology |
| gynécomastie | gynecomastia |
| gyrus | gyrus |
| habitude | habit |
| habituel | usual |
| haleine | breath |
| halitose | halitosis |
| hallucination | delusion; hallucination |
| hallucinogène | hallucinogen |
| hallux | hallux |
| hamartome | hamartoma |
| hamatum | uncinate bone |
| hanche | hip |
| haploïde | haploid |
| haptène | hapten |
| hasard au | at random |
| haschisch | cannabis |
| hauteur | height |
| haut-le-cœur | retching |
| hebdomadaire | weekly |
| hébéphrénie | hcbcphrenia |
| hédonisme | hedonism |
| héliothérapie | heliotherapy |
| hélium | helium |
| helminthe | helminth |
| helminthiase | helminthiasis |
| hémagglutinine | hemagglutinin |
| hémangiome | hemangioma |
| hémarthrose | hemarthrosis |
| hématémèse | hematemesis |
| hématie granuleuse | reticulocyte |
| hématine | hematin |
| hématinique | hematinic |
| hématocèle | hematocele |
| hématocrite | hematocrit |
| hématome | hematoma |
| hématome extradural | epidural hematoma |
| hématome rétroplacentaire | abruptio placentae |

| French | English |
| --- | --- |
| hématome sous-dural | subdural hematoma |
| hématomètre | hematometra |
| hématomyélie | hematomyelia |
| hématoporphyrine | hematoporphyrin |
| hématosalpinx | hematosalpinx |
| hématozoaire | hematozoa |
| hématurie | hematuria |
| hème | heme |
| héméralopie | hemeralopia (nigh blindness) |
| hémianopsie | hemianopsia |
| hémianopsie bitemporale | bitemporale hemianopsia |
| hémiballisme | hemiballismus |
| hémicolectomie | hemicolectomy |
| hémicrânie | hemicrania |
| hémiparésie | hemiparesia |
| hémiplégie | hemiplegia |
| hémiptère | bug |
| hémisphère | hemisphere |
| hémizygote | hemizygote |
| hémochromatose | hemochromatosis |
| hémoconcentration | hemoconcentration |
| hémocytomètre | hemocytometer |
| hémodialyse | hemodialysis |
| hémoglobine | hemoglobin |
| hémoglobinurie | hemoglobinuria |
| hémolyse | hemolysis |
| hémolytique | hemolytic |
| hémopéricarde | hemopericardium |
| hémopéritoine | hemoperitoneum |
| hémophile | hémophiliac |
| hémophilie | hemophilia |
| hémophtalmie | hemophthalmia |
| hémopoïèse | hemopoiesis |
| hémopoïétine | hemopoietin |
| hémoptysie | hemoptysis |
| hémorragie | hemorrhage |
| hémorragie cérébrale | cerebral hemorrhage |
| hémorragie intracérébrale | intracerebral hemorrhage |
| hémorragie occulte | occult bleeding |
| hémorragie sous-durale | subdural hemorrhage |
| hémorragie utérine | uterine bleeding |
| hémorroïdectomie | hemorrhoidectomy |

| French | English |
|---|---|
| hémorroïdes | hemorrhoids |
| hémostase | hemostasis |
| hémothorax | hemothrorax |
| héparine | heparin |
| hépatectomie | hepatectomy |
| hépatique | hepatic |
| hépatite | hepatitis |
| hépatocyte | hepatocyte |
| hépatome | hepatoma |
| hépatomégalie | hepatomegaly |
| hépatosplénomégalie | hepatosplenomegaly |
| héréditaire | hereditary |
| hermaphrodite | hermaphrodite |
| hernie diaphragmatique | diaphragmatic hernia |
| hernia discale | herniated disc |
| hernia hiatale | hiatus hernia |
| herniorraphie | herniorrhaphy |
| héroïne | heroin |
| herpangine | herpangina |
| herpès | herpes |
| herpès génital | genital herpes |
| herpétiforme | herpetiform |
| herpétique | herpetic |
| hétérogène | heterogenous |
| hétérotropie | heterotropia |
| hétérozygote | heterozygous |
| hidradénite | hidradenitis |
| hidrose | hidrosis |
| hilaire | hilar |
| hile | hilum |
| hippocampe | hippocampus |
| hippocrastisme digital | clubbing |
| hirsutisme | hirsutism |
| histamine | histamine |
| histidine | histidine |
| histiocyte | histiocyte |
| histochimie | histochemistry |
| histoire | story |
| histologie | histology |
| histoplasmose | histoplasmosis |
| Holter ECG | ambulatory electrocardiographic monitoring |
| homéopathie | homeopathy |

| French | English |
|---|---|
| homéostasie | homeostasis |
| homicide | homicide |
| homme | man |
| homogreffe | homograft |
| homolatéral | ipsilateral |
| homologue | homologous |
| homosexualité | homosexuality |
| homozygote | homozygous |
| honteux | pudendal |
| hôpital | hospital |
| hoquet | hiccup |
| hormone | hormone |
| humain | human |
| humanité | mankind |
| humérus | humerus |
| humeur aqueuse | aqueous humor |
| humide | moist |
| hurler | yell |
| hyalin | hyaline |
| hyaloïde | hyaloid |
| hybride | hybrid |
| hydarthrose | hydarthrosis |
| hydatiforme | hydatiform |
| hydratation | hydration |
| hydrocèle | hydrocele |
| hydrocèle vaginale | scrotal hydrocele |
| hydrocéphalie | hydrocephalus |
| hydrocortisone | hydrocortisone |
| hydrolyse | hydrolysis |
| hydronéphrose | hydronephrosis |
| hydrophobie | hydrophobia |
| hydropisie | hydrops |
| hydropneumothorax | hydropneumothorax |
| hydrosalpinx | hydrosalpinx |
| hydrothorax | hydrothorax |
| hygiène de la grossesse | prenatal care |
| hygroma | hygroma |
| hygroscopique | hygroscopic |
| hymen | hymen |
| hyménotomie | hymenotomy |
| hyperacidité | hyperacidity |
| hyperactivité | hyperactivity |

| French | English |
|---|---|
| hyperaldostéronisme | aldosteronism |
| hyperalgésie | hyperalgesia |
| hyperbare | hyperbaric |
| hyperbilirubinémie | hyperbilirubinemia |
| hypercalcémie | hypercalcemia |
| hypercapnie | hypercapnia |
| hypercholestérolémie | hypercholesterolemia |
| hyperchromie | hyperchromia |
| hyperémie | hyperemia |
| hyperéphidrose | hyperhidrosis |
| hyperesthésie | hyperesthesia |
| hyperextension | hyperextension |
| hyperflexion | hyperflexion |
| hyperglycémie | hyperglycemia |
| hyperglycémie provoquée, test d' | glucose tolerance test |
| hypergonadisme | hypergonadism |
| hyperkaliémie | hyperkalemia |
| hyperkératose | hyperkeratosis |
| hyperkinésie | hyperkinesis |
| hyperlaxité articulaire | arthrochalasis |
| hyperlipémie | hyperlipidemia |
| hypermétrope | longsighted |
| hypermétropie | hypermetropia |
| hypermnésie | hypermnesia |
| hypermyotonie | hypermyotonia |
| hypernéphrome | hypernephroma |
| hyperonychose | hyperonychia |
| hyperparathyroïdie | hyperparathyroidism |
| hyperphagie | hyperphagia |
| hyperphorie | hyperphoria |
| hyperpituitarisme | hyperpituitarism |
| hyperplasie | hyperplasia |
| hyperpnée | hyperpnea |
| hyperpyrexie | hyperpyrexia |
| hypersensibilité | hypersensitivity |
| hypersplénisme | hypersplenism |
| hypertension | hypertension |
| hypertension artérielle | arterial hypertension |
| hypertension maligne | malignant hypertension |
| hyperthermie | hyperthermia |
| hyperthyroïdie | hyperthyroidism |
| hypertonie | hypertonia |

| French | English |
|---|---|
| hypertonique | hypertonic |
| hypertrichose | hypertrichosis |
| hypertrophie | hypertrophy |
| hyperventilation | hyperventilation |
| hypervolémie | hypervolemia |
| hypnotique | hypnotic |
| hypnurie | nocturia |
| hypocalcémie | hypocalcemia |
| hypochrome | hypochromic |
| hypocondre | hypochondrium |
| hypocondriaque | hypochondriac |
| hypocondrie | hypochondriasis |
| hypodermite | panniculitis |
| hypoesthésie | hypoesthesia |
| hypofibrinogénémie | hypofibrinogenemia |
| hypogastre | hypogastrium |
| hypogastrique | hypogastric |
| hypoglycémie | hypoglycemia |
| hypogonadisme | hypogonadism |
| hypokaliémie | hypokalemia |
| hypolipémiant | lipid-lowering agent |
| hypomanie | hypomania |
| hyponatrémie | hyponatremia |
| hypoparathyroïdie | hypoparathyroidism |
| hypophorie | hypophoria |
| hypophosphatasie | hypophosphatasia |
| hypophyse | hypophysis; pituitary gland |
| hypophysectomie | hypophysectomy |
| hypopion | hypopyon |
| hypotituiarisme | hypopituitarism |
| hypoplasie | hypoplasia |
| hyposécrétion | hyposecretion |
| hypospadias | hypospadias |
| hypostase | hypostasis |
| hypotension | hypotension |
| hypotension orthostatique | orthostatic hypotension |
| hypothalamus | hypothalamus |
| hypothermie | hypothermia |
| hypothyroïdie | hypothyroidism |
| hypotonie | hypotonia |
| hypoxie | hypoxia |
| hystérectomie | hysterectomy |

| French | English |
|---|---|
| hystérie | hysteria |
| hystérographie | hysterography |
| hystéromyomectomie | hysteromyomectomy |
| hystéropexie | hysteropexy |
| hystérosalpinographie | hysterosalpingography |
| hystérotomie | hysterotomy |
| iatrogène | iatrogenic |
| ichtyose | ichthyosis |
| ictère | icterus |
| ictère nucléaire | kernicterus |
| ictus | seizure |
| ictus amnésique | amnesiac stroke |
| idée fixe | monomania |
| idiopathique | idiopathic |
| iléite | ileitis |
| iléocolite | ileocolitis |
| iléocolostomie | ileocolostomy |
| iléon | ileum |
| iléorectal | ileorectal |
| iléorectostomie | ileoproctostomy |
| iléostomie | ileostomy |
| iléus | ileus |
| iliaque | iliac |
| ilio-coccygien | iliococcygeal |
| ilion | ilium |
| ilot | islet |
| imagerie par résonance magnétique | magnetic resonance imaging (MRI) |
| immobilisation | immobilization |
| immun | immune |
| immunisation | immunization |
| immunité croisée | cross-immunity |
| immunochimie | immunochemistry |
| immunodéficience | immunodeficiency |
| immuno-électrophorèse | immunoelectrophoresis |
| immunoglobuline | immunoglobulin |
| immunosuppression | immunosuppression |
| impatiences | restless legs |
| imperforé | imperforate |
| impétigo bulleux | bullous impetigo |
| impétigo sycosiforme | sycosis |
| implant | implant |
| impliqué | involved |

| French | English |
|---|---|
| impossibilité d'avaler | aglutition |
| impuissance | impotence |
| inadaptation | maladjustment |
| inanition | inanition |
| inarticulé | inarticulate |
| inattendu | unexpected |
| incapacité | disability |
| inceste | incest |
| incipiens | incipient |
| incision | incision |
| incisive | incisor |
| incisure | incisure |
| inclusion cellulaire | inclusion body |
| incohérent | incoherent |
| inconnu | unknown |
| inconscience | unconsciousness |
| incontinence | incontinence |
| incontinence urinaire | urinary incontinence |
| incoordination | incoordination |
| incubateur | incubator |
| incurie | malpractice |
| indigestion | indigestion |
| indolent | indolent |
| induit | induced |
| induration | induration |
| inefficace | ineffective |
| inertie | inertia |
| inévitable | inevitable |
| infantile | infantile |
| infarci | infarcted |
| infarcissement | infarction |
| infarctus myocardique | myocardial infarction |
| infectieux | infectious |
| infection bactérienne | sepsis |
| infection du liquide d'ascite | ascitic fluid infection |
| infection du système nerveux central | central nervous system infection |
| infection nosocomiale | nosocomial infection |
| infection opportunistes | opportunistic infection |
| inférieur | inferior |
| infestation | infestation |
| infirme moteur cérébral | cerebral palsy |
| inflammation | inflammation |

| French | English |
|---|---|
| influx nerveux | nerve impulse |
| infra-épineux | infraspinous |
| infundibulum | infundibulum |
| infusion | infusion |
| ingestion | ingestion |
| inguinal | inguinal |
| inhalation | inhalation |
| inhibiteur calcique | calcium channel blocker |
| inhibiteur de la monoamine oxydase | monoamine oxidase inhibitor (MAOI) |
| inhibiteurs de l'enzyme de conversion | angiotensin converting enzyme inhibitors (ACEI) |
| injection | injection |
| inné | congenital |
| innervation | innervation |
| innominé | innominate |
| inoculation | inoculation |
| insensible | insensible |
| insertion | insertion |
| insidieux | insidious |
| insomnie | insomnia |
| inspiration | inspiration |
| instable | unsteady |
| insuffisance aortique | aortic insufficiency |
| insuffisance cardiaque | cardiac failure |
| insuffisance cardiaque congestive | congestive heart failure |
| insuffisance mitrale | mitral regurgitation |
| insuffisance rénale | renal failure |
| insuffisance respiratoire | respiratory insufficiency |
| insuffisance vertébrobasilaire | verteobrobasilar insufficiency |
| insuline | insulin |
| insulinome | insulinoma |
| intensif | intensive |
| interaction médicamenteuse | medication interactions |
| interarticulaire | interarticular |
| intercellulaire | intercellular |
| intérieur | inside |
| intermittent | intermittent |
| interne | internal |
| internement | confinement |
| interosseux | interosseous |
| interrogatoire | history taking |
| interstitiel | interstitial |

| French | English |
|---|---|
| intertrigo | intertrigo |
| intertrochantérien | intertrochanteric |
| intervalle entre les prises | dosing interval |
| interventriculaire | interventricular |
| intestin | intestine |
| intestinal | intestinal |
| intoxication alimentaire | food poisoning |
| intoxication par le monoxyde de carbone | carbon monoxide poisoning |
| intra-abdominal | intraabdominal |
| intra-articulaire | intraarticular |
| intracellulaire | intracellular |
| intracérébral | intracerebral |
| intracrânien | intracranial |
| intradermique | intradermal |
| intradural | intradural |
| intramédullaire | intramedullary |
| intramusculaire | intramuscular |
| intra-osseux | intraosseous |
| intrapéritonéal | intraperitoneal |
| intrathécal | intrathecal |
| intra-utérin | intrauterine |
| intraveineux | intravenous |
| intubation | intubation |
| inuline | inulin |
| invagination | intussusception |
| involucre | involucrum |
| iode | iodine |
| iodisme | iodism |
| ipsilatéral | ipsilateral |
| iridectomie | iridectomy |
| iridocyclite | iridocyclitis |
| iridoplégie | iridoplegia |
| iridotomie | iridotomy |
| iris | iris |
| irradiation | irradiation |
| ischémie | ischemia |
| ischio-jambiers | hamstrings |
| ischion | ischium |
| isoanticorps | isoantibody |
| isolement | isolation |
| isotope radioactif | radioactive isotope |
| isotopique | radionuclide |

| French | English |
|---|---|
| isthme | isthmus |
| ivresse | inebriation |
| jalon | milestone |
| jambe | leg |
| jauge | gauge |
| jaune | yellow |
| jaunisse | jaundice |
| jéjunectomie | jejunectomy |
| jéjunostomie | jejunostomy |
| jeun à | fasting |
| jeune | young |
| jeûne | fasting |
| jeunesse | youth |
| joue | cheek |
| jugulaire | jugular |
| jumeaux | twins |
| jumeaux hétérozygotes | dizygotic twins |
| jumeaux homozygotes | identical twins |
| juridique | forensic |
| juste | fair |
| juxta-articulaire | juxta-articular |
| kala-azar | kala-azar |
| kaposi, sarcome de | kaposi's sarcoma |
| Keith et Flack, nœud de | sinoatrial node |
| kératectasie | keratectasia |
| kératectomie | keratectomy |
| kératine | keratin |
| kératomalacie | keratomalacia |
| kératome | keratoma |
| kératose | keratosis |
| kinase | kinase |
| kinésithérapie | physical therapy |
| Köhler, maladie de | Köhler's disease |
| koïlonychie | koilonychia |
| Koplik, taches de | Koplik's spots |
| Krebs, cycle de | Krebs cycle |
| kwashiorkor | kwashiorkor |
| kyste dermoïde | dermoid cyst |
| kyste hydatique | hydatid cyst |
| kyste thyréoglosse | thyroglossal cyst |
| kystectomie | cystectomy |
| labial | labial |

| French | English |
| --- | --- |
| labile | labile |
| laboratoire | laboratory |
| labrum | labrum |
| labyrinthe | labyrinth |
| labyrinthite | labyrinthitis |
| lâche | loose |
| lâcher | blurt out |
| lacrymal | lacrimal |
| lactalbumine | lactalbumin |
| lactase | lactase |
| lactate | lactate |
| lactation | lactation |
| lactique | lactic |
| lactoflavine | riboflavin |
| lactose | lactose |
| lacunes cérébrales (AVC) | lacunar cerebral infarcts |
| lait de vache | cow's milk |
| lambdoïde | lambdoid |
| lambeau | flap |
| lame | slide |
| lame de bistouri | scalpel |
| lame quadrijumelle | tectum mesencephali |
| lame de rasoir | razor blade |
| lamelle | lamella |
| laminectomie | laminectomy |
| lancette | lancet |
| langue | tongue |
| langue noire | lingua nigra |
| laparoscope | laparoscope |
| laparotomie | laparotomy |
| largeur | width |
| larme | tear |
| larmoiement | lacrimation |
| larmoyant | weepy |
| larva migrans cutanées | cutaneous larva migrans |
| larva migrans viscérales | visceral larva migrans |
| laryngé | laryngeal |
| laryngectomie | laryngectomy |
| laryngite | laryngitis |
| laryngite striduleuse | laryngismus stridulus |
| laryngologie | laryngology |
| laryngopharynx | laryngopharynx |

| French | English |
| --- | --- |
| laryngospasme | laryngospasm |
| laryngosténose | laryngostenosis |
| laryngotomie | laryngotomy |
| larynx | larynx |
| Lassa, fièvre de | Lassa fever |
| Lassègue, manœuvre | straight leg raising test |
| latéral | lateral |
| lavage gastrique | gastric lavage |
| lavage vaginal | douche |
| lavement | enema |
| lavement baryté | barium enema |
| laxité | laxity |
| LCR | CSF |
| lécithine | lecithin |
| léger | slight |
| légionnaires, maladie des | legionnaires' disease |
| leishmaniose | leishmaniasis |
| lent | slow |
| lenticulaire | lenticular |
| lentigo | lentigo |
| lentille | lens |
| lentille de contact | contact lens |
| leontiasis ossea | leontiasis ossea |
| lèpre | leprosy |
| léprome | leproma |
| leptoméningite | leptomeningitis |
| leptospirose | leptospirosis |
| lesbienne | lesbian |
| lésion cutanée | skin lesion |
| lésion par souffle | blast injury |
| létal | lethal |
| léthargie | lethargy |
| leucémie | leukemia |
| leucémie lymphoïde | lymphocytic leukemia |
| leucine | leukine |
| leucinose | leucinosis; maple syrup urine disease |
| leucocyte | leukocyte |
| leucocythémie | leukocythemia |
| leucocytolyse | leukocytolysis |
| leucocytose | leukocytosis |
| leucocytose monocytaire | monocytosis |
| leucodermia | leukodermia |

| French | English |
|---|---|
| leuconychie | leukonychia |
| leucopénie | leukopenia |
| leucopoïèse | leukopoiesis |
| leucorrhée | leukorrhea |
| lévocardie | sinistrocardia |
| lévorotation | sinistrotorsion |
| lèvre | labium; lip |
| lévulose | levulose |
| lévulosurie | fructosuria |
| levure | yeast |
| l'hypertrophie ventriculaire gauche | left ventricular hypertrophy |
| libération, hormone de | releasing hormone |
| libération, prolongée | sustained release |
| liberté | freedom |
| libido | libido |
| libre | free |
| lichen | lichen |
| lieu | site |
| ligament de Chopart | bifurcate ligament |
| ligament de Cooper | pectineal ligament |
| ligament large de l'utérus | broad ligament of uterus |
| ligament rond | round ligament |
| ligature | ligature |
| ligne médiane | midline |
| limbe | limbus |
| liminaire | liminal |
| limitation des naissances | birth control |
| lingual | glossal |
| lipase | lipase |
| lipémie | lipemia |
| lipide | lipid |
| lipo-atrophie | lipoatrophy |
| lipochondrodystrophie | lipochondrodystrophy |
| lipocyte | lipocyte |
| lipodystrophie | lipodystrophy |
| lipoïdique | lipoid |
| lipoïdose | lipoidosis |
| lipome | lipoma |
| lipoprotéine | lipoprotein |
| liposoluble | fat soluble |
| lipotrope substance | lipotrophic substance |
| liquide amniotique | amniotic fluid |

| French | English |
| --- | --- |
| liquide céphalorachidien (LCR) | cerebrospinal fluid (CSF) |
| liquide intra-oculaire | intraocular fluid |
| liquide synovial | synovial fluid |
| lit | bed |
| lithagogue | lithagogue |
| lithiase | calculus (stone) |
| lithiase rénale | nephrolithiasis |
| litholapaxie | litholapaxy |
| lithotomie | lithotomy |
| lithotriteur | lithotritor |
| litre | liter |
| livedo reticularis | livedo reticularis |
| livrer | deliver |
| lobaire | lobar |
| lobe | lobe |
| lobectomie | lobectomy |
| Lobo, maladie de | Lobo's disease |
| lobotomie | lobotomy |
| lobule | lobule |
| localisation | localization |
| localisé | localized |
| lochies | lochia |
| loculaire | loculated |
| lombaire | lumbar |
| lombalgie | low back pain |
| longue date de | long-standing |
| longueur | length |
| lordose | lordosis |
| lourd | heavy |
| lubrifiant | lubricant |
| luette | uvula |
| lumbago | lumbago |
| lumen | lumen |
| lumière | light |
| lunatum | lunate bone |
| lunettes de protection | goggles |
| lunule | lunula |
| lupus érythémateux | lupus erythematosous |
| lutéinisante hormone | luteinizing hormone (LH) |
| lutéotrope | luteotropic |
| luxation | dislocation |
| lymphadénite | lymphadenitis |

| French | English |
|---|---|
| lymphangiectasie | lymphangiectasis |
| lymphangiome | lymphagioma |
| lymphangite | lymphangitis |
| lymphangite endémique tropicale | elephantiasis |
| lymphatique | lymphatic |
| lymphe | lymph |
| lymphocyte | lymphocyte |
| lymphocythémie | lymphocytemia |
| lymphocytopénie | lymphocytopenia |
| lymphoctyose | lymphoctyosis |
| lymphoïde | lymphoid |
| lymphome | lymphoma |
| lymphopénie | lymphocytopenia |
| lymphoréticulose bénigne d'inoculation | cat scratch fever |
| lymphosarcome | lymphosarcoma |
| lyse | lysis |
| lysine | lysine |
| lysosomial | lysosomal |
| lysozyme | lysozyme |
| lytique | lytic |
| mâcher | chew |
| mâchoire | jaw |
| macrocéphale | macrocephalus |
| macrochéilie | macrocheilia |
| macrocytaire | macrocytic |
| macrocyte | macrocyte |
| macrodactylie | macrodactyly |
| macroglobulinémie | macroglobulinemia |
| macroglossie | macroglossia |
| macromastie | macromastia |
| macromélie | macromelia |
| macrophage | macrophage |
| macrostomie | macrostomia |
| macula | macula |
| maculopapulaire | maculopapular |
| magnétique | magnetic |
| maigre | thin |
| maigreur extrême | maramus |
| main | hand |
| main en griffe | clawhand |
| mains-pieds-bouche, syndrome | hand-foot-mouth disease |
| mal | disease |

| French | English |
|---|---|
| mal des montagnes | altitude sickness |
| mal de tête | headache |
| malacie | malacia |
| malade | patient |
| malade sexuellement transmissible (MST) | sexually transmitted disease (STD) |
| malade vénérienne | venereal disease |
| malaire os | zygomatic bone |
| malaria | malaria |
| malentendant | hard of hearing |
| malgré | despite |
| malin | malignant |
| malléole | malleolus |
| malleus | malleus |
| malnutrition | malnutrition |
| maltose | maltose |
| malversation | malpractice |
| mamelon | nipple |
| mamillaire | mammillary |
| mammaire | mammary |
| mammectomie | mastectomy |
| mammographie | mammography |
| mammoplastie | mammaplasty |
| mandibulaire | gnathic |
| mandibule | mandible |
| manger | eat |
| manie | mania |
| manifeste | overt |
| manœuvre de Hallpike | Hallpike maneuver |
| manœuvre de Valsalva | Valsalva's maneuver |
| manomètre | manometer |
| manubrium sternal | manubrium sterni |
| marasme | marasmus |
| Marie-Sainton, syndrome de | cleidocranial dysostosis |
| marijuana | marijuana |
| marmonner | mumble |
| marsupialisation | marsupialization |
| marteau | malleus |
| martelage | pounding |
| masculinisation | virilization |
| masse | mass |
| mastectomie | mastectomy |
| mastication | mastication |

219

| French | English |
|---|---|
| mastite | mastitis |
| mastocyte | mast cell |
| mastodynie | mastodynia |
| mastoïde | mastoid |
| mastoïdectomie | mastoidectomy |
| mastoïdite | mastoiditis |
| matelas | mattress |
| matériel | equipment |
| maxillaire inférieur | mandible |
| maxillaire supérieur | maxilla |
| méat | meatus |
| mèche | wick; drain |
| méconium | meconium |
| médecin | physician |
| médecine | medicine |
| médecine dentaire | odontology |
| médecine nucléaire | nuclear medicine |
| médecine périnatale | perinatology |
| médial | medial |
| médianoscopie | medianoscopy |
| médiastin | mediastinum |
| médicament | medication |
| médicochirurgical | medicosurgical |
| médullaire | medullary |
| médulloblastome | medullobastoma |
| médullosurrénale | adrenal medulla |
| mégacaryocyte | megakaryocyte |
| mégacéphalie | megacephaly |
| mégacôlon | megacolon |
| mégaloblaste | megaloblast |
| mégalomanie | megalomania |
| meilleur | best |
| méiose | meiosis |
| mélancolie | melancholia |
| mélanine | melanin |
| mélanome | melanoma |
| membrane cellulaire | cell membrane |
| membrane du tympan | tympanic membrane |
| membre supérieur | upper limb |
| mémoire | memory |
| menaçant la vie du patient | life-threatening |
| ménarche | menarche |

220

| French | English |
|---|---|
| méningé | meningeal |
| méningiome | meningioma |
| méningisme | meningism |
| méningite | meningitis |
| méningocèle | meningocele |
| méningococcémie | meningococcemia |
| méniscectomie | meniscectomy |
| ménisque | meniscus |
| ménopause | menopause |
| ménorragie | menorrhagia |
| menstruation | menstruation |
| mental | mental |
| menton | chin |
| mésartérite | mesarteritis |
| mésencéphale | mesencephalon; midbrain |
| mésenchyme | mesenchyme |
| mésentère | mesentery |
| méso-appendice | mesoappendix |
| mésocôlon | mesocolon |
| mésoderme | mesoderm |
| mésonéphrome | mesonephroma |
| mésosalpinx | mesosalpinx |
| mésothéliome | mesothelioma |
| mésovarium | mesovarium |
| métabolique | metabolic |
| métacarpe | metacarpal |
| métacarpophalangien | metacarpophalangeal |
| métaphore | metaphore |
| métaphyse | metaphysis |
| métaplasie | metaplasia |
| métatarsalgie | metatarsalgia |
| métatarsien | metatarsal |
| météorisme | flatulence |
| méthémoglobine | methemoglobin |
| méthionine | methionine |
| mètre | meter |
| métrorragie | metrorrhagia |
| microbe | microbe |
| microbiologie | microbiology |
| microcéphale | microcephalic |
| microcyte | microcyte |
| micrognathie | micrognathia |

| French | English |
|---|---|
| microgramme | microgram |
| micromètre | micrometer |
| micro-organisme | microorganism |
| microphtalmie | microphthalmos |
| microscope | microscope |
| microscopie électronique | electron microscopy |
| microsphérocytose héréditaire | hereditary spherocytosis |
| miction | micturition; urination |
| midi | noon |
| migraine | migraine |
| miliaire | miliary |
| milligramme | milligram |
| millilitre | milliliter |
| millimètre | millimeter |
| millimètre cube | cubic millimeter |
| Milroy, maladie de | Milroy's disease |
| Minkkowski=Chauffard, maladie de | hereditary spherocytosis |
| minuscule | minute |
| miroir | mirror |
| mise en œuvre | implementation |
| mitochondrie | mitochondria |
| mitose | mitosis |
| mitral | mitral |
| modiolus | modiolus |
| moelle épinière | spinal cord |
| moelle osseuse | bone marrow |
| moignon | stump |
| moins | less |
| moitié | half |
| molaires | molar teeth |
| molalité | molality |
| molécule | molecule |
| mollet | calf |
| monitorage | monitoring |
| monoblaste | promonocyte |
| monoclonal | monoclonal |
| monocyte | monocyte |
| monocytose | monocytosis |
| mononévrite | mononeuritis |
| mononucléaire | mononuclear |
| mononucléose | mononucleosis |
| monoplégie | monoplegia |

| French | English |
|---|---|
| montant | amount |
| mont de Vénus | mons pubis |
| morbide | morbid |
| morgue | morgue |
| moribond | moribund |
| morphine | morphine |
| morphologie | morphology |
| morsure de tique | tick bite |
| mort cérébrale | brain death |
| mort subite dunourrisson | sudden infant death syndrome |
| mort-né | stillborn |
| morue | cod |
| morula | morula |
| moteur | motor |
| moteur oculaire externe nerf | abducens nerve |
| moteur oculomoteur commun nerf | oculomotor nerve |
| mou | soft |
| mouche tsé-tsé | tsetse fly |
| mouillé | wet |
| moule | cast |
| mourir | die, to |
| mousse | foam |
| moustiquaire | mosquito net |
| mouvement oculaire rapide | Rapid Eye Movement |
| mucilage | mucilage |
| mucine | mucin |
| mucocèle | mucocele |
| mucoïde | mucoid |
| mucolytique | mucolytic |
| mucopurulent | mucopurulent |
| mucoviscidose | cystic fibrosis |
| mucus | mucus |
| muet | mute |
| muguet | aphthous stomatitis |
| multigeste | multigravida |
| multiloculaire | multilocular |
| multipare | multipara |
| muqueuse | mucosa |
| murmure | murmur |
| murmure vésiculaire | breath sound |
| muscle | muscle |
| musculaire | muscular |

| French | English |
|---|---|
| mutation | mutation |
| mutisme | mutism |
| myalgie | myalgia |
| myasthénie | myasthenia gravis |
| mycétome | mycetoma |
| mycose | mycosis |
| mycotoxine | mycotoxin |
| mydriase | mydriasis |
| myéline | myelin |
| myélite | myelitis |
| myélocèle | myelocele |
| myélogramme | myelogram |
| myéloïde | myeloid |
| myélomatose | myelomatosis |
| myélome | myeloma |
| myéloméningocèle | myelomeningocele |
| myélopathie | myelopathy |
| myéloplaxe | osteoclast |
| myocarde | myocardium |
| myocardique | myocardial |
| myocardite | myocarditis |
| myoglobine | myoglobin |
| myome | myoma |
| myomectomie | myomectomy |
| myomètre | myometrium |
| myopathie | myopathy |
| myope | myope |
| myopie | myopia |
| myocarcome | myosarcoma |
| myosine | myosin |
| myosis | myosis |
| myosite | myositis |
| myosite ossifiante | myositis ossificans |
| myotique | myotic |
| myotomie | myotomy |
| myotonie atrophique | myotonia dystrophica |
| myringite | myringitis |
| myringoplastie | myringoplasty |
| myringotomie | myringotomy |
| myxœdème | myxedema |
| myxome | myxoma |
| myxosarcome | myxosarcoma |

224

| French | English |
|---|---|
| nævus | nevus |
| nain | dwarf |
| naissance | birth |
| narcissisme | narcissism |
| narcolepsie | narcolepsy |
| narcose | narcosis |
| narcotique | narcotic |
| narine | nostril |
| nasal | nasal |
| nasolacrymal | nasolacrimal |
| nasopharynx | nasopharynx |
| nausée | nausea |
| naviculaire | navicular |
| né | born |
| nébulisation | nebulizer treatment |
| nébuliseur | nebulizer |
| nécropsie | necropsy |
| nécrose | necrosis |
| nécrotique | necrotic |
| nématode | nematode |
| néonatal | neonatal |
| néoplasme | neoplasm |
| néphélion | nebula |
| néphrectomie | nephrectomy |
| néphrite | nephritis |
| néphroblastome | nephroblastoma |
| néphrocalcinose | nephrocalcinosis |
| néphrocarcinome | renal adenocarcinoma |
| néphrolithotomie | nephrolithotomy |
| néphrome | nephroma |
| néphron | nephron |
| néphropathie | nephropathy |
| néphropexie | nephropexy |
| néphroptose | nephroptosis |
| néphrosclérose | nephrosclerosis |
| néphrose | nephrosis |
| néphrostomie | nephrostomy |
| néphrotique | nephrotic |
| néphrotomie | nephrotomy |
| nerf | nerve |
| neural | neural |
| neurapraxie | neurapraxia |

| French | English |
|---|---|
| neurasthénie | neurasthenia |
| neurectomie | neurectomy |
| neurilemme | neurilemma |
| neurinome de l'acoustique | acoustic neuroma |
| neuroblastome | neuroblastoma |
| neurochirurgie | neurosurgery |
| neuro-épithélium | neuroepithelium |
| neurofibromatose | neurofibromatosis |
| neurofibrome | neurofibroma |
| neuroleptique | neuroleptic |
| neurologie | neurology |
| neurologue | neurologist |
| neurone | neuron |
| neuropathie | neuropathy |
| neuropathique | neuropathic |
| neurosyphilis | neurosyphilis |
| neurotmésis | neurotmesis |
| neurotomie | neurotomy |
| neurotransmetteur | neurotransmitter |
| neutropénie | neutropenia |
| neutrophile | neutrophil |
| névralgie | neuralgia |
| névralgie faciale | trigeminal neuralgia |
| névrectomie | neurectomy |
| névrite | neuritis |
| névrite optique rétrobulbaire | retrobulbar optic neuritis |
| névrodermite | neurodermatitis |
| névroglie | neuroglia |
| névrome | neuroma |
| névrose | neurosis |
| névrosé d'angoisse | anxiety neurosis |
| nexus | tight junction |
| nez | nose |
| nier | deny |
| nocif | detrimental |
| nocturne | nocturnal |
| nodosité | nodule |
| nodosité d'Heberden | Heberden's node |
| nodule | nodule; tubercle |
| nœud | knot |
| noir | black |
| nom | name |

| French | English |
|---|---|
| nom de famille | surname |
| nom de jeune fille | maiden name |
| noma | cancrum oris |
| nombril | umbilicus |
| noradrénaline | norepinephrine |
| normoblaste | normoblast |
| normocyte | normocyte |
| nosologie | nosology |
| nosophobie | nosophobia |
| nourrisson (jusqu' à 12 mois) | infant |
| nouveau-né | neonate |
| noyade | drowning |
| noyau arqué | arcuate nucleus |
| noyau rouge | red nucleus |
| noyaux gris centraux | basal ganglia |
| nucléaire | nuclear |
| nucléique acide | nucleic acid |
| nucléoprotéine | nucleoprotein |
| nuisible | noxious |
| nullipare | nullipara |
| numération formule sanguine | complete blood count |
| nummulaire | nummulated |
| nuque | neck |
| nutation | nutation |
| nutriment | nutrient |
| nutrition | nutrition |
| nycturie | nocturia |
| nystagmus | nystagmus |
| nystagmus à ressort | resilient nystagmus |
| nystagmus pendulaire | oscillating nystagmus |
| obésité | obesity |
| obligatoire | mandatory |
| obscurci | dimmed |
| observance | compliance |
| obsession | obsession |
| obstétrical | obstetric |
| obstétricien | obstetrician |
| obstétrique | midwifery |
| obstrué | obstructed |
| obturateur | obturator |
| occipital | occipital |
| occlusion intestinale | intestinal obstruction |

| French | English |
| --- | --- |
| oculaire | ocular |
| oculogyre | oculogyric |
| ocytocine | oxytocin |
| ocytocique | oxytocic |
| odeur | odor |
| odontalgie | odontalgia |
| odontoïde | odontoid |
| odontologie | odontology |
| œdémateux | edematous |
| œdème | edema |
| œdème aigu du poumon | acute pulmonary edema |
| œdème angioneurotique | angioneurotic edema |
| œdème des membres inférieurs | lower extremity edema |
| œdème de Quincke | angioneurotic edema |
| œdème papillaire | papilledema |
| œsophage | esophagus |
| œsophagectomie | eosphagectomy |
| œsophagien | esophageal |
| œsophagoscopie | esophagoscopy |
| œstrogène | estrogen |
| œuf | egg |
| oignon | bunion |
| olécrâne | olecranon |
| olfactif | olfactory |
| oligodendroglie | oligodendroglia |
| oligoménorrhée | oligomenorrhea |
| oligospermie | oligospermia |
| oligotrophie | oligotrophia |
| oligurie | oliguria |
| olive cérébelleuse | dentatum |
| ombilic | umbilicus |
| ombiliqué | umbilicated |
| omentopexie | omentopexy |
| omentum | omentum |
| omoplate | scapula |
| omphalite | omphalitis |
| omphalocèle | omphalocele |
| Organisation mondiale de la santé (OMS) | World Health Organization (WHO) |
| onction | inunction |
| onde alpha | alpha wave |
| ondulant | undulant |
| ongle | nail |

| French | English |
|---|---|
| ongle incarné | onychocryptosis |
| onguent | ointment |
| onychie | onychia |
| onychogryphose | onychogryphosis |
| onychomycose | onychomycosis |
| onyxis | onychia |
| oocyte | oocyte |
| oogenèse | oogenesis |
| oophorectomie | oophorectomy |
| oophorite | oophoritis |
| oophorosalpingectomie | oophorosalpingectomy |
| ophtalmie | ophthalmia |
| ophtalmique | ophthalmic |
| ophtalmologie | opthalmology |
| ophtalmologiste | opthalmologist |
| ophtalmoplégie | ophthalmoplegia |
| ophtalmoscope | opthalmoscope |
| opiacé | opiate |
| opioïde | opioid |
| opisthotonos | opisthotonos |
| opium | opium |
| opposant | opponens |
| opsonine | opsonin |
| opticien | optician |
| optique | optic |
| optométrie | optometry |
| or | gold |
| oral | oral |
| orbiculaire | orbicular |
| orbitaire | orbital |
| orbite | orbit |
| orchidectomie | orchidectomy |
| orchidopexie | orchidopexy |
| orchi-épididymite | orchiepididymitis |
| orchite | orchitis |
| ordonnance | prescription |
| oreille | ear |
| oreille externe | external ear |
| oreille interne | internal ear |
| oreille moyenne | middle ear |
| oreiller | pillow |
| oreillette | atrium |

| French | English |
| --- | --- |
| oreillons | mumps |
| organe | organ |
| orgelet | hordeolum |
| orifice | orifice; foramen |
| ORL | ENT |
| ornithose | ornithosis |
| oropharynx | oropharynx |
| orteil | hallux |
| orteil en marteau | hammer toe |
| orthèse | orthosis |
| orthodontie | orthodontics |
| orthopédie | orthopedics |
| orthophoniste | speech therapist |
| orthostatique | orthostatic |
| os | bone |
| os scaphoïde | navicular bone |
| osmolalité | osmolality |
| osmole | osmole |
| osmose | osmosis |
| osmotique | osmotic |
| osselet | ossicle |
| osseux | osseous |
| ossification | ossification |
| ostéite | osteitis |
| ostéo-arthropathie | ostoarthropathy |
| ostéo-arthrose | osteoarthrosis |
| ostéoblaste | osteoblast |
| ostéocartilagineux | osteochondral |
| ostéochondrite | osteochondritis |
| ostéochondrome | osteochondroma |
| ostéoclasie | osteoclasis |
| ostéoclaste | osteoclast |
| ostéoclastome | osteoclastoma |
| ostéocyte | osteocyte |
| ostéodystrophie | osteodystrophy |
| ostéogenèsis | osteogenesis |
| ostéolytique | osteolytic |
| ostéomalacie | osteomalacia |
| ostéomyélite | osteomyelitis |
| ostéopathie | osteopathy |
| ostéopétrose | osteopetrosis |
| ostéophonie | osteophony |

| French | English |
|---|---|
| ostéophyte | osteophyte |
| ostéoporose | osteoporosis |
| ostéosarcome | osteosarcoma |
| ostéosclérose | osteosclerosis |
| ostéo-tendineux réflexe | deep tendon reflex |
| ostéotomie | osteotomy |
| ostium | ostium |
| otalgie | otalgia |
| otite | otitis |
| otite moyenne adhésive | glue ear |
| otite moyenne aiguë | acute otitis media |
| otolithe | otolith |
| otologie | otology |
| otomycose | otomycosis |
| otorhinolaryngologie (ORL) | otolaryngologist |
| otosclérose | otosclerosis |
| otoscope | otoscope |
| ototoxique | ototoxic |
| ouate | cotton wool |
| ouïe | hearing |
| ourantie | uvulitis |
| ouraque | urachus |
| ourlien | mumps |
| ouverture | aperture |
| ouvre-bouche | gag |
| ovaire | oophoron; ovary |
| ovariectomie | oophorectomy |
| ovariosalpingectomie | oophorosalpingectomy |
| ovarite | ovaritis |
| oviducte | oviduct |
| ovocyte | oocyte |
| ovogenèse | oogenesis |
| ovulation | ovulation |
| ovule | ovule |
| oxalurie | oxaluria |
| oxycéphalie | oxycephaly |
| oxydation | oxidation |
| oxygénation | oxygenation |
| oxygène | oxygen |
| oxygénothérapie | oxygen therapy |
| oxyhémoglobine | oxyhemoglobin |
| oxymètre | oximeter |

| French | English |
|---|---|
| oxyure | pinworm |
| oxyurose | enterobiasis |
| ozène | ozena |
| ozone | ozone |
| pachydermie | pachydermia |
| pachyméningite | pachymeningitis |
| palais | palate |
| palatoplégie | palatoplegia |
| pâleur | pallor |
| palisyllabie | stuttering |
| palliatif | palliative |
| pallidectomie | pallidectomy |
| pallidum | globus pallidus |
| palmaire | palmar |
| palmier | palm |
| palpation | plapation |
| palpitation | palpitation |
| paludisme | malaria (paludism) |
| panaris | whitlow |
| panarthrite | panarthritis |
| pancardite | pancarditis |
| pancréas | pancreas |
| pancréatectomie | pancreatectomy |
| pancréatite | pancreatitis |
| pancréozymine | pancreozymin |
| pandémique | pandemic |
| panhypopituitarisme | panhypopituitarism |
| panique, attaque de | panic attack |
| panniculite | panniculitis |
| panophtalmie | panophthalmia |
| panotite | panotitis |
| pansement | dressing |
| pansement occlusif | occlusive dressing |
| papille optique | optic disk |
| papillite | papillitits |
| papillome | papilloma |
| papule | papule |
| para-aminobenzoïque acide (PABA) | para-aminobenzoic acid |
| para-aminohippurique acide | para-aminohippuric acid (PAH) |
| paracentèse | paracentesis |
| paracentèse tympanique | myringotomy |
| paracétamol | acetaminophen |

| French | English |
|---|---|
| paracousie | paracusia |
| parage | wound care |
| paralysé | cripple |
| paralysie agitante | paralysis agitans |
| paralysie bulbaire | bulbar palsy |
| paralysie diaphragmatique | phrenoplegia |
| paralysie faciale | facial paralysis |
| paralysie pseudobulbaire | pseudobulbar palsy |
| paralytique | paralytic |
| paramédian | paramedian |
| paramédical | paramedical |
| paramètre | parametrium |
| paramétrite | parametritis |
| paramnésie | paramnesia |
| paranasal | paranasal |
| paranoïa | paranoia |
| paranoïde | paranoid |
| paraphimosis | paraphimosis |
| paraplégie | paraplegia |
| pararectal | pararectal |
| parasite | parasite |
| parasympathique | parasympathetic |
| parathormone | parathormone |
| parathyroïde | parathyroid |
| paravertébral | paravertebral |
| parenchyme | parenchyma |
| parentéral | parenteral |
| parésie | paresis |
| paresthésie | paraethesia |
| pariétal | parietal |
| parité | parity |
| Parkinson, maladie de | Parkinson's disease |
| parodontopathie | peridontal disease |
| paroi cellulaire | cell wall |
| paroi thoracique | chest wall |
| paronychie | paronychia |
| parosmie | parosmia |
| parotide | parotid |
| parotidite | parotiditis |
| paroxysmal | paroxysmal |
| parthénogenèse | parthenogenesis |
| partie centrale | core |

| French | English |
|---|---|
| partigène | hapten |
| partout | throughout |
| parturition | parturition |
| passif | passive |
| pâte | paste |
| patellectomie | patellectomy |
| pathétique nerf | trochlear nerve |
| pathogène | pathogenic |
| pathogenèse | pathogenesis |
| pathogénique | pathogenic |
| pathognomonique | pathognomonic |
| pathologie | pathology |
| pathologique | pathological |
| patient | patient |
| patient en fin de vie | terminally ill patient |
| paume | palm |
| paupière | eyelid; palpebra |
| pavillon de l'oreille | auricle |
| peau | skin |
| pectoral | pectoral |
| pédiatre | pediatrician |
| pédiatrie | pediatrics |
| pédicule | pedicle |
| pédiculé | pediculated |
| pédiculose | pediculosis |
| pédicure | chiropodist |
| pédoncule | peduncle |
| pédoncule cérébelleux | brachium cerebelli |
| peigne | comb |
| peine | sorrow |
| pellagre | pellagra |
| pellicules | dandruff |
| pelvien | pelvic |
| pelvimétrie | pelvimetry |
| pelvis | pelvis |
| pemphigus | pemphigus |
| pénétration | penetration |
| pénicilline | penicillin |
| pénis | penis |
| pentosurie | pentosuria |
| pepsine | pepsin |
| pepsique | peptic |

| French | English |
|---|---|
| peptide | peptide |
| peptique | peptic |
| perceuse | drill |
| percussion | percussion |
| percutané | transdermal |
| perdu de vue | lost to follow-up |
| perforation | perforation |
| perfusion intraveineuse | intravenous infusion |
| périamygdalien | peritonsillar |
| périartérite noueuse | polyarteritis nodosa |
| périarthrite | periarthritis |
| péricarde | pericardium |
| péricardique | pericardial |
| péricardite | pericarditis |
| périchondre | perichondrium |
| périchondrite | perichondritis |
| péricolite | pericolitis |
| périlymphe | perilymph |
| périmé | outdated |
| périnéal | perineal |
| périnée | perineum |
| périnéorraphie | perineorrhaphy |
| périnéphrétique | perinephric |
| périostal | peristeal |
| périoste | periosteum |
| périostique | periosteal |
| périostite | periostitis |
| périphérique | peripheral |
| périproctite | periproctitis |
| péristaltisme | peristalsis |
| péritoine | peritoneum |
| péritomie | peritomy |
| péritonéal | peritoneal |
| péritonite | peritonitis |
| périurétral | periurethral |
| perméabilité du foramen ovale | patent foramen ovale |
| pernicieux | pernicious |
| péroné | fibula |
| péronier | peroneal |
| personnes âgées | elderly |
| perspiration | perspiration |
| perte de connaissance | loss of consciousness |

| French | English |
|---|---|
| pertes blanches | leukorrhea |
| pèse-bébé | baby-scale |
| pessaire | pessary |
| peste bubonique | bubonic plague |
| pet | fart |
| pétéchie | petechia |
| petit juif | funny bone |
| petite enfance | infancy |
| pétreux | petrous |
| pétrissage | petrissage |
| phagocyte | phagocyte |
| phagocytose | phagocytosis |
| pharmacie | pharmacy |
| pharmacien | pharmacist |
| pharmacocinétique | pharmacokinetics |
| pharmacodépendance | drug dependence |
| pharmacologie | pharmacology |
| pharyngé | pharyngeal |
| pharyngectomie | pharyngectomy |
| pharyngite | pharyngitis |
| pharyngolaryngectomie | pharyngolaryngectomy |
| pharynx | pharynx |
| phénomènes cadavériques | post-mortem changes |
| phénotype | phenotype |
| phénylcétonurie | phenylketonuria |
| phlébectomie | phlebectomy |
| phlébite | phlebitis |
| phlébographie | venography |
| phlébothrombose | phlebothrombosis |
| phlegmatia | phlegmasia |
| phlegmatia alba doens | phlegmasia alba dolens |
| phlycténulaire | phlyctenular |
| phobie | phobia |
| phonation | phonation |
| phoniatrie | phoniatrics |
| phosphatase acide | acid phosphatase |
| phosphaturie | phosphaturia |
| phospholipide | phospholipid |
| phosphonécrose | phosphonecrosis |
| photochimiothérapie | photochimiotherapy |
| photomètre à flamme | flame photometer |
| photophobie | photophobia |

| French | English |
|---|---|
| photosensibilisation | photosensitization |
| phrénicectomie | phrenicectomy |
| phrénique | phrenic |
| phrénoplégie | phrenoplegia |
| phtiriase | pediculosis |
| physicien | physicist |
| physiologie | physiology |
| physiothérapie | physiotherapy |
| pian | framboesia; yaws |
| pica | pica |
| picotement | tingling |
| pied bot | talipes |
| pied bot talus | talipes calcaneus |
| pied varus équin | talipes equinus |
| pied creux | pes cavus |
| pied plat | pes valgus |
| pied tombant | drop foot |
| pie-mère | pia mater |
| pigment biliaire | bile pigment |
| pileux | hairy |
| pilule | pill |
| pince | forceps |
| pincement articulaire | joint space narrowing |
| pinces | tongs |
| pinguécula | pinguecula |
| pinocytose | pinocytosis |
| pipette | pipet |
| piqûre | injection; puncture |
| piqûre d'abeille | bee sting |
| pityriasis rosé de Gibert | pityriasis rosea |
| placenta | placenta |
| placenta praevia | placenta praevia |
| placentaire | placental |
| plagiocéphalie | plagiocephaly |
| plaie | wound |
| plaie par arme blanche | stab wound |
| plainte | complaint |
| plainte actuelles | current (chief) complaint |
| plan | scheme |
| planche anatomique | anatomical chart |
| planification familiale | family planning |
| plantaire | plantar |

| French | English |
|---|---|
| plante du pied | sole |
| plaque motrice | motor end plate |
| plaquette | platelet |
| plasmaphérèse | plasmapheresis |
| plasmocyte | plasma cell |
| plasmocytose | plasmacytosis |
| plat | flat |
| plathelminthe | flatworm |
| plâtre | plaster |
| pléomorphisme | pleomorphism |
| pléthore | plethora |
| pléthysmographe | plethysmograph |
| pleurésie | pleurisy |
| plèvre | pleura |
| plexus brachial | brachial plexus |
| plexus solaire | solar plexus |
| pli cutané | skin fold |
| plicature | plica |
| plomb | lead |
| plongée | diving |
| plus grand que la normale | greater than normal |
| plus vieux | older |
| pneumatocèle | pneumoatocele |
| pneumaturie | pneumaturia |
| pneumoconiose | pneumoconiosis |
| pneumocoque | pneumococcus |
| pneumogastrique nerf | vagus nerve |
| pneumonectomie | pneumonectomy |
| pneumonie | pneumonia |
| pneumopéritoine | pneumoperitoneum |
| pneumothorax | pneumothorax |
| poche pharyngée | pharyngeal pouch |
| poids corporel | body weight |
| poignet | wrist |
| poïkilocytose | poikilocytosis |
| poil | hair |
| poing | fist |
| pointe du cœur | apex of heart |
| poison | poison |
| poisson | fish |
| poitrine | chest |
| polioencéphalite | polioencephalitis |

238

| French | English |
|---|---|
| poliomyélite | polymyelitis |
| polyarthrite rhumatoïde | rheumatoid arthritis |
| polychondrite | polychondritis |
| polycythémie | polycythemia |
| polycactylie | polydactyly |
| polydipsie | polydipsia |
| polyglobulie | polycythemia |
| polyglobulie essentielle | polycythemia vera |
| polykystique | polycystic |
| polyménorrhée | polymenorrhea |
| polymyosite | polymyositis |
| polyneuropathie | polyneuropathy |
| polynévrite | polyneuritis |
| polyopie | polyopia |
| polyoside | polysaccharide |
| polype | polypus |
| polypose | polyposis |
| polysialie | polysialia |
| polytraumatisme | polytrauma |
| polyurie | polyuria |
| pommade | ointment |
| pommade camphrée | camphor ointment |
| pomme d'Adam | Adam's apple |
| pompholyx | pompholyx |
| ponction ascite | paracentesis |
| ponction cisternale | cisternal puncture |
| ponction lombaire | lumbar puncture |
| ponction pleurale | thoracentesis |
| ponction-biopsie | needle biopsy |
| pontage | bypass |
| poplité | popliteal |
| porphyrie | porphyria |
| porphyrine | porphyrin |
| portail | portal |
| porte-aiguille | needle holder |
| positif | positive |
| position debout | upright |
| position genupectorale | knee elbow position |
| posologie | dose regimen |
| post-abortum | postaboral |
| post-charge | after-load |
| postérieur | posterior |

| French | English |
| --- | --- |
| post-maturité | postmaturity |
| post-mictionnel | postvoiding |
| postural | postural |
| potassium | potassium |
| potentiel d'action | action potential |
| potentiel de repos | resting potential |
| potentiel évoqué | evoked potential |
| pou du pubis | crab louse |
| pouce | thumb |
| poudre | powder |
| pouls | pulse |
| pouls alternant | pulsus alternans |
| poumon | lung |
| poumon du fermier | farmer's lung |
| pourpre rétinien | rhodopsin |
| poussée | flare |
| poussière | dust |
| poux | lice |
| préalable au | beforehand |
| préauriculaire | preauricular |
| précancéreux | precancerous |
| précipitine | precipitin |
| précordialgie | precordialgia |
| précordium | precordium |
| prélèvement de moelle osseuse | bone marrow puncture |
| prématuré | premature |
| prémenstruel | premenstrual |
| premiers secours | first aid |
| prémolaire | premolar |
| prénatal | prenatal |
| prépuce | foreskin |
| presbyacousie | presbyacusia |
| presbyophrénie | presbyophrenia |
| presbytie | presbyopia |
| prescripteur | prescriber |
| prescription | prescription |
| présentation de la face | face presentation |
| présentation frontale | brow presentation |
| préservatif | condom |
| pression artérielle | blood pressure |
| présystole | presystole |
| priapisme | priapism |

| French | English |
|---|---|
| primipare | primipara |
| prise en charge | management |
| privation | deprivation |
| problème | problem |
| prochain | next |
| proche | near |
| procidence | prolapse |
| proctalgie | proctalgia |
| proctectomie | proctectomy |
| proctite | proctitis |
| proctocèle | proctocele |
| proctoscopie | proctoscopy |
| procubitus | prone |
| proenzyme | zymogen |
| profond | deep |
| progéniture | offspring |
| progérie | progeria |
| progestérone | progesterone |
| proglottis | proglotttis |
| progressif | progressive |
| prolactine | prolactin |
| prolapsus | prolapse |
| prolongé | extended |
| promonocyte | promonocyte |
| promontoire | promontory |
| pronation | pronation |
| pronostic | prognosis |
| prophylaxie | prophylaxis |
| propriocepteur | proprioceptor |
| prostacycline | prostacyclin |
| prostaglandine | prostaglandin |
| prostate | prostate |
| prostatectomie | prostatectomy |
| protéine | protein |
| protéinurie | proteinuria |
| protéolyse | proteolysis |
| prothèse | prosthesis |
| prothèse acoustique | hearing aid |
| prothrombine | prothrombin |
| protocole opératoire | operative note |
| protocole thérapeutique | treatment regimen |
| protoplasme | protoplasm |

| French | English |
|---|---|
| protoxyde d'azote | nitrous oxide |
| protozoaire | protozoa |
| protrusion oculaire | proptosis oculi |
| protubérance annulaire | pons |
| protubérantiel | pontine |
| provisions | supplies |
| provoquer | provoke |
| proximal | proximal |
| prurit | pruritis |
| pseudarthrose | pseudarthrosis |
| pseudo-méningite | meningism |
| psittacose | psittacosis |
| psoïtis | psoitis |
| psoriasis | psoriasis |
| psorique | scabietic |
| psychasthénie | psychasthenia |
| psychiatrie | psychiatry |
| psychologie | psychology |
| psycholgue | psychologist |
| psychonévrose | psychoneurosis |
| psychopathologie | psychopathology |
| psychose | psychosis |
| psychose maniacodépressive | manic-depressive psychosis |
| psychose puerpérale | postpartum psychosis |
| psychosomatique | psychosomatic |
| psychothérapie | psychotherapy |
| ptérigion | pterygium |
| ptose | ptosis |
| ptyaline | ptyalin |
| ptyalisme | polysialia |
| puanteur | fetor |
| puberté | puberty |
| pubis | pubis |
| puce | flea |
| puceron | aphid |
| pudendal | pudendal |
| puerpéralité | puerperium |
| puerpérum | puerperium |
| puissance | potency |
| pulmonaire | pulmonary |
| pulpe | pulp |
| pulpite | pulpitis |

| French | English |
|---|---|
| pulsatile | throbbing |
| pulsation | pulsation |
| pulvérisation | spray |
| punaise de lit | bedbug |
| pupille | pupil |
| purpura | purpura |
| purpura rhumatoïde | Henoch purpura |
| purulent | purulent |
| pus | pus |
| putréfaction | putrefaction |
| pycnique | pyknic |
| pycnose | pyknosis |
| pyélite | pyelitis |
| pyélographie | pyelography |
| pyélolithotomie | pyelolithotomy |
| pyémie | pyemia |
| pylore | pylorus |
| pylorique | pyloric |
| pyloroplastie | pyloroplasty |
| pyodermite | pyoderma |
| pyogène | pyogenic |
| pyonéphrose | pyonephrosis |
| pyorrhée | pyorrhea |
| pyosalpinx | pyosalpinx |
| pyramidal | pyramidal |
| pyrexie | pyrexia |
| pyridoxine | pyridoxine |
| pyrogène | pyrogen |
| pyrosis | pyrosis |
| pyurie | pyuria |
| quadriceps | quadriceps |
| quadriplégie | quadriplegia |
| qualifier | qualify |
| quarantaine | quarantine |
| quatre pattes à | on all fours |
| quel que soit | regardless of |
| quérulence | querulousness |
| queue de cheval | cauda equina |
| quinquinisme | cinchonism |
| quinte de toux | coughing fit |
| quotidien | every day |
| quotient intellectuel | intelligence quotient (IQ) |

| French | English |
|---|---|
| raccourcissement | shortening |
| racémeux | racemose |
| rachidien nerf | spinal nerve |
| rachis | spine |
| rachitisme | rickets |
| racine | root |
| racine antérieure | anterior root |
| racine carrée | square root |
| racine dorsale | dorsal root |
| raclement de gorge | clearing of throat |
| radial | radial |
| radiation | radiation |
| radicotomie | rhizotomy |
| radiculite | radiculitis |
| radioactif | radioactive |
| radiobiologie | radiobiology |
| radiographie | radiography |
| radiologie | radiology |
| radiologiste | radiologist |
| radiomucite | radioepithelitis |
| radionucléide | radionuclide |
| radiosensibilité | radiosensitivity |
| radiothérapie | radiotherapy |
| radon 219 | actinon |
| rage | rabies |
| raideur de la nuque | stiff-neck |
| râle | rale |
| râle sous-crépitant | subcrepitant rale |
| rameau | ramus |
| ramollissement | malacia |
| rang | grade |
| ranula | ranula |
| rapport sexuel | sexual intercourse |
| rash | rash |
| rate | spleen |
| ration | intake |
| ration alimentaire | oral intake |
| rauque | hoarse |
| Raynaud, syndrome de | Raynaud's syndrome |
| rayon gamma | gamma ray |
| rayonnement ionisant | ionizing radiation |
| rayons ultraviolets | ultraviolet rays |

| French | English |
|---|---|
| réactif | reactive; reagent |
| réaction d'arrêt | arousal response |
| réaction d'immunofluorenscence | fluorescent antibody test |
| réaction médicamenteuse | drug reaction |
| rebond | rebound |
| rebouteux | bonesetter |
| récepteur | receptor |
| récessif | recessive |
| rechute | relapse |
| réclamation | complaint |
| rectal | rectal |
| rectite | proctitis |
| rectocèle | rectocele |
| rectocolite ulcéro-hémorragique | ulcerative colitis |
| rectoscopie | rectoscopy |
| rectosigmoïdectomie | rectosigmoidectomy |
| rectus abdominis muscle | rectus abdominis muscle |
| recueil | compendium |
| réduction | reduction |
| réflexe achilléen | Achilles tendon reflex |
| réflexe bicipital | biceps reflex |
| réflexe cutané abdominal | abdominal reflex |
| réflexe de préhension | grasp reflex |
| réflexe du canif | clasp knife reflex |
| réflexe gastrocolique | gastrocolic reflex |
| réflexe médullaire | spinal reflex |
| réflexe nauséeux | gag reflex |
| réflexe rotulien | knee jerk reflex |
| réflexe tendineux | tendon reflex |
| réflexe tricipital | triceps reflex |
| regard | gaze |
| régime alimentaire | diet |
| régime pauvre en graisses | low-fat diet |
| région précordiale | precordium |
| règles | menses |
| régurgitation | regurgitation |
| rein | kidney |
| rein en fer à cheval | horseshoe kidney |
| relâchement | looseness |
| relation | relation; intercourse |
| relaxine | relaxin |
| releveur | levator |

| French | English |
| --- | --- |
| rémission | remission |
| rénal | renal |
| rendez-vous | appointment |
| reniflement | sniffing |
| rénine | renin |
| repas baryté | barium enema |
| repli | plica |
| réponse immunologique | immune response |
| repos | rest |
| résection | resection |
| résidu vésical | residual urine |
| résine | resin |
| résistance globulaire, épreuve de la | osmotic fragility test |
| résonance magnétique nucléaire | nuclear magnetic resonance (NMR) |
| respirateur | respirator |
| respiration de Kussmaul | Kussmaul respiration |
| respiratoire | respiratory |
| résultat de laboratoire | lab result |
| retenir son souffle | hold one's breath |
| réticulaire | reticular |
| réticulocyte | reticulocyte |
| réticulocytose | reticulocytosis |
| réticulo-endothélial | reticulo-endothelial |
| réticulosarcome | reticulum cell sarcoma |
| réticulum endoplasmique | endoplasmic reticulum |
| rétine | retina |
| rétinite | retinitis |
| rétinoblastome | retinoblastoma |
| rétinopathie | retinopathy |
| rétinopathie diabétique | diabetic retinopathy |
| retour de couches | resumption of menses |
| rétracteur | retractor |
| rétraction | retraction |
| rétrécissement aortique | aortic stenosis |
| rétrécissement mitral | mitral stenosis |
| rétrécissement pulmonaire | pulmonary stenosis |
| rétrograde | retrograde |
| rétropéritonéal | retroperitoneal |
| rétropharyngé | retropharyngeal |
| réussite | success |
| rêve | dream |
| réveil | awakening |

| French | English |
|---|---|
| rhagade | rhagade |
| rhinite | rhinitis |
| rhinite allergique | allergic rhinitis |
| rhinopharyngien | nasopharyngeal |
| rhinopharyngite aiguë | acute nasopharyngitis |
| rhinoplastie | rhinoplasty |
| rhinorrhée | rhinorrhea |
| rhinoscopie | rhinoscopy |
| rhizomère | dermatome |
| rhizotomie | rhizotomy |
| rhodopsine | rhrodopsin |
| rhomboïde | rhomboid |
| rhumatismal | rheumatic |
| rhumatisme | rheumatism |
| rhumatisme articulaire aigu | rheumatic fever |
| rhume des foins | hay fever |
| riboflavine | riboflavin |
| ribonucléique acide | ribonucleic acid |
| ricin | castor bean |
| rickettsie | rickettsia |
| rictus sardonique | risus sardonicus |
| rigidité cadavérique | rigor mortis |
| rigidité décérébration | decerebrate rigidity |
| rire | laugh, to |
| robe | gown |
| robinet | tap |
| rocher | petrous bone |
| Roentgen | Roentgen |
| ronchus | rhonchus |
| ronfler | snore, to |
| ronger | abrade, to |
| rongeur | rodent |
| rotation | rotation |
| rotule | patella |
| roue dentée | cog wheel |
| rougeole | measles |
| rougeur | flush |
| rougir | blush, to |
| rubéfiant | rubefacient |
| rubéole | German measles (rubella) |
| rugine | rugine |
| rupia | rupia |

| French | English |
|---|---|
| rupture | rupture |
| rythme | rhythm |
| rythme circadien | circadian rhythm |
| rythme de galop | cantering rhythm |
| sacralisation | sacralization |
| sac à urine | urinary drainage bag |
| sac de colostomie | colostomy bag |
| sacré | sacral |
| sacrum | sacrum |
| sage | wise |
| sage-femme | midwife |
| saignement | bleeding |
| saillant | buldging |
| Saint-Guy, danse de | Saint Vitus' dance |
| sale | dirty |
| salidiurétique | saluretic |
| salin | saline |
| salivation | salivation |
| salive | saliva |
| salle d'hôpital | ward |
| salpingectomie | salpingectomy |
| salpingite | salpingitis |
| salpingographie | salpingography |
| salpingostomie | salpingostomy |
| sang | blood |
| sanglot | sob |
| sangsue | leech |
| sans objet | irrelevant |
| sans signification | meaningless |
| sans-abri | homeless |
| santé | health |
| saphène | saphena |
| saponification | saponify |
| saprophyte | saprophyte |
| sarcoïde | sarcoid |
| sarcoïdose | sarcoidosis |
| sarcolemme | sarcolemme |
| sarcome | sarcoma |
| sartorius muscle | sartorius muscle |
| saturation | saturation |
| saturnisme | lead poisoning |
| saveur | taste |

| French | English |
|---|---|
| savon | soap |
| scabies | scabies |
| scalp | scalp |
| scalpel | scalpel |
| scaphocéphalie | scaphocephaly |
| scaphoïde carpien | scaphoid bone |
| scaphoïdite tarsienne | Köhler's disease |
| scapulaire | scapula |
| scapulalgie | scapulalgia |
| scarification | scarification |
| scarlatine | scarlet fever |
| scellés | seals |
| schistocyte | schistocyte |
| Schistosoma | Bilharzia |
| schistosomiase | schistosomiasis |
| schizocyte | schistocyte |
| schizophrénie | schizophrenia |
| Schwann, gaine de | neurilemma |
| sciatalgie | sciatica |
| scie | saw |
| scintigraphie osseuse | bone scan |
| scissure | fissure |
| sclérite | scleritis |
| sclérodactylie | sclerodactylia |
| sclérodermie | scleroderma |
| sclérodermie circonscrite | morphea |
| sclérose en plaques | multiple sclerosis |
| sclérose latérale amyotrophique | amyotrophic lateral sclerosis |
| sclérotique | sclera |
| sclérotomie | sclerotomy |
| scolex | scolex |
| scoliose | scoliosis |
| scopophilie | scopophilia |
| scorbut | scurvy |
| scotome | scotoma |
| scrotal | scrotal |
| scrotum | scrotum |
| scybales | scybalum |
| sébacé | sebaceous |
| séborrhée | seborrhea |
| sec | dry |
| secousse musculaire | twitch |

| French | English |
|---|---|
| sécrétine | secretin |
| sécrétion | secretion |
| sédatif | sedative |
| segment de Fowler | segmentum apicale |
| segmentation | cleavage |
| sein | breast |
| sel | salt |
| selles | feces |
| selles noires | black stools |
| selon | according to |
| sels biliares | bile salts |
| semi-lunaire os | lunate bone |
| séminoma | seminoma |
| sénescence | senescence |
| sénile | senile |
| sénilité | senility |
| sens des aiguilles d'une montre dans le | clockwise |
| sensation | sensation |
| sensé | sensible |
| sensibilisation | sensitization |
| sensibilisé | sensitized |
| sensibilité | sensibility |
| sensitif nerf | sensory nerve |
| séparation | parting |
| séparé | apart |
| sepsie | sepsis |
| septicémie | septicemia |
| septicopyohémie | pyemia |
| septique | septic |
| septum | septum |
| séquelle | sequela |
| séquestre | sequestrum |
| séreux | serous |
| série | series |
| sérié | serial |
| seringue | syringe |
| serment d'Hippocrate | Hippocratic oath |
| sérotonine | serotonin |
| serpigineux | serpiginous |
| sérum | serum |
| sérum physiologique | physiological saline |
| serviette hygiénique | feminine pad |

| French | English |
|---|---|
| sessile | sessile |
| seuil rénal | renal threshold |
| seul | single |
| sevrage | withdrawal |
| sexe | sex |
| shunt | shunt |
| sialadénite | sialadenitis |
| sialagogue | sialogogue |
| sialolithe | sialolith |
| sialorrhée | polysialia; pytalism |
| SIDA | AIDS |
| sidération médullaire | spinal shock |
| sidérophiline | iron binding protein |
| sidérose | siderosis |
| sieste | nap |
| sifflement | whistle |
| sifflement respiratoire | wheeze |
| sigmoïde | sigmoid |
| sigmoïdoscopie | sigmoidoscopy |
| sigmoïdostomie | sigmoidostomy |
| signe du lacet | capillary fragility test |
| signes cliniques | clinical signs |
| signes vitaux | vital signs |
| silencieux | silent |
| silicose | silicosis; grinders's disease |
| sillon | sulcus |
| simulation | malingering |
| simulie | black fly |
| simultané | simultaneous |
| sinistrocardie | sinistrocardia |
| sino-auriculaire | sinoatrial |
| sinus caverneux | cavernous sinus |
| sinus de la face | paranasal sinus |
| sinus pilonidal | pilonidal cyst |
| sinus sphénoïdal | sphenoidal sinus |
| sinusite | sinusitis |
| sinusite aiguë | acute sinusitis |
| sinusoïdal | sinusoid |
| sirop | syrup |
| siroter | sip, to |
| situation matrimoniale | marital status |
| smegma | smegma |

| French | English |
|---|---|
| système nerveux central (SNC) | central nervous system (CNS) |
| sodoku | rat bite fever |
| soif | thirst |
| soignant | caregiver |
| soins infirmiers | nursing care |
| soins intensif | intensive care |
| soléaire muscle | soleus muscle |
| solide | firm |
| solution salée | saline |
| solvant | solvent |
| somatique | somatic |
| sommeil | sleep |
| sommeil, maladie du | sleeping sickness |
| sommeil à mouvements oculaires rapides (MOR) | REM (rapid eye movement) sleep |
| sommet | apex |
| somnambulisme | somnambulism |
| somnifère | hypnotic |
| somnolence | somnolence |
| sondage | probing |
| sonde à ballonnet | cuffed tube |
| sonde à demeure | indwelling catheter |
| sonde naso-œsophagienne | nasogastric tube |
| soporifique | soporific |
| souci | worry |
| souffle cardiaque | heart murmur |
| souffle carotidien | carotid bruit |
| souffle de vie | mouth to mouth resuscitation |
| souffrance fœtale | fetal distress |
| souffrir | suffer, to |
| soufre | sulfur |
| soulagement | relief |
| soulagement de la douleur | pain relief |
| soulager | relieve, to |
| soulever | lift, to |
| soupir | sigh, to |
| sourcil | eyebrow; supercilium |
| sourd | deaf |
| sourd-muet | deaf-mute |
| sous | under; infra |
| sous-alimentation | malnutrition |
| sous-arachnoïdien | subarachnoid |
| sous-clavier | subclavian |

| French | English |
|---|---|
| sous-diaphragmatique | subphrenic |
| sous-dural | subdural |
| sous-épineux | infraspinous |
| sous-jacent | underlying |
| sous-maxillaire | submaxillary |
| soutenu | sustained |
| souvenir | recollection |
| sparadrap | adhesive tape |
| spasme carpopédal | carpopedal spasm |
| spasme de torsion | torsion spasm |
| spasmolytique | spasmolytic |
| spasticité | spasticity |
| spastique | spastic |
| spécifique | specific |
| spécimen | specimen |
| spectrométrie | spectrometry |
| spectroscope | spectroscope |
| spéculum | speculum |
| spermatocèle | spermatocele |
| spermatogenèse | spermatogenesis |
| spermatozoïde | spermatozoon |
| sperme | sperm |
| spermicide | spermicide |
| spermogramme | semen analysis |
| sphérocyte | spherocyte |
| sphérocytose | spherocytosis |
| sphinctérotomie | sphincterotomy |
| sphygmomanomètre | sphygmomanometer |
| spica | spica |
| spicule | spicule |
| spinal | spinal |
| spirographe | spirograph |
| spiromètre | spirometer |
| splanchniques nerfs | splanchnic nerves |
| spleen | spleen |
| splénectomie | splenectomy |
| splénique | splenic |
| splénomégalie | splenomegaly |
| spondylarthrite anklyosante | ankylosing spondylitis |
| spondylite | spondylitis |
| spondylolisthésis | spondylolisthesis |
| spndylolyse | spondylolysis |

253

| French | English |
| --- | --- |
| spongieux os | cancellous bone |
| spongiose | spongiosis |
| spontané | spontaneous |
| sporotrichose | sporotrichosis |
| spume | foam |
| squame | squama |
| squameux | squamous |
| squelette | skeleton |
| squirrhe | scirrhus |
| stadification | staging |
| stapédectomie | stapedectomy |
| stapedius muscle | stapedius muscle |
| stapes | stapes |
| staphylome | staphyloma |
| staphylorraphie | staphylorrhaphy |
| stase | stasis |
| statique | static |
| status | status |
| statut nutritionnel | nutritional status |
| statut vaccinal | vaccine status |
| stéatome | steatoma |
| stéatorrhée | steatorrhea |
| stéatose | steatosis |
| Steinert, maladie de | myotonia dystrophica; Steinert's disease |
| stellaire ganglion | stellate ganglion |
| sténose | stenosis |
| steppage | drop foot gait |
| stercobiline | stercobilin |
| sterocolithe | sterocolith |
| stéréognosie | stereognosis |
| stérile | sterile |
| stérilet | intrauterine contraceptive device |
| stérilisation | sterilization |
| stérilité féminine | acyesis |
| sternal | sternal |
| stérol | sterol |
| stéthoscope | stethoscope |
| stimulateur cardiaque | pacemaker |
| stomatite aphteuse | aphthous stomatitis |
| stomatite gangreneuse | cancrum oris |
| strabisme | strabismus |
| strabisme convergent | convergent strabismus |

| French | English |
|---|---|
| stratum granulosum | granular layer |
| stricture | stricture |
| strie Z | Z band |
| stroma | stroma |
| stupéfiant | narcotic |
| stupeur | stupor |
| stylet | stylet |
| subaigue | subacute |
| subérose | suberosis |
| sublingual | sublingual |
| substance blanche | white matter |
| substance grise | gray matter |
| substance grise périaqueducale | periaqueductal gray matter |
| suc gastrique | gastric secretions |
| succion | sucking |
| succussion | succussion |
| sucre | sugar |
| sudamina | sudamina |
| sueur | sweat |
| suicide | suicide |
| suintement | oozing |
| suite de couches | puerperium |
| sulcus | sulcus |
| sulfamide | sulfonamide |
| superfécondation | superfecundation |
| supérieur | superior |
| supination | supination |
| suppositoire | suppository |
| suppuration | suppuration |
| suppuré | purulent |
| suppurer | fester |
| sural | sural |
| surcharge pondérale | overweight |
| surdité | deafness |
| surdose | overdose |
| surface corporelle | body surface area |
| surfactant | surfactant |
| surjet | running suture |
| surrénale glande | adrenal gland |
| surrénalectomie | adrenalectomy |
| surrénalien | adrenal |
| sus-orbitaire | supraorbital |

| French | English |
|---|---|
| sus-pubien | suprapubic |
| suture | suture |
| suture coronale | coronal suture |
| suture dentée | serrated suture |
| suture sagittale | sagittal suture |
| sycosis trichophytique | barber's itch |
| symbiose | symbiosis |
| symétrie | symmetry |
| sympathectomie | sympathectomy |
| symptôme | symptom |
| symptôme révélateur | presenting symptom |
| synapse | synapse |
| synarthrose | synarthrosis |
| synchondrose | synchondrosis |
| syncope | syncope |
| syncope par hyperexitabilité du sinus carotidien | carotid sinus syncope |
| syndrome canalaire | entrapment neuropathy |
| syndrome de chasse | dumping syndrome |
| syndrome de l'anse borgne | blind loop syndrome |
| syndrome d'écrasement | crush syndrome |
| syndrome d'immunodéficience acquise (SIDA) | Acquired Immunodeficiency Syndrome (AIDS) |
| syndrome du cimeterre | scimitar syndrome |
| syndrome du vol de la sous-clavière | subclavian steal syndrome |
| syndrome prémenstruel | presmenstruel syndrome |
| synéchie | synechia |
| synovectomie | synovectomy |
| synovite | synovitis |
| syphilis | syphilis |
| syringomyélie | syringomelia |
| système ABO | ABO system |
| système métrique | metric system |
| système nerveux autonome | autonomic nervous system |
| système sympathique | sympathetic nervous system |
| systole | systole |
| systolique | systolic |
| tabagisme | smoking |
| tabatière anatomique | anatomical snuff-box |
| tablette | tablet |
| tablier | apron |
| tabouret | stool |
| tache | macula |

| French | English |
| --- | --- |
| tâche | task |
| tache aveugle | blind spot |
| tache de rousseur | ephelis; freckle |
| tacheture | mottling |
| tachycardie | tachycardia |
| tactile | tactile |
| tænia | tapeworm |
| taille | height |
| talon | heel |
| talus | talus |
| tampon d'ouate | pledget |
| tamponnade | tamponade |
| tapis roulant | treadmill |
| tardif | late |
| tarsal | tarsal |
| tarsalgie | tarsalgia |
| tarse | tarsus |
| tarsectomie | tarsectomy |
| tarsien | tarsal |
| tarsoplastie | tarsoplasty |
| tarsorraphie | tarsorrhaphy |
| tartre dentaire | dental calculus |
| taurocholique acide | taurocholic acid |
| taux de natalité | birth rate |
| taux de survie à un an | one year survival rate |
| taxinomie | taxinomy |
| tégument | integument |
| teigne | tinea |
| teinture | tincture |
| télangiectasie | telangiectasis |
| télémétrie | telemetry |
| température | temperature |
| temps de saignement | bleeding time |
| tendinite | tendinitis |
| tendinite de la coiffe des rotateurs | impingement syndrome |
| tendon | tendon |
| ténesme | tenesmus |
| ténoplastie | tenoplasty |
| ténorraphie | tenorrhaphy |
| ténosynovite | tenosynovitis |
| ténotomie | tenotomy |
| tension artérielle | blood pressure |

| French | English |
|---|---|
| tente à oxygène | oxygen tent |
| tératogène | teratogen |
| tèratome | teratoma |
| térébrant | terebrant |
| terme à | full-term |
| terminaison d'un nerf afférent | end organ |
| terreur nocturne | night terror |
| tertiaire | tertiary |
| test à l'antiglobuline | antiglobulin test (Coombs' test) |
| test de fixation du complément | complement fixation test |
| test percutané | patch test |
| testicule | testicle |
| testostérone | testosterone |
| tétanie | tetany |
| tétanos | tetanus |
| tête | head |
| tétracycline | tetracycline |
| tétradactyle | tetradactylous |
| tétraplégie | quadriplegia |
| thalamus | thalamus |
| thalassémie | thalassemia; Mediterranean anemia |
| thalidomide | thalidomide |
| thécome | thecoma |
| thèque | theca |
| thermalisme | balneology |
| thermomètre | thermometer |
| thiamine | thiamine |
| thoracique | thoracic |
| thoracentèse | thoracentesis |
| thoracoplastie | thoracoplasty |
| thoracoscopie | thoracoscopy |
| thoracotomie | thoracotomy |
| thorax | thorax |
| thorax en carène | pigeon chest |
| thorax en entonnoir | funnel chest |
| thréonine | threonine |
| thrombectomie | thrombectomy |
| thrombine | thrombin |
| thrombangéite | thromboangiitis |
| thromboartérite | thromboarteritis |
| thrombocyte | platelet |
| thrombocytopénie | thrombocytopenia |

258

| French | English |
|---|---|
| thrombophlébite | thrombophlebitis |
| thrombose | thrombosis |
| thymectomie | thymectomy |
| thymie | mood |
| thymine | thymine |
| thymoanaleptique | antidepressant |
| thymocyte | thymocyte |
| thymome | thymoma |
| thymus | thymus |
| thyréotoxicose | thyrotoxicosis |
| thyréotrope hormone | thyroid stimulating hormone (TSH) |
| thyroïde | thyroid |
| thyroïdectomie | thyroidectomy |
| thyroxine | thyroxine |
| tibia | tibia |
| tibial | cnemial |
| tiède | tepid |
| tinnitus | tinnitus |
| tirer | pull, to |
| tissu conjonctif lâche | areolar tissue |
| titubant | staggering |
| tocophérol | tocopherol |
| toise | tape measure |
| toit | tectum |
| tomodensitométrie | CT scan |
| tomographie par émission de positons | PET scan |
| tonomètre | tonometer |
| tonsillectomie | tonsillectomy |
| tonsillite | tonsillits |
| torpeur | torpor |
| torpide | indolent |
| torsade de pointe | torsade de pointe (ventricular cardiac rhythm disturbance) |
| torse | torso |
| torsion | torsion |
| torticolis | torticollis |
| toucher rectal | rectal digital examination |
| tour de hanches | hip girth |
| tournesol | litmus |
| tourniquet | tourniquet |
| tous les deux jours | every other day |
| toux | cough |

| French | English |
|---|---|
| toxémie | toxemia |
| toxicologie | toxicology |
| toxicomanie | addiction |
| toxicomanie à la colle | glue sniffing addiction |
| toxicose alimentaire | food poisoning |
| toxidermie | drug eruption |
| toxine | toxin |
| toxique | toxic |
| toxoplasmose | toxoplasmosis |
| trabécule | trabecule |
| trabéculotomie | trabeculotomy |
| trachée | trachea |
| trachéite | tracheitis |
| trachélorraphie | trachelorrhaphy |
| trachéobronchite | tracheobronchitis |
| trachéostomie | tracheostomy |
| trachéotomie | tracheotomy |
| trachome | trachoma |
| tractus uvéal | uveal tract |
| tragus | tragus |
| traitement | treatment |
| tranche | slice |
| tranchées utérines | after-pains |
| tranquillisant | tranquilizer |
| transabdominal | transabdominal |
| transaminase | transaminase |
| transdermique | transdermal |
| transfusion | transfusion |
| transplant | transplant |
| transplantation | transplantation |
| transports, mal des | motion sickness |
| transsudation | transudation |
| trapèze | trapezium |
| trapézoïde | trapezoid |
| trauma | trauma |
| traumatisme crânien | head trauma |
| trématode | trematoda |
| tremblement | tremor |
| tremblement intentionnel | intention tremor |
| trépanation | trephining |
| triangle | trigone |
| triangle de Scarpa | femoral triangle |

| French | English |
|---|---|
| triceps | triceps |
| trichiasis | trichiasis |
| trichinose | trichinosis |
| trichocéphale | whipworm |
| trichophytie | trichophytosis |
| trigéminal | trigeminal |
| trigone | trigone |
| trijumeau nerf | trigeminal nerve |
| triplégie | triplegia |
| triplés | triplets |
| triploïde | triploid |
| trismus | trismus; lockjaw |
| trisomie | trisomy |
| trisomie 21 | trisomy 21; Down's syndrome |
| tristesse | sadness |
| trocart | trocar |
| trochanter | trochanter |
| trochléaire | trochlear |
| trochlée | trochlea |
| trompe d'Eustache | pharyngotympanic tube |
| tronc artériel brachiocéphalique | innominate artery |
| tronc cérébral | brain stem |
| tronculaire | truncal |
| trophoblaste | trophoblast |
| trou de Botal | foramen ovale |
| trou nourricier | nutrient foramen |
| trou occipital | foramen magnum |
| trou pratiqué avec une fraise | burr hole |
| trouble de l'alimentation | eating disorder |
| trouble du comportement | behavior disorder |
| trouble thymique | affective disorder |
| troubles cognitifs | cognitive disorders |
| trypanosomiase | trypanosomiasis |
| trypsine | trypsin |
| trypsinogène | trypsinogen |
| tryptophane | tryptophan |
| tubage | intubation |
| tubaire | tubal |
| tube digestif | gastrointestinal tract |
| tubercule | tubercle |
| tubercules quadrijumeaux | quadrigeminal bodies |
| tuberculeux | tuberculous |

| French | English |
|---|---|
| tuberculine | tuberculin |
| tuberculome | tuberculoma |
| tuberculose | tuberculosis |
| tubérosité | tuberosity |
| tubes séminifères | seminiferous tubules |
| tubo-ovarien | tubo-ovarian |
| tubulaire | tubular |
| tularémie | tularemia |
| tuméfaction | tumefaction |
| tumeur | tumor |
| tumeur à myéloplaxes | osteoclastoma |
| tunique | tunica |
| turbinectomie | turbinectomy |
| turgescence | turgor |
| turgescent | turgid |
| tympan | tympanic membrane |
| tympanique | tympanic |
| tympanite | myringitis |
| tympanoplastie | tympanoplasty |
| typhoïde fièvre | typhoid fever |
| typhus | typhus fever |
| typhus exanthématique | mite fever |
| tyrosine | tyrosine |
| ulcératif | ulcerative |
| ulcération | canker |
| ulcère | ulcer |
| ulcère gastro-duodénal | gastroduodenal ulcer |
| ultrason | ultrasound |
| ultrasonographie | ultrasonography |
| unciforme | unciform |
| uncinariose | uncinariasis |
| unicellulaire | unicellular |
| unilatéral | unilateral |
| uniovulaire | uniovular |
| unipare | uniparous |
| unipolaire | monopolar |
| unité de soins intensifs | intensive care unit |
| unité motrice | motor unit |
| urate | urate |
| urée | urea |
| uréique | urea |
| urémie | uremia |

| French | English |
| --- | --- |
| urétéral | ureteral |
| uretère | ureter |
| urétérectomie | ureterectomy |
| urétérique | ureteral |
| urétérite | ureteritis |
| urétérocèle | ureterocele |
| urétérolithe | ureterolith |
| urétérolithotomie | ureterolithotomy |
| urétérovaginal | ureterovaginal |
| urétérovésical | ureterovesical |
| urétral | urethral |
| urètre | urethra |
| urétrite | urethritis |
| urétrocèle | urethrocele |
| urétrography | urethrography |
| urétroplastie | urethroplasty |
| urétroscope | urethroscope |
| urétrotomie | urethrotomy |
| urgence | emergency |
| urinaire | urinary |
| urine | urine |
| urines à odeur de sirop d'érable, maladie des | maple syrup urine disease |
| urines du milieu du jet | midstream urine |
| urinomètre | urinometer |
| urique | uric |
| urobiline | urobilin |
| urobilinogène | urobilinogen |
| urochrome | urochrome |
| urogénital | urogenital |
| urographie | urography |
| urolithe | urolith |
| urologie | urology |
| urticaire | urticaria |
| usage unique | single use |
| utérin | uterine |
| utérovésical | uterovesical |
| utérus | uterus |
| utérus rétrofléchi | retroflexed uterus |
| utricule | utricle |
| uvée | uveal tract |
| uvéite | uveitis |
| uvula | uvula |

| French | English |
|---|---|
| uvulectomie | uvulectomy |
| uvulite | uvulitis |
| vaccin | vaccine |
| vaccination | vaccination |
| vaccine | cowpox; vaccinia |
| vache folle, maladie de la | mad cow disease |
| vacuole | vacuole |
| vagal | vagal |
| vagin | vagina |
| vaginal | vaginal |
| vaginisme | vaginismus |
| vaginite | colpitis; vaginitis |
| vagissement | vagitus |
| vagotomie | vagotomy |
| vague nerf | vagus nerve; pneumogastric nerve |
| vaisseau coronaire | coronary vessel |
| valgus | valgus |
| valine | valine |
| valve aortique | aortic valve |
| valve mitrale | mitral valve |
| valvule iléo-cæcale | ileocecal valve |
| valvule tricuspide | tricuspid valve |
| valvulotomie | valvulotomy |
| vaporisateur | nebulizer |
| varice | varix |
| varicelle | varicella; chickenpox |
| varicocèle | varicocele |
| variole | smallpox; variola |
| variqueux | varicose |
| varus | varus |
| vasculaire | vascular |
| vascularite | vasculitis |
| vasectomie | vasectomy |
| vasoconstriction | vasoconstriction |
| vasodilatation | vasodilatation |
| vasomoteur | vasomotor |
| vasopressine | vasopressin |
| vasospasme | vasospasm |
| vasovagal | vasovagal |
| vecteur | vector |
| végétation | vegetation |
| végétations adénoïdes | adenoids |

| French | English |
| --- | --- |
| veine basilique | basilic vein |
| veineux | venous |
| veinographie | venography |
| veinotonique | phlebotonic |
| veinule | venula |
| venin | venom |
| ventilation | ventilation |
| ventilation assistée | assisted ventilation |
| ventral | ventral |
| ventre de bois | wooden belly |
| ventricule | ventricle |
| ventriculographie | ventriculography |
| ver | worm |
| ver de Guinée | guinea worm |
| verge | penis |
| vergeture | stria |
| vérifier | check for, to |
| vérité | truth |
| vermifuge | anthelmintic |
| vermineux | verminous |
| vérole | pox |
| verouillage, syndrome de | locked-in syndrome |
| verrue | verruca |
| verrue plantaire | plantar wart |
| vers le bas | down |
| vertèbre | vertebra |
| vertex | vertex |
| vertige | vertigo |
| vertige paroxystique positionnel bénin | benign paroxysmal vertigo |
| vésical | vesical |
| vésicovaginal | vesicovaginal |
| vésicule biliaire | gallbladder |
| vésicule urine | urinary bladder |
| vésiculite | vesiculitis |
| vessie | urinary bladder |
| vestibulaire | vestibular |
| vestigial | vestigial |
| viable | viable |
| vibration | vibration |
| vide | empty |
| vieillesse | old age |
| vieillissement | aging |

| French | English |
|---|---|
| vigueur | stamina |
| VIH | HIV |
| villeux | villous |
| villosité | villus |
| villosité chorionique | chorionic villus |
| viol | rape |
| violet de gentiane | gentian violet |
| virologie | virology |
| virulence | virulence |
| virus APC | adenovirus |
| viscère | viscera |
| viscomètre | viscometer |
| vision | vision |
| vision trouble | blurred vision |
| visqueux | viscous |
| vitamine B2 | riboflavin |
| vitamine C | ascorbic acid |
| vitamine D | calciferol |
| vitellin | vitelline |
| vitesse de sédimentation | blood sedimentation rate (ESR) |
| vitré | vitreous |
| vivisection | vivisection |
| vocal | vocal |
| voies biliaires | hepatic ducts |
| voies cordonales postérieures | posterior columns |
| voie extrapyramidale | extrapyramidal tract |
| voie orale | orally |
| voies respiratoires supérieures | upper respiratory tract |
| voie urinaires | urinary tract |
| voile | velum |
| voile noir | blackout |
| voix | voice |
| volémie | blood volume |
| volume courant | tidal volume |
| volume de réserve expiratoire | expiratory reserve volume |
| volume de réserve inspiratoire | inspiratory reserve volume |
| volume d'éjection | stroke volume |
| volume expiratoire maximal par seconde (VEMS) | forced expiratory volume per second (FEV1) |
| volume résiduel | residual volume (RV) |
| sanguin | blood volume |
| volvulus | volvulus |

| French | English |
|---|---|
| vomir | vomit, to |
| vomissement | emesis; vomiting |
| vomissement acétonémique | cyclical vomiting |
| voûte crânienne | calvaria |
| vraisemblance | likelihood |
| vulvaire | pudendal |
| vulve | pudendum muliebre vulva |
| vulvectomie | vulvectomy |
| vulvite | vulvitis |
| vulvovaginite | vulvovaginitis |
| xanthine | xanthine |
| xanthochromie | xanthochromia |
| xanthome | xanthoma |
| xérodermie | xerodermia |
| xérophtalmie | xerophthalmia |
| xéroradiographie | xeroradiography |
| xérostomie | xerostomia |
| yoyo | grommet |
| zéiose | zeiosis |
| zéro | zero |
| zézaiement | lisping |
| zinc | zinc |
| zona | herpes zoster; shingles |
| zonule | zonula |
| zoologie | zoology |
| zoonose | zoonosis |
| zoopsie | zoopsia |
| zygote | zygote |
| zymogène | zymogen |
| zymotique | zymotic |

|  | English | French |
|---|---|---|
| **Introduction** | How are you? | Comment ça va? |
| | Good morning, good afternoon, good evening | Bonjour, Bon après midi, Bon soir |
| | My name is ... | Je m'appelle ... |
| **Demographics** | What is your name? | Comment vous appelez-vous? Commet t'appelles-tu? |
| | What province do you live in ? | Quelle province habitez-vous? |
| | Are you married? | Est-ce que vous êtes maries? |
| | What is your age? | Quel âge avez-vous? |
| **Chief complaint** | What is your health concern? | Quel problème avez-vous? |
| | When did this problem start? | A quelle date ce problème est-il apparu? |
| | Are you in pain now? | Sentez-vous la douleur maintenant? |
| | Is the pain severe? | Est-ce que la douleur est sévère? |
| | Sharp or dull? | Vive ou atténuée? |
| | Touch the spot with one finger. | Touchez l'endroit avec un doigt. |
| | What makes it better? | Qu'est-ce qui l'améliore? |
| | What makes it worse? | Qu'est-ce qui l'aggrave? |
| | When do you get the pain... | Quand est-ce que vous sentez la douleur... |
| | at night, before meals, after meals? | la nuit, avant le repas, après le repas? |
| | Have you been in the hospital before? | Avez-vous été à l'hôpital avant? |
| | What were you treated for? | Quelle plainte présentez-vous? |
| **Past medical history** | Are you being treated for any chronic health problem? | Avez-vous prendre les médicaments pour un problème chronique? |
| | Do you have a history of... | Avez-vous souvent souffert... |
| | asthma | d'asthme |
| | epilepsy | épilepsie |
| | hypertension | hypertension |
| | thyroid disease | les maladie de thyroïdiennes |
| | diabetes | diabète |
| | hepatitis | hépatite |
| | cancer | cancer |
| | HIV/AIDS | VIH/SIDA |
| | Date starting ARV? | Date de début des ARV's? |
| | Date and value of last CD4? | Date et quantité de CD4 derniers? |
| | Have you had pneumonia or meningitis? | Avez-vous contracté la pneumonie ou la méningite? |
| **Past surgical history** | Have you had surgery in the past? | Est-ce que vous avez déjà été opéré? |

| | English | French |
|---|---|---|
| | What surgery was done? | Quelle opération avez-vous reçu? |
| | What year was the surgery? | En quelle année avez-vous subi cette opération? |
| **Medications** | Do you take medication at home? | Prenez-vous le médicament chez vous? |
| | Have you taken drugs (illegal) recently? | Avez-vous pris de la drogue récemment? |
| | Are you taking bactrim? | Etes-vous en train de prendre Bactrim? |
| | I want to see the medication bottle. | Je voudrais voir la bouteille des médicaments. |
| **Allergies** | Have you had reactions to medications? | Aviez-vous allergie des médicaments? |
| **Family history** | Is your mother living? | Est-ce que votre (ta) mère est encore vivante? |
| | Is your father living? | Est-ce que votre (ton) père est encore vivant? |
| | Do your brothers/sisters have health problems? | Est-ce que votre frère/sœur a un problème e de santé? |
| **Social history** | Do you drink alcohol? | Est-ce que tu prends de l'alcool? |
| | How many drinks per day? | Buvez-vous combien de fois par jour? |
| | Do you drink every day? | Bois-tu (buvez-vous) tous les jours? |
| | Do you smoke? | Fume-tu? |
| **Review of systems** | Do you have skin problems? | Vous avez mal à la peau? |
| **Lymphatic** | Do you have lymph node enlargement or pain? | Vous avez mal à la ganglion lymphe? |
| **Bone** | Do you have bone pain? | Avez-vous du mal aux os? |
| | Do you have joint pain? | Avez-vous des douleurs articulaires? |
| | Do you have joint swelling? | Avez-vous des gonflements articulaires? |
| **Blood** | Do you have bleeding problems? | Avez-vous un problème de saignement? |
| **Endocrine** | Do you urinate frequently? | Urinez-vous fréquemment? |
| | Are you thirsty all the time? | Avez-vous toujours de la soif? |
| | Has your weight decreased? | Avez-vous maigri? Avez-vous perdu le poids? |
| **Head** | Have you suffered from head trauma? | Avez-vous souffert de traumatisme de la tête? |
| | Do you have vertigo, syncope? | Avez-vous vertige, syncope? |
| **Eyes** | Do you have vision loss? | Avez-vous eu une perte de vue? |
| | Do you have double vision? | Avez-vous une vue double? |
| | Do you have blurred vision? | Avez-vous une vue brumeuse? |
| | Do you have pain in bright light? | Avez-vous du mal à la lumière vive? |

| | English | French |
|---|---|---|
| **Ears** | Have you had a hearing problem recently? | Aviez-vous les problèmes d'entendre récemment? |
| | Do you have drainage from the ears? | Avez-vous des problèmes de drainage de l'oreille? |
| **Nose** | Do you have epistaxis? | Souffrez-vous de l'épistaxis? |
| **Mouth** | Do you have a toothache? | Orage de dent? |
| **Throat** | Do you have hoarseness? | Enroué voix enrouée? |
| | Do you have a sore throat? | Avoir mal à la gorge? |
| **Neck** | Do you have neck stiffness? | Est-ce que vous avez mal au cou de raideur? |
| **Breast** | Have you noticed breast lumps? | Avez-vous grosseurs du sein? |
| | Do you have nipple discharge? | Avez-vous décharge du mamelon? |
| **Respiratory** | Do you have difficulty breathing? | Avez-vous du mal à essouffler? |
| | Do you sit up at night to breathe? | Vous-vous asseyez pendant la nuit pour respirer? |
| | Do you have pain when you take a deep breath? | Avez-vous mal quand vous respirez profondément? |
| | Do you have wheezing? | Avez-vous le wheezing? |
| | Do you have a cough? | Avez-vous la toux? |
| | How long have you had the cough? | Depuis quand avez-vous la toux? |
| | Do you have a lot of sputum? | Crachez-vous souvent? |
| | Do you have bloody sputum? | Crachez-vous le sang? |
| | What color is your sputum? | Quelle est la couleur de votre crachat? |
| | Have you had tuberculosis? | Avez-vous eu la tuberculose? |
| **Cardio-vascular** | Do you have chest pain? | Souffrez-vous à la poitrine? |
| | Do you have palpitations? | Avez-vous des palpitations? |
| | Do you have leg edema? | Vous avez mal les jambes gonflées? |
| | Have you been weak? | Vous n'avez pas de forces? |
| **Gastro-intestinal** | Do you have abdominal pain? (Do you have pain in your belly?) | Est-ce que vous avez mal au ventre? |
| | ...after you eat, with certain foods? | ...après avoir mangé? Avec certain aliment? |
| | When did this problem start? | Depuis quand avez-vous ce problème? |
| | Has it been weeks, months years? | Il y a des semaines, des mois, des années? |
| | Are you in pain now? | Sentez-vous la douleur maintenant? |
| | Touch the spot? | Touchez la ou vous sentez la douleur? |
| | Is the pain better than yesterday? | La douleur serait plus grave que celle d'hier? |
| | Do you have ...fever? | Avez-vous la fièvre? |
| | ...night sweats? | transpirations nocturnes? |
| | ...chills? | des frissons? |
| | How is your appetite? | Avez-vous l'appétit? |

| English | French |
|---|---|
| Have you vomited? | Avez-vous des vomissements? |
| Are you nauseated? | Avez-vous la nausée? |
| Did you have a stool today? | Avez-vous caca aujourd'hui? |
| When was your last stool? | Quand es-tu allé à selle la dernière fois? |
| Do you have constipation? | Avez-vous la constipation? |
| Do you have diarrhea? | Avez-vous la diarrhée? |
| How many times per day? | Combien de fois par jour? |
| Is the stool black or bloody? | Les selles sont noires ou sanglants? |
| What color was the stool? | De quelle couleur sont des selles? |
| Do you have pain with swallowing? | Avez-vous des problèmes d'avaler? |
| Do you have difficulty swallowing? | Avez-vous des difficultés à avaler? |
| Do you have burning pain in the stomach? | Sentez-vous la douleur brûlante dans l'estomac? |
| Have you had a gastroscopy before? | Avez-vous connu la gastroscopie au paravent? |
| **Genitourinary** Do you have burning on urination? | Sentez-vous la douleur brûlante quand vous urinez? |
| Have you had penile discharge? | Avez-vous senti la décharge du pénis? |
| Do you have sores on the penis? | Y-il des ulcères sur votre pénis? |
| How often do you void at night? | Combien do fois videz-vous par nuit? |
| Is the urine stream slow? | Est-ce que le jet des urines est lent ou rapide? |
| Do you have blood in the urine? | Y-il du sang dans les urines? |
| **Women's health** Are you pregnant? | Etes-vous enceinte? |
| Are your periods regular? | Etes-vous en règles normalement? |
| Are your periods painful? | Connais-tu des règles douloureuse? |
| Do you have heavy periods? | Y a-t-il beaucoup sang? |
| When did your last period start? | Quand ont-ils commencé les dernières règles? |
| Do you have vaginal itching? | Avez-vous démangeaisons vaginal? |
| Do you vaginal pain? | Sentez-vous la douleur dans le vagin? |
| Do you have unusual discharge from the vagina? | Avez-vous des sécrétions vaginales extraordinaires? |
| ...a lot or a little? | ...beaucoup ou peu? |
| How many times have you been pregnant? | Combien de fois avez-vous conçu? |
| How many children do you have? | Avez-vous combien d'enfants? |
| Are you taking any medicine at home? | Tu prends des médicaments à la maison? |
| What is the name of the medicine? | Quel est le nom de ces médicaments? |
| What is your blood type? | Quel est ton groupe sanguine? |
| Are you in labor? | Tu es en travail? |

| | English | French |
|---|---|---|
| **Peripartum/ neonatal** | When did your labor start? | Depuis combien de temps es-tu en travail? |
| | Is this your first baby? | C'est votre première enfant? |
| | Do you feel the baby move? | Sens-tu l'enfant remuer? |
| | Did your water break? | As-tu perdu les eaux? |
| | Were you ill before the delivery? | Avez-vous un autre problème avant l'accouchement? |
| | What was the baby's birth weight? | Son enfant avait combien de poids à la naissance? |
| | How many times have you been pregnant? | Combien de grossesse avait-vous? |
| | How many children do you have? | Combien d'enfants avez-vous eu? |
| | Is the baby nursing well? | Est-ce qu'il tété bien? |
| | Has the baby had any convulsions? | Cet enfant a eu la convulsion? |
| | Apgar at 1 minute. | Apgar à 1 minute. |
| | Apgar at 5 minutes. | Apgar à 5 minutes. |
| | Moro reflex. | Réflexe de moro. |
| | Fontanelle. | Fontanelle. |
| **Amniotic fluid** | clear fluid | liquide clair |
| | colored fluid | liquide teinté |
| | meconium stained | liquide meconial |
| **Pediatrics** | Is he (she) drinking ok? | Est-ce qu'il (qu'elle) boit bien? |
| | Is he (she) eating ok? | Est-ce qu'il (qu'elle) mange bien? |
| | Have you seen worms in the vomit or the stool? | Avez-vous vu les vers dans les vomissements ou dans les selles? |
| **Neurologic** | Do you have: facial weakness? | Avez-vous: la faiblesse de la face? |
| | facial numbness? | engourdissement de la figure? |
| | leg weakness? | faiblesse des jambes? |
| | leg numbness? | engourdissement des jambes? |
| | arm weakness? | faiblesse des bras? |
| | arm numbness? | engourdissement des bras? |
| | Have you been unconscious? | Est-ce que vous avez perdu connaissance? |
| | Have you had tremors? | Avez-vous eu des tremblements? |
| | Have you had recent vision loss in one eye? | Avez-vous des difficultés à voir d'un œil récemment? |
| | Have you had problems with your balance? | Avez-vous des difficultés à maintenir votre équilibre? |
| **Psychiatric** | Do you have anxiety? | Avez-vous mal a la anxiété? |
| | Do you have depression? | Avez-vous mal a la dépression? |
| **Physical exam** | appearance, height | aspect, taille |
| **General** | pulse    bp    resp<br>temp    wt | pouls    T/A    FR<br>temp.    poids |

| | English | French |
|---|---|---|
| | skin | peau |
| **HEENT** | visual acuity | visuel acuité |
| | conjunctiva, sclera | conjonctive, sclérotique |
| | pupils | pupille |
| | optic disc | disque optique |
| | ear canal, tympanic membrane | tympan |
| | nasal mucosa | muqueuse du nasal |
| | sinuses | sinus |
| | mouth, gums, dental, uvula "open your mouth" | bouche, gencive, dent, uvula "ouvrez la bouche" |
| | "stick out your tongue" | "montrez la langue" |
| | "say ahh" | "dites ahh" |
| **Pulmonary** | auscultation "breathe deep" | auscultation "respire profond" |
| | percussion | percussion |
| **Back** | Lie on your left side. | Couchez-vous sur le côté gauche. |
| | Lie on your right side. | Couchez-vous sur le côté droit. |
| | tenderness "does it hurt here?" | sensible "sentez-vous la douleur ici? |
| | cva tenderness | douleur (à la palpation) angle costovertebral |
| **Cardio-vascular** | heart rate, rhythm "breathe normally" | fréquence cardiaque "respire normalement" |
| | heart murmur? | souffle cardiaque? |
| | carotid "hold your breath" | carotide "ne respirez pas" |
| | jugular venous distention | jugulaire veineux distendu |
| **Breasts** | nipple discharge | évacuation du téton |
| | tenderness "Does it hurt here?" | sensible "Sentez-vous la douleur ici?" |
| | mass | masse |
| **Vascular** | carotid, radial, aortic pulsation | carotide, radial, aortique pulsation |
| | femoral, dorsalis pedis, posterior tibial | fémoral, dos du pied, le postérieure du tibia |
| | leg edema | gonflement du jambes |
| **Abdomen** | Lie down. | Couchez-vous. |
| | umbilicus | ombilic |
| | hernia, inguinal | hernie, inguinal |
| | palpation | palpation |
| | auscultation | auscultation |
| | fluid wave, superficial abdominal veins? | onde liquide, les veines abdominales superficielle? |
| **Maternal/gyn** | uterine height (cm) | HU haut utérine |
| | Fetal heart rate | BCF bruit de cœur fœtal |
| | urine sample | CU culot urine |
| | presentation | présentation |
| | head presentation | présentation céphalique |

273

| | English | French |
|---|---|---|
| | breech presentation | présentation siège |
| | transverse presentation | présentation transverse |
| | speculum exam | spéculum |
| | vaginal exam | TV toucher vaginal |
| | gestational age | âge gestationnel |
| | amniotic fluid | liquide amniotique |
| **Genitourinary ; male** | circumcised? | circoncis? |
| | genital herpes? | herpès génital |
| | testicles | testicules |
| **Rectal exam** | hemorrhoids, nodules,　prostate? | hémorroïdes, nodosité, prostate? |
| | "I want to check your rectum (for hemorrhoids), bend over please." | "J'ai besoin examiner votre rectum (pour hémorroïdes), penchez-vous s'il vous plaît." |
| | guaiac; positive or negative | guïac; positif ou négatif |
| **Neurologic Cranial nerves** | N1 olfactory: coffee, peppermint? | olfactif:　café, pastille de menthe? |
| | N2 optic: snellen, confrontation | optique: "Suivre au doigt." |
| | N3,4, 6, oculomotor, trochlear, abducens: EOM's "Follow my finger" | moteur oculomoteur commun, pathétique, abducens: "Suivre mon doigt." |
| | N5 trigeminal | trigéminal |
| | "Clench your jaw." | "Serre la mâchoire." |
| | "Move your jaw back and forth." | "Agitez votre mâchoire comme ci comme ça." |
| | forehead (ophthalmic) cheek(maxillary) chin (mandibular) "Do you feel this?" | front, joue, menton "Vous avez sensé ce?" |
| | N7 facial: "Raise your eye brows." | facial: "Elevez au sourcils" |
| | "Close your eyes tightly, smile big." | "Ferme votre yeux, sourire a la bouche largement." |
| | N8 acoustic: whisper, rinne | auditif: chuchoterie, épreuve de Rinne |
| | "Can you hear this?" | "Pouvez-vous entendre ce?" |
| | "Tell me when you can't feel vibration" | "Dit moi qui ne sentir pas a la vibration." |
| | N9 glossopharyngeal: swallow, (hoarseness), "Swallow now." | glossopharyngien: (enrouement) "Avalez maintenant." |
| | N10 vagus: swallow, soft palate, gag reflex | vague: avalement, voile du palais, réflexe pharyngé |
| | "Stick out your tongue." | "Montrez moi la langue." |
| | N11 accessory nerve: "Turn your head, shrug your shoulders." | accessoire: "Tourne a la tête, détenir les épaules." |
| | N12 hypoglossal: tongue midline | hypoglosse: langue médiane |

| | English | French |
|---|---|---|
| **Glasgow coma score** | opens eyes to: spontaneous (4),to speech (3), to pain (2), none (1) | échelle de Glasgow: les yeux s'ouvrent spontanément (4), les yeux s'ouvrent à la voix (3), les s'ouvrent à la douleur (2), ne s'ouvrent pas du tout (1) |
| | best motor "Hold up 2 fingers." obeys commands (6), localizes (5), withdraws (4), abnormal flexion (3), abnormal extension (2), none (1) | motricité meilleur: "Détenir deux doigts." on obéit aux ordres pour faire l'action (6), on peut localiser la douleur (5), on peut retire de la douleur (4), flexion: position anormale (3), extension: position anormale (2), on ne fait pas de mouvement ni position (1) |
| | best verbal: clear (5), confused (4), inappropriate (3), garbled (2), none (1) | langage meilleur: on est conscient (5), on peut parler, mais on est confus (4), on ne fait pas le sens (3), on fait les mots incompréhensible (2), on ne fait pas un son (1) |
| **Motor** | Motor function | Motricité |
| | biceps brachii, elbow flexion | (C-5) biceps brachial |
| | "pull your arm up" | "tirez au bras" |
| | wrist extensors | (C-6) poignet extenseur |
| | "bend your wrist up" | "plier au poignet" |
| | triceps brachii, elbow extension | (C-7) triceps brachial, coude extenseur |
| | "straighten your arm out" | "redressez au bras" |
| | finger flexors, distal phalanx middle finger | (C-8) doigt fléchisseur, articulation phalangette, doigt du milieu |
| | "bend the tip of this finger" | "plier au bout de doigt" |
| | finger abduction, little finger | (T-1) petit doigt, doigt abducteur |
| | "hold the small finger tightly" | "tenir au doigt petit fort" |
| | iliopsoas, hip flexors | (L-2) psoas-iliaque, hanche fléchisseur |
| | "move your knee to your chest" | "mouvoir votre genou à la poitrine" |
| | quadriceps, knee extensors | (L-3) quadriceps, genou extenseur |
| | "straighten your leg out" | "redressez à la jambe" |
| | tibialis anterior, ankle dorsiflexors | (L-4) tibiale antérieure, dorsiflexion |
| | "pull your foot up" | "remontez à la pied" |
| | extensor hallucis longus, long toe extension | (L-5) extenseur commun des orteils |
| | "raise your toe up" | "tinez au orteil grande" |
| | gastrocnemius, ankle plantar flexors | (S-1) gastrocnémien, cheville plantaire fléchisseur |
| | "push your foot down" | "poussez à la pied" |
| **Sensory** | Sensation "can you feel this?" | "dite 'oui' si vous pouvez sentir ce" |
| | C-4 (top of acromioclavicular joint) | C-4 (en haut d'articulation acromio-claviculaire) |

| | English | French |
|---|---|---|
| | C-5 (lateral side of antecubital fossa) | C-5 (aspect latérale, pli de coude) |
| | C-6 (thumb) | C-6 (pouce) |
| | C-7 ( middle finger) | C-7 (doigt (m) du milieu) |
| | C-8 (little finger) | C-8 (petit doigt) |
| | T-4 (nipple line) | T-4 (mamelon) |
| | T-10 (umbilicus) | T-10 (ombilic) |
| | L-2 (mid-anterior thigh) | L-2 (moyenne face antérieure de la cuisse) |
| | L-3 (medial femoral condyle) | L-3 (interne condyle fémoral) |
| | L-4 (medial malleolus) | L-4 (interne du tarse) |
| | L-5 (dorsum of the foot, at third MTP joint) | L-5 (dos du pied, troisième articulation métatarso-phalangienne) |
| | S-1 (Lateral heel) | S-1 (aspect latérale, calcanéum) |
| | S-2 (popliteal fossa of the knee, in the midline) | S-2 (aspect médiane, postérieur, genou) |
| | S-3 (ischial tuberosity) | S-3 (épine sciatique) |
| | S4-5 (perianal area) | S4-5 (la région périanal) |
| reflex | Reflexes | Réflexe |
| | triceps right and left | tricipital, droit et gauche |
| | biceps, right and left | bicipital, droit et gauche |
| | patella, right and left | rotulien, droit et gauche |
| | ankle, right and left | achilléen, droit et gauche |
| | babinski, right and left (great toe extension= positive) | signe de Babinski, droit et gauche (gros orteil extension= positif) |
| screen | Tandem walk | Marcher en tandem |
| | "Walk like this, one foot in front of other." | "Marchez ce manière, un pied avant l'autre pied." |
| | heel walk, toe walk, | épreuve marcher talons, épreuve marcher orteils |
| | "Walk on your heels, now on toes." | "Marchez au talons, maintenant marche au orteils." |
| | romberg "Stand up, hold your arms out, close your eyes." | épreuve de Romberg "Debout tenir, élevez les bras, fermez les yeux." |
| Coordination | rapid alternating movement (2nd finger, thumb) "Do this, fast". | épreuve rapide alternatif mouvement "Faire cet rapide." |
| | heel-shin "Move your right heel from your left knee to the ankle with your eyes shut." | épreuve talon-tibia "Mouvoir à la talon de la genou à cheville avec les yeux ferme." |
| | finger nose finger "Touch my finger with your finger then touch your nose." | épreuve doigt-nez-doigt "Touchez mon doigt avec votre doigt, ensuite touchez votre nez." |
| Discriminative | stereognosis (key, pencil, cup) "Close your eyes; what is this in your hand?" | stéréognosie (clé, crayon, tasse) "Ferme les yeux, que est-ce que la main?" |

276

| | English | French |
|---|---|---|
| | graphesthesia (draw #3 in hand) "Close your eyes, what is the number written in your hand?" | dermolexie "Ferme les yeux; que est-ce que la nombre d'écris dans votre mains?" |
| | point localization: "Close your eyes, tell me what part of your body is being touched." | pointe localisation "Ferme les yeux, vous me dites que est-ce que partie de le corps je touche?" |
| **Counseling:** | You need to go for an x ray. | Tu dois aller aux rayons X. |
| **Pulmonary** | I have the result of your sputum. | J'ai le résultat de ton cas. |
| | You have... | Vous avez... |
| | tuberculosis | tuberculose |
| | pneumonia | pneumonie |
| | Your lungs are... | Tes poumons sont atteints... |
| | one is affected, the other is healthy. | un seul est malade, l'autre est sain. |
| | Your illness can be healed. | Ta maladie peut se soigner. |
| **Gastro-enterology** | There is an ulcer in your stomach. | Il y a ton estomac un ulcère. |
| | You need to quit drinking beer completely. | Tu dois t'abstenir complètement de bière. |
| **Surgery** | You need to have an operation today. | Tu dois te faire opérer aujourd'hui même. |
| | You need to have this wound sewed up (sutured). | Tu feras coudre cette blessure. |
| | When did you last eat and drink? | Quand as-tu mangé et bu pour la dernière fois? |
| | You need to rest at the hospital a few days. | Tu dois rester à l'hôpital peu de jours. |
| **Pharmacy** | You take this medicine two (one, three, four)times per day. | Vous prenez ce médicament deux (une, trois, quatre) fois par jour. |
| | Do not stop this medication! | N'arrêtez pas ce médicament! |
| | Take this medication only if you want to. | Vous prenez ce médicament si vous en avez besoin. |
| | Take this medication before eating. | Vous prenez ce médicament avant les repas. |
| | Take this medication with food. | Vous prenez ce médicament avec les repas. |
| | Take this medication after meals. | Vous prenez ce médicament après les repas. |
| **Maternity** | The nurse is on her way. | L'infirmière va venir. |
| | She will help with the delivery. | Elle va venir faire ton accouchement. |
| **Laboratory/ imaging** | I need a... 1) urine sample 2) stool sample 3) blood sample 4) sputum specimen. | J'ai besoin 1) d'un échantillon d'urine 2) de selles 3) d'un échantillon de sang 4) de crachat |
| **Procedures** | I need to put this tube in your nose. | Je dois introduire ce tube dans votre nez. |
| | I need to start an IV. | Je dois commencer une perfusion. |

| English | French |
| --- | --- |
| I need to give you a shot 1) in the arm 2) in the leg. | Je dois vous faire une piqûre 1) dans le bras 2) dans la jambe. |

CPSIA information can be obtained at www.ICGtesting.com
Printed in the USA
LVOW070027150312

273176LV00006B/115/P

9 781450 589680